Pharmaceutical Medicine
second edition

PHARMACEUTICAL MEDICINE
second edition

Edited by

Denis M. Burley, FRCP, FFPM
Formerly Director, Centre for Pharmaceutical Medicine,
Woking and President, Faculty of Pharmaceutical Medicine

Joan M. Clarke, MBChB, MD, FFPM
European Safety Director, Syntex Development Research,
Maidenhead

Louis Lasagna, MD
Director and Chairman of the Board, Center for the Study of
Drug Development, Tufts University, Boston, Massachusetts

with foreword by Professor Sir Abraham Goldberg

Edward Arnold
A member of the Hodder Headline Group
LONDON   BOSTON   MELBOURNE   AUCKLAND

© 1993 Denis M. Burley, Joan M. Clarke and Louis Lasagna

First published in Great Britain 1993
Distributed in the Americas by Little, Brown and Company,
34 Beacon Street, Boston, MA 02108

British Library Cataloguing in Publication Data

Pharmaceutical Medicine. – 2Rev. ed
  I. Burley, D. M.   II. Binns, T. B.
  III. Clarke, Joan   IV. Lasagna, Louis
  615

  ISBN 0–340–52517–7

Typeset in 10/11 pt Palatino by Anneset, Weston-super-Mare, Avon.
Printed in Great Britain for Edward Arnold, a division of Hodder
Headline PLC, Mill Road, Dunton Green, Sevenoaks, Kent TN13 2YA
by St. Edmundsbury Press.
Bound by Hartnolls Ltd, Bodmin, Cornwall.

Contents

Foreword

In my Foreword to the first edition of 'Pharmaceutical Medicine' in 1985 I sought evidence to justify a textbook on this subject – and this easily presents itself. Perhaps the most cogent proof for such a justification is the emergence of the second edition. Further milestones in the development of the subject are the relatively greater expansion of the numbers of pharmaceutical physicians in the UK than of other specialists in the 25 years up to 1987; the inauguration of the Faculty of Pharmaceutical Medicine of the three Royal Colleges of Physicians in 1989; and the publication now of two journals of pharmaceutical medicine.

A considerable recasting of chapters and changes of authorship reflect the changes in the various topics. Each chapter has evoked in me a special response; the scrupulous care taken in the quality of the products in the development of medicines, even to the consideration of temperature changes in transport of medication from one country to another; the preclinical toxicity testing carried out to the limits of contemporary knowledge; clinical trials – elaborate, sophisticated yet requiring to conform to the simple adage: 'you only get a focused answer when you ask a focused question'; the unfolding of adverse reactions in postmarketing surveillance studies; the emergence of pharmacoepidemiology; and all these topics rendered scientifically acceptable by statistics, gently introduced and later more robustly considered by Win Castle and Alan Ebbutt.

The drug regulatory changes of the European Community and the dominating importance of pharmaceutical regulation in the USA have required a total reconstruction of these topics. The issues of economics and ethics are common threads that are part of the tapestry of every contemporary human endeavour and pharmaceutical medicine is no exception. Dr Grebmer and Dr Marsh, in their respective chapters, have mobilized, with disarming simplicity, all the important aspects of these topics. The chapter on 'The Pharmaceutical Physician' is an ideal introduction by a senior pharmaceutical officer to a neophyte, recalling the sage advice of Polonius to his son Laertes in Act 1 Scene III of Hamlet. The legal aspects of pharmaceutical medicine have, in recent years, donated a range of topics, some of which have fascinated the media and the public. Diana Brahams, a barrister experienced in such presentations to medical readers, rivets attention.

My feelings on reading the second edition of the book are mixed – pride to have been associated with the subject from the early days, delight that Joan Clarke and Louis Lasagna are involved in its editing, but sadness above all that Denis Burley, who initiated the work with Terry Binns and who has done much for pharmaceutical medicine throughout his professional life, died in 1992 before the publication of this book and before the completion of his Presidency of the Faculty of Pharmaceutical Medicine.

The quality of this second edition stands as a memorial to his work.

June 1993
Professor Sir Abraham Goldberg

Preface

The tremendous growth of drug research and the increasing availability of new and effective remedies have changed the whole face of medicine in the past 35 years. One consequence has been the development of the academic discipline of clinical pharmacology, often described as 'the scientific study of drugs in man'. There is now an abundant literature on this subject with several textbooks and numerous journals.

It is more difficult to define Pharmaceutical Medicine. It has much in common with clinical pharmacology, but it includes the medical aspects of the work of the pharmaceutical industry which discovers and develops almost all of the new drugs. It also includes insight into the social and legal aspects of medicines and particularly the involvement of government through the regulatory authority and through various controls on labelling, prices and promotion.

Thus it could be said that pharmaceutical medicine occupies the area of common ground between the medical profession, the pharmaceutical industry and government. Its boundaries are hazy but the principal areas are indicated by the chapter headings of this book which is designed to complement but not compete with those on related disciplines such as clinical pharmacology and statistics. The first edition of this textbook on Pharmaceutical Medicine was put together mainly for the benefit of doctors working in the pharmaceutical industry in the UK to assist in postgraduate education for the Diploma of Pharmaceutical Medicine which was set up in 1976 jointly by the three Royal Colleges of Physicians in the UK. Now there are probably about 5000 pharmaceutical physicians working worldwide, and a large proportion of them in the USA. This second edition has therefore been expanded to include larger chapters and additional material more relevant to the needs of North American pharmaceutical physicians in their own medical and regulatory environment.

Also in Europe, the period since the first edition was published has seen considerable change in the regulatory picture. The Multi-State and so-called 'high-tech' registration procedures are now well in place; debate begin currently focused on the relative merits of mutual recognition as opposed to a centralized European registration authority.

Dr Joan Clarke has taken over from Dr Terry Binns who has now retired and Dr Louis Lasagna has kindly agreed to join the editorial team. We believe that this book will now have much wider value in all areas of the world where pharmaceutical research and development and clinical testing is carried out. Large sections will be of interest not only to medical doctors, but also to those many other groups who are concerned with various aspects of pharmaceutical medicine: clinical research associates, monitors, statisticians, information and regulatory personnel as well as many staff in research, marketing and management.

Despite its great contribution to health care over many years, there is still remarkable ignorance about the industry, even among people whose work brings them into contact with it. It is hoped that this book will find its way into the libraries of medical and pharmacy schools and postgraduate centres. Not only do most doctors regularly prescribe the industry's products, but an increasing number of doctors and pharmacists are involved in clinical testing, in teaching and as members of expert committees at local or national level. Finally we hope that the staff of regulatory authorities will find the book useful.

The information it contains could doubtless be found scattered in the literature. It is not otherwise available under a single cover.

No expert can be expected to be expert in so many disparate fields, but many people, especially pharmaceutical physicians, should have sufficient knowledge of them to be able to converse intelligently and constructively with the experts.

We should like to thank the contributors, their secretaries and our secretaries for their cooperation, hard work and forbearance.

1993
Denis M. Burley
Joan M. Clarke
Louis Lasagna

Although Denis Burley did not live to see the second edition completed, he had made an enormous contribution to it before his sad and untimely death in 1992.

1993
Joan M. Clarke
Louis Lasagna

List of contributors

Diana Brahams, Barrister, Lincoln's Inn, London, UK; Editor, Medico-Legal Journal; Correspondent to the Lancet.

Roger W. Brimblecombe, PhD, DSc, FRCPath, FIBiol, Chairman, Vanguard Medica Ltd., Codicote, UK.

Denis M. Burley, FRCP, FFPM, Formerly Director, Centre for Pharmaceutical Medicine, Woking, UK; President, Faculty of Pharmaceutical Medicine of the Royal College of Physicians of the United Kingdom.

Win M. Castle, MD, MFCM, FFPM, MIS, Vice-President, International Drug Surveillance, Glaxo Inc., Research Triangle Park, North Carolina, USA.

Anthony D. Dayan, MD, FRCP, FRCPath, FFPM, FIBiol, Professor of Toxicology, St Bartholomew's Hospital Medical College, London, UK.

Alan F. Ebbutt, PhD, BSc, Head of Medical Statistics, Glaxo Group Research, London, UK.

Klaus von Grebmer, PhD, Head of Plant Protection Communication, Ciba-Geigy Ltd, Basle, Switzerland.

Peter Barton Hutt, BA, LLB, LLM, Partner, Covington and Burling, Washington, USA.

Juhana E. Idänpään-Heikkilä, MD, DMSC, Chief Medical Officer for Drug Evaluation, Health Directorate of Finland, Helsinki, Finland; Deputy Director, Drug Management and Policies, World Health Organization, Geneva, Switzerland.

David B. Jefferys, BSc, MD, FRCP, FFPM, Head of New Drugs and European Licensing, MCA, London, UK.

Gerald Jones, BA, MSc, PhD, FRCP, Senior Principal Medical Officer, DH, London, UK.

Judith K. Jones, PhD, MD, President, Drug Safety Research and Information, The Degge Group Ltd; Director of Education and Research, PERI, Arlington, Virginia, USA.

Louis Lasagna, MD, Dean, Sackler School of Graduate Biomedical Sciences; Academic Dean of the Medical School; Director and Chairman, Center for the Study of Drug Development, Tufts University, Boston, USA

Don Maclean, PhD, BSc, MRPharmS, Regulatory Affairs Manager-Europe, Syntex Development Research, Maidenhead, UK.

Brian T. Marsh, BA, MB BS(Hnrs), DRCOG, FFPM, Consultant in Pharmaceutical Medicine; formerly Chairman, British Association of Pharmaceutical Physicians; Chairman, ABPI Medical Committee, London; Medical Director, Leo Laboratories Ltd, Princes Risborough, UK.

Brian B. Newbould, BPharm, FPS, PhD, MCPP, Director, International Research Affairs, ICI Corporate Research and Technology, Macclesfield, UK.

John M. Padfield, BPharm, PhD, FRPharmS, CChem, FRSC, Managing Director, Glaxo Manufacturing Services, Uxbridge, UK.

Karen Summers, MB, BS, MFPM, Vice-President and Director, Medical Research-Europe, Syntex Development Research, Maidenhead, UK.

1

How are medicines discovered?
Brian B. Newbold

In 1934 the British Pharmaceutical Codex contained approximately 1000 monographs. Of these over 900 were inorganic chemicals or substances derived from plants. Less than 100 were synthetic organic chemicals with claimed medicinal properties. The number of these which we would recognize as having utility today is less than 10 and includes acetylsalicylic acid, phenobarbitone, procaine and the anaesthetics – ether and chloroform.

The medical profession of that time struggled heroically to prevent premature death and alleviate pain and suffering but a stroll through any graveyard and observation of the tombstones recording the age at which loved ones died reveals that many people passed away prematurely. This is understandable, given the paucity of medicines to effectively treat infections and life-threatening diseases of organic dysfunction. The general physician was not alone in having few effective medicines to satisfy patient needs. Surgeons and anaesthetists had to operate with explosive or liver-damaging anaesthetics and few medicaments were available to relax muscles with precision, control blood pressure or combat postoperative infection.

Since 1934 there has been a remarkable revolution in the number and different types of synthetic medicines made available to the medical profession (Fig. 1.1). An important stimulus was undoubtedly the invention of Prontosil by Klarer and Mietzsc in 1932 and the reports by Domagk,[1,2] 1935, that mice with streptococcal and other infections could be protected by this azo-dye which contained a sulphonamide group. By the time the first supplement to the British Pharmaceutical Codex was published in 1940, four sulphonamides were listed – sulphacetamide, sulphanilamide, sulphapyridine and sulphathiazole. Subsequently many sulphonamides were invented, some of which are still in use today. The early clinical results with Prontosil and its active metabolite p-amino-benzene sulphonamide (sulphanilamide), reported by Colebrook and Kenny[3] and Buttle et al.[4] in 1936, brought hope where previously there had been fear and despair. The trials also demonstrated that certain bacterial diseases could be cured – without harming the patient, thus heralding the important era of selective toxicity.

This breakthrough in the successful treatment of many bacterial diseases with synthetic chemicals undoubtedly acted as a stimulus to research workers in the then fledgling pharmaceutical industry, encouraging them to broaden their horizons. Much attention was understandably focused in these early years on parasitic diseases, since in many cases the cause was

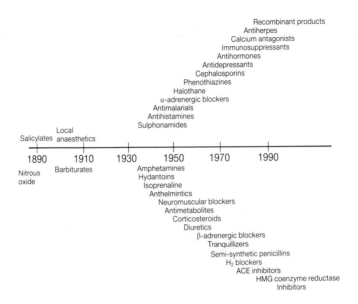

Fig. 1.1 Major classes of synthetic medicines introduced since 1850. First letter approximates to year of introduction. H$_2$, histamine-2; ACE, angiotensin converting enzyme; HMG, 3-hydroxy-3-methylglutaryl.

known and, with imagination and skill, test systems could be created in the test tube and/or laboratory animal to evaluate the potential utility of the many chemicals being synthesized by medicinal chemists or isolated from natural sources. Thus, in the 1940s the range of medicines made available to the physicians and patients was rapidly extended, and included synthetic antimalarials, antihistamines, α-adrenergic blockers, amphetamines, anticonvulsant hydantoins and neuromuscular blockers, as well as an exciting range of antibiotics such as penicillin, chlortetracycline, choramphenicol, streptomycin, etc.

Whilst this explosion of interest and success in the treatment of parasitic diseases and some diseases of organic dysfunction was underway, scientists in academe were painstakingly continuing to put together many jigsaws that would ultimately reveal the complex functioning of many important physiological processes. Others were beginning to understand the aetiology and pathogenesis of a wider range of diseases of organic dysfunction. From the late 1940s onwards the symbiosis between scientists in academe and those in industry was to have a profound effect on the discovery and development of new medicines.

The discovery phase

A chemical does not become a medicine until the potential utility observed in the laboratory has been proven in clinical trials and regulatory agencies have accepted the results of exhaustive tests for efficacy, safety and quality. Because of this, the discovery of a new medicine is an integral part of its development. However, the two phases are so different that they will be dealt with separately.

In an earlier edition of this book, Dr Miles Weatherall[5] detailed elegantly and exhaustively the choice of laboratory test systems used to discover new chemical entitites and outlined the thought processes that led to the invention of many of today's medicines. The value and relevance of that text has not changed with time and is well worth reading. In addition, Dr Barry Cox,[6] in the Science Chairman's Address at the 1989 British Pharmaceutical Conference gave a fascinating account of key events in the discovery of the angiotensin converting enzyme inhibitors (ACEIs) and why there is currently a surge of interest in chemicals that interfere with 5-hydroxytryptamine (5-HT) at its many receptors.

Rather than replay these and similar accounts, attention will be focused on certain principles. However, these principles can only be illustrative, since as pointed out by Nayak and Kettingham[7] in their enthralling book *Breakthroughs!*: 'The many intangible elements that affect a breakthrough make it impossible to extrapolate a sure-fire success formula'.

A young bioscientist venturing into industry from academe some 30 years ago, as I did, would quickly find that the expectations of his colleagues in chemistry were centred on the need to elaborate a simple and rapid sequence of laboratory tests to mimic as closely as possible some aspect of the disease or condition to which the bioscientist had been assigned. These tests would then be used to 'screen', at high throughput, many chemical compounds of different chemical types. Some of these would be the result of careful and imaginative thought, the remainder would be available from other programmes. When a 'lead' emerged, the power and intellect of the synthetic chemists would be brought to bear to 'optimize' the properties of the lead compound and produce a compound for development. This approach had proved immensely successful in the 1940s and 1950s in the hunt for antihistamines, antibacterials, antimalarials and even very potent and selective semisynthetic corticosteroids. However, because of the paucity of knowledge about the aetiology and pathogenesis of most diseases of organic dysfunction, many of the tests could only mimic some facet of the human condition, e.g. localized inflammation in rodents as model for inflammation of the joints in patients with rheumatoid arthritis or constriction of the bronchi in guinea pigs as a model of one of the distressing symptoms of asthma. Some of the models developed would have seemed to an outsider to be rather remote but many have resulted in the discovery of valuable new medicines such as indomethacin,[8] ibuprofen[9] and salbutamol.[10]

This type of approach is still used today, when knowledge of the aetiology and pathogenesis of the human condition is sparse.

A quite different approach is illustrated by the success of Sir James Black, Nobel Laureate, in the discovery of the β-adrenergic receptor blockers,[11,12] which represented a major advance in the treatment of cardiovascular disorders and the histamine-2 (H_2) blockers[13] for the inhibition of gastric acid secretion and the treatment of gastric and duodenal ulcers. Although bioassays were required in the search for these two classes of compounds, the discovery process was initiated to prove a hypothesis.

In the case of β-blockers, Dale,[14] 1906, had shown that certain actions of adrenaline could be blocked by the ergot alkaloids. However it was not until 1948 that Ahlquist[15] suggested that there were two distinct types of adrenotropic receptors, which he designated α (shown by others to be blocked by ergot alkaloids) and β, which could not be blocked by any chemical of natural or synthetic origin then available. Black's hypothesis was that if a chemical could be found to block the β-receptors, it would not only prove their existence but also have utility in the treatment of ischaemic heart disease. He and his colleagues in chemistry were gloriously successful.

In the case of H_2 blockers, it was known that histamine injected intravenously resulted in an increase in secretion of gastric juice in animals, including humans. Available antihistamines did not block the increased secretion caused by histamine, hence Black postulated there must be a second receptor capable of being blocked by a chemical of different structure to those available at that time. Although the concepts were, with hindsight, simple and 'obvious', intense and dedicated collaboration with medicinal chemists and other scientists was required to prove the hypotheses and ultimately develop marketable products.

There is no doubt that as fundamental knowledge continues to accumulate, this more sophisticated approach to the discovery of new chemical entities is likely to be increasingly successful. In this context it is noteworthy that an increasing number of preliminary evaluations for new chemical entities are now being conducted against isolated enzymes which have been shown or are thought to be important in the pathogenesis of certain diseases. This, in part, has been responsible for the encouraging decline in the number of animals used in research during the last 10 years (Fig. 1.2).

Research to discover new medicines requires above all, bright, knowledgeable and imaginative individuals with the ability and capability to pursue, without diversion, an obsession. However, whilst ideas come from individuals, multidisciplinary teams of colleagues are required to help pursue the ideas with a productive team spirit and towards agreed decision points. These include a technical information support group, which can intelligently sift and process on demand the world's knowledge base; expert patent agents who can effectively protect the intellectual property resulting from the many years of expensive research; and well equipped support groups in pharmaceutical research, information systems, computer technology, physical methods and general support services. It also requires patient, sensitive, enlightened and astute management in the research, medical, development and commercial functions.

Whereas many references have been made to the important rôle of the medicinal chemists in the search for new chemical entities, it would be remiss to conclude this section without reference to the exciting opportunities presented by those engaged in biotechnology.

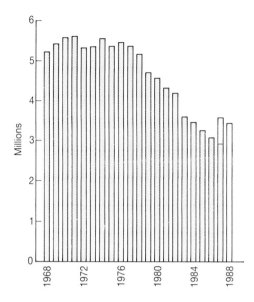

Fig. 1.2 Number of experiments (■) or scientific procedures (□), as classified by the 1876 or 1986 Acts, commenced each year from 1968 to 1988. (Based on Home Office Statistics.[16])

The discovery by Watson and Crick[17] of the structure of DNA in 1952 eventually resulted in scientists being able to synthesize genes that could be inserted into micro-organisms to instruct them to produce human proteins of use in the laboratory and clinic. During the last 10 years, biotechnology departments, with their bright and imaginative 'genetic engineers', have become an integral and important part of the search for new chemical entities in many companies. Biotechnology is currently a means to an end, in that those skilled in the science of genetic engineering are able to make micro-organisms and mammalian cells produce active proteins that medicinal chemists have not been able to synthesize or have only been able to synthesize with great difficulty in small amounts. The first protein to be made commercially available for human use by genetic engineering was human insulin.[18] Subsequently, human growth hormone[19] for the treatment of dwarfism, tissue plasminogen activating factor[20] for dissolving fibrin clots and erythropoietin[21] for the stimulation of red cell production have also been approved for human use. Many other exciting molecules are currently in development, including Factor VIII for the treatment of haemophilia and a variety of colony stimulating factors for improving the levels of granulocytes, macrophages and other cell types.

It is extremely sad that the availability of genetically engineered human growth hormone and Factor VIII was just too late to save a generation of haemophiliacs and youngsters with growth hormone deficiency being infected with the AIDS virus. Had these products of genetic engineering been available only a few years earlier, it is probable that they would have quickly replaced the proteins derived, with difficulty, from human pituitaries and human blood – some samples of which we now know to have been disastrously contaminated with this disease-causing virus.

Proteins synthesized by modified micro-organisms have also been of great value in the facilitation of research in many therapeutic areas, e.g. the production of human renin,[22] which hitherto had to be extracted in minute amounts from human kidneys for research on novel antihypertensive therapies and the production of a variety of receptors to permit test-tube assays.

Although biotechnology is *currently* a means to an end, there can be no doubt that in the not too distant future the prospects of manipulating genes in the human body could have a profound effect on the treatment of conditions like cancer, where abhorrent genes need to be switched on or switched off to cause cells to revert to their normal healthy state. Advances such as these will also rely heavily on the developing skills of imaginative pharmacists and allied scientists who have already mastered the controlled release of certain polypeptides, e.g. luteinizing hormone releasing hormone agonists,[23] and who in the future will be required to develop novel, targeted delivery systems to facilitate the interaction of novel medicines with specific cell types in the human body.

Finally, we must not forget when considering the discovery process the rôle of the astute physician. There will always be limitations to the accuracy with which scientists in the laboratory can predict efficacy in humans. However, the rôle of the physician does not end when efficacy is proven at the proving trial stage, since some medicines introduced for the treatment of one disease state have subsequently been observed to be of value in unrelated diseases. The list given in Table 1.1[24] is testimony to the prowess of physicians with acute and fertile minds who, having prescribed a medicine for the treatment of one disease, have observed 'other effects' that have subsequently proven to be of immense importance in other disease states – states totally unrelated to the original indication!

Lest all should appear sweetness and light regarding the discovery of new medicine, it is important to recognize that scientists throughout the world are subjected to a plethora of increasing controls that divert them from their principal task of preventing premature death and alleviating suffering. In the UK, for example, recent legislation associated with the control of ionizing radiation, the control of substances hazardous to health, the release of micro-organisms in the environment, the Animal Procedures Act 1986, etc., etc., all mitigate against the speedy discovery and development of new medicines.

It is difficult to object to virtue but care will be required by those promulgating future legislation to understand the realities of the medicine discovery process and to take into account the need for as much freedom as possible to allow scientists time to think about new and exciting opportunities rather than spending the majority of their time worrying about whether they are complying fully with the multiplicity of the laws governing the conduct of science.

Table 1.1 Additional uses of medicines discovered during clinical usage

Drug	Initial use	Additional or new primary use
Allopurinol	Antineoplastic	Treatment for gout
Amphetamine	Stimulant	Hyperkinesis in children
Benziodarone	Anti-anginal	Uricosuric
Chlorpromazine	Anthelmintic	Antischizophrenic
Oestrogens	Replacement therapy	Contraception
Imipramine	Sedative	Antidepressant
Lignocaine	Local anaesthetic	Anti-arrhythmic
Chlordiazepoxide	Muscle relaxant	Tranquillizer
Amantadine	Antiviral	Antiparkinson
Penicillamine	Copper chelating agent for Wilson's disease	Antirheumatic
Adrenergic blockers	Anti-arrhythmic/ anti-anginal	Antihypertensive
Metronidazole	Antitrichomonal	Antibacterial-anaerobic organisms
Chloroquin	Antimalarial	Antirheumatic
Anturan	Uricosuric	Secondary prevention of myocardial infarction; inhibitor of platelet aggregation

The development phase

The transition from the research phase to the development phase is recognized to be one of the most difficult and complex decisions that senior management has to make.

Whereas millions may have been spent on nurturing a research team to the point where they are convinced they have a chemical with potentially valuable medicinal properties, the decision to develop will commit the company to a complex, tedious and lengthy development programme and to expenditure which could exceed £100 million. Those making the decision must therefore have a full and detailed understanding of why the bioscience is considered to have exciting medical implications and what are the excitements and concerns of the medicinal and process development chemists, the patent experts, the pharmacists and those engaged in preliminary safety evaluation. In addition, views are required from the medical advisers about the nature and complexity of the eventual clinical research and proving trials and also from those skilled in forecasting the commercial value of the potential new medicine. Essentially, the decision makers have to form a view of the likely technical outcome of the project; whether the continued high investment is likely to yield an appropriate commercial return; and what is the likely impact at the end of development of competitor activity.

Although the 6 years or more of the discovery phase has changed little over the last 30 years, the time span of the development phase has become increasingly protracted.

In the period up to the mid 1960s, it rarely took more than 3 years or so from the time of invention for the public to receive the benefits.[25] It now takes in excess of 6 years for a chemical destined for the therapy of acute conditions to become a medicine and in excess of 10 years for one targeted for the treatment of chronic disease states. The reasons for these lengthening development times can be traced to an increase in preclinical safety evaluation tests in the late 1960s and early 1970s,[26] followed by an increased requirement for more clinical efficacy and safety data in the 1980s.

During the 1960s the serious adverse teratogenic effects associated with the introduction of thalidomide stimulated scientists in industry and those working for regulatory authorities to consider how such disastrous events could, in the future, be avoided. In consequence, during the late 1960s and throughout the 1970s, there was an escalation in the number and type of tests required to be conducted at the preclinical evaluation stage and an increase in the number of animals deemed necessary to confer statistical validity. The length of time over which the tests were conducted was also extended and inevitably the amount of data to be analysed and reported increased enormously. By the mid to late 1970s it was rare for the preclinical safety evaluation phase to be completed in less than 3 years, even with the most careful planning and with the maximum acceptance of risk, by conducting tests in parallel rather than sequentially.

In addition, during the late 1970s, it became mandatory for laboratories to conduct all preclinical safety evaluation tests in accordance with standards prescribed in Good Laboratory Practice (GLP) regulations.[27] This initiative did not extend the period of preclinical evaluation but it did require the recording and archiving of many more data and the storage for at least 10 years of all tissues and organs sampled for histological examination, together with the microscopy slides used in the evaluation of the study. All these initiatives were accommodated by industry in the interests of patient safety and data integrity. However, the increased costs associated with the employment of more people and the construction of more buildings were considerable.

The period of clinical evaluation has always been dependent on whether the potential medicine is destined for the treatment of acute or chronic conditions. However, a feature of the 1980s is that there has been a striking increase in the number of clinical trials required by the regulatory authorities and an increase in the number of patients to be involved in those trials. All studies are now expected to be conducted in accordance with the principles of Good Clinical Research Practice,[28] which in turn reflects on the nature and quantity of data which is required to be analysed and archived. Furthermore, the development of more effective postmarketing surveillance (PMS) techniques, which are of value to all involved in establishing safety profiles, add to the data banks which have to be analysed and archived.

The compilation of documents detailing the work conducted at the pre-clinical and clinical stages of development is a formidable task, involving many years of effort. The data are now so voluminous that specialist 'quality assurance teams' are required to examine final documents for accuracy and consistency. Furthermore, in order to facilitate the eventual appraisal of the documentation by regulatory authorities, it is now necessary for the manufacturer to provide 'Expert Summaries' covering the important issues embodied within the documents relating to chemistry and pharmacy, pharmacology and toxicology and, finally, the clinical sections of the submission.

The amount of paper submitted to 25 registration authorities in association with four products was recently highlighted by Cox.[6] In 1976/1977 the pile was *c.* 50 m in height. By 1989/1990 it was almost the height of the Eiffel Tower (Fig. 1.3)!

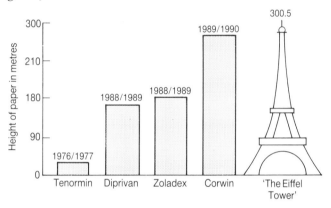

Compound submitted and approximate date of marketing

Fig. 1.3 Amount of paper submitted to the 25 'First Wave' registration authorities. (From Cox.[6])

All the changes referred to have been developed with and accepted by industry in an effort to assure doctors and patients that the discovery and development of a chemical into a medicine is a thorough and highly professional process. It cannot guarantee complete safety but should permit an improved analysis of risk/benefit at the different stages of development. However, the consequence of increased development time scales is a serious erosion of effective patent life (Fig. 1.4).

Reflections

The discovery of a chemical with potential medicinal properties and its development to the point where it can be made available to people throughout the world for preventing premature death or alleviating suffering is a challenging, lengthy and very costly process. Although much has been achieved during my lifetime – much remains to be accomplished. There is no shortage of 'targets', e.g. AIDS, senile dementia, rheumatoid

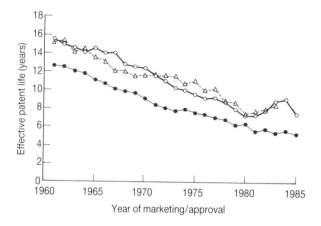

Fig. 1.4   Pharmaceutical patent erosion – a comparison of the UK (● — ●), USA (△ - - - △) and former West Germany (○—○) shown as a 3-year moving average.

arthritis, Parkinson's disease, many many different types of cancer, and improved treatments for cardiovascular and circulatory disorders, acute and chronic schizophrenia, motor neurone diseases, muscular dystrophy, disseminated sclerosis, diabetes, etc., etc., etc. – the list is endless. It is essential that those involved and associated with the search for new medicines recognize that of the many factors involved there are three that are paramount.

1. 'State-of-the-art', imaginative and obsessive researchers in bioscience, chemistry, medicine and cognate sciences.
2. Visionary sponsors in academe and industry with appropriate patience.
3. Regulators who are dedicated to achieving the international harmonization of preclinical and clinical data requirements to enable life-saving new medicines discovered in the future by dedicated scientists to become available to physicians and patients internationally, as quickly and as efficiently as possible.

References

1. Domagk G (1935). Ein beitrag zur chemotherapie der bakteriellen infectionen. *Deutsche Medizinische Wochenschrift* **61**: 250.
2. Domagk G (1935). Eine neue klasse von desinfektonsmittein. *Deutsche Medizinische Wochenschrift* **61**: 829.
3. Colebrook L, Kenny M (1936). Treatment of human puerperal infections and of experimental infections in mice with Prontosil. *Lancet* **1**: 1279.
4. Buttle GAH, Gray WH, Stephenson D (1936). Protection of mice against streptococcal and other infections by p-aminobenzene sulphonamide and related substances. *Lancet* **1**: 1286.
5. Weatherall M (1985). How are drugs discovered? In Burley DM, Binns TB (eds.) *Pharmaceutical Medicine*. London: Edward Arnold: 1–17.

6. Cox B (1980). Strategies for drug discovery: structuring serendipity. *Pharmaceutical Journal* **243**: 329.
7. Nayak PR, Kettingham JM (1986). *Breakthroughs!* New York: Rawson Associates.
8. Shen TY, Winter CA (1977). Chemical and biological studies on indomethacin, sulindac and their analogues. *Advances in Drug Research* **12**: 90.
9. Adams SS, Buckler JW (1979). Ibuprofen and flurbiprofen. *Clinical Rheumatic Diseases* **5**: 359.
10. Cullum VA, Farmer JB, Jack D *et al.* (1969). Salbutamol; a beta-adrenoceptive receptor stimulant. *Journal of Pharmacology* **35**: 141.
11. Black JW, Stephenson JS (1962). Pharmacology of a new adrenergic beta-receptor-blocking compound (nethalide). *Lancet* **ii**: 311.
12. Black JW, Crowther AF, Shanks RG *et al.* (1964). A new adrenergic beta-receptor antagonist. *Lancet* **i**: 1080.
13. Black JW, Duncan WAM, Durant CJ *et al.* (1972). Definition and antagonism of histamine H_2-receptors. *Nature* **236**: 385.
14. Dale HH (1906). On some physiological actions of ergot. *Journal of Physiology* **34**: 163.
15. Ahlquist RP (1948). A study of the adrenotropic receptors. *American Journal of Physiology* **153**: 586.
16. Home Office (1988). *Statistics of Scientific Procedures on Living Animals; Great Britain 1988*. London: HMSO.
17. Watson JD, Crick FHC (1953). Molecular structure of nucleic acids. Genetical implications of the structure of deoxyribonucleic acid. *Nature* **171**: 737.
18. Johnson IS (1983). Human insulin from recombinant DNA technology. *Science* **219**: 632.
19. Ross MJ, Olson KC, Geier MD *et al.* (1986). Recombinant DNA synthesis of human growth hormone. In Raiti S, Tolman RA (eds.) *Human Growth Hormone*. New York: Plenum: 241.
20. Grossbard EB (1987). Recombinant tissue plasminogen activator: a brief review. *Pharmacological Research* **4**: 375.
21. Egrie JC, Stickland TW, Lane J *et al.* (1986). Characterization and biological effects of recombinant human erythropoietin. *Immunobiology* **172**: 213.
22. Haas E, Goldblatt H, Gipson EC (1965). Extraction, purification and acetylation of human renin and the production of antirenin to human renin. *Archives of Biochemistry and Biophysics* **110**: 534.
23. Hutchinson FG, Furr BJA (1987). Biodegradable carriers for the sustained release of polypeptides. *Trends in Biotechnology* **5**: 102.
24. Newbould BB (1987). *Pharmaceuticals – Focus on R&D* London: National Economic Development Office: 28.
25. Newbould BB (1987). *Pharmaceuticals – Focus on R&D*. London: National Economic Development Office: 14.
26. Newbould BB (1981). *Risk–benefit Analysis in Drug Research*. Lancaster: MTP Press Ltd.
27. DoH (1989). *Good Laboratory Practice. The United Kingdom Compliance Programme (1989)*. London: Department of Health.
28. ABPI (1988). *Guidelines On Good Clinical Research Practice*. London: The Association of the British Pharmaceutical Industry.

2

Preclinical toxicity testing

*Roger W. Brimblecombe and
Anthony D. Dayan*

Before starting to investigate a potential new medicine in humans, it is necessary to carry out preclinical studies to explore the biological activities of the compound in terms of its potential efficacy and safety.

Studies relevant to proposed therapeutic or prophylactic use vary considerably with the class of drug concerned. This chapter is not concerned with that aspect but rather with safety studies which tend to be more stereotyped. Even so, there are differences according to such factors as the chemical nature and therapeutic class of the drug, its pharmaceutical formulation, route of administration, anticipated duration of use and the type of patient to be treated.

Although the investigations described here are conventionally and conveniently described as 'safety' studies, it is important to emphasize that their purpose is not to establish that a drug is *safe* – absolute safety is unachievable and the common term 'safety evaluation' refers to a judgement based on experimentation – but rather to determine the nature and degree of the risk likely to be associated with use of the drug. There has been regrettably little attempt to review the correlation between preclinical 'safety' studies and clinical observations, but general experience suggests it is reasonable.[1-3]

The degree of risk can be estimated very approximately by dividing the effective dose or the anticipated therapeutic dose into the maximum dose tolerated without adverse effects in animal toxicity studies. If all doses are expressed per kg body weight, a therapeutic ratio or risk/benefit ratio may be obtained. It is imprecise and varies with many factors, but the ratio does give some basis for comparison between drugs. It is, appropriately, becoming more common to express the ratio in terms of blood levels achieved rather than dose administered. The acceptable ratio might be much lower, for example, for a drug for use in a life-threatening condition than for one designed to alleviate symptoms of a relatively trivial complaint.

The nature of the risk can be assessed by careful appraisal of the results of animal toxicity studies. One aim should be to determine the likely target organ(s) for adverse effects of high doses of the drug and to establish whether the effects are reversible. Particular attention can then be paid to monitoring the function of such organs in early clinical studies and, if appropriate, when the drug is eventually released for widespread use.

The studies described in this chapter are generally applicable to most drugs. All exceptions cannot be mentioned, and neither can the individual requirements of regulatory agencies around the world. If a dossier were prepared along the lines suggested here, it is anticipated that the strictly scientific requirements of agencies in most countries would be satisfied. It should be noted that the newly formed 'International Conference on Harmonisation', which comprises representatives of regulatory agencies and the pharmaceutical industry is trying to regularize drug testing regimes by obtaining general acceptance of simplified protocols for the principal types of non-clinical testing which will be acceptable in all major countries. So far there has been agreement about replacement of the LD_{50} test by 'limit dose' and similar procedures and about the acceptability of 6-month instead of 12-month tests in rodents.[4]

General aspects of toxicity testing

The basic format of the test is to expose animals or *in vitro* systems to a range of doses or concentrations of the drug in circumstances in which either it is considered likely that relevant actions will be detectable, or in which precedent has shown them to occur. (For a general review see Barnes and Denz[5] and Paget;[6] for an example of regulatory interpretation in Europe see the Committee on Proprietary Medicinal Products;[7] for a listing of regulatory demands see Alder and Zbinden;[8] and for a recent general review see Dayan.[9])

A wide range of observations is made in order to detect any effect and its consequences, predicted from prior knowledge of the pharmacological properties and chemical structure of the compound and using a standard set of general techniques to detect and explore as many actions as possible.

The general features implicit in the experiments merit separate discussion.

Choice of test

Different types of experiment are necessary to reveal different types of effects: acute and chronic toxicity tests in animals to reveal general and organ-specific actions; the very prolonged carcinogenicity tests in animals to show any potential for producing tumours; effects on reproductive processes in tests involving fertilization of animals, as well as by studies on the developing foetus and on postnatal development of the young; various *in vitro* and *in vivo* techniques to detect mutagenicity, i.e. the possibility that a substance might affect DNA; and for substances to be applied topically, the study of local effects as well as any general activity of absorbed material. As either the desired therapeutic or unwanted toxic actions may be due to the parent substance or to a metabolite, absorption, distribution, metabolism and excretion must also be examined, and this knowledge may help to validate other tests by relating plasma levels and metabolism in the test species and humans. Last, if prior biological or chemical knowledge of the test material, or experience of it or close analogues in humans, suggests the likelihood of special types of toxicity, then specific tests should be employed to investigate their occurrence and importance, e.g. the possibility of sensitization, of general depression or enhancement of immune responses, of physical dependence (addiction), of interaction with the pharmacological actions or metabolism of other medicines, of any influence of genotypic differences, such as acetylator status, etc.

A topic under current debate concerns compounds containing chiral centres. Such compounds should be regarded as mixtures of two or more enantiomers. The attitude of regulatory agencies is hardening against the development of such racemates unless evidence can be provided to indicate that there is no penalty, especially in terms of safety, of developing them rather than single enantiomers. Toxicity studies, in conjunction with other investigations, would be required to justify such development.

In general terms, the preclinical investigation of biologicals and biotechnology products follows a similar pattern, but it should be modified to take account of the unique properties of these agents, their immunogenicity and their common species specificity.[10]

Nature of tests in animals

The majority of toxicity tests are firmly based on studies in whole animals, because only in them is it possible to approach the complexity of organization of body systems in humans, to explore any consequences of variable absorption, metabolism and excretion, and to reveal not only direct toxic effects but also those of a secondary or indirect nature due to induced abnormalities in integrative mechanisms, or distant effects of a toxic metabolite produced in one organ that acts on another, e.g. the consequences of the hypothyroid state produced by sulphonamides, or the crystal nephropathy that follows conversion of swallowed ethylene glycol to oxalate in the liver. Studies in animals, too, permit many general investigative procedures to be employed, often identical to those used in humans, e.g. clinical observation, change in weight, blood biochemistry, etc. *In vitro* techniques tend to be far more restricted and so are better adapted to precise analysis of discrete actions previously identified by less specific means, e.g. *in vitro* enzyme assays to determine the consequences of exposure to a cholinesterase or cyclo-oxygenase inhibitor, or study of the tissue transport mechanisms that may underlie the nephrotoxicity of the aminoglycoside antibiotics.

The privilege and opportunity to carry out studies in animals brings with it the responsibility of ensuring that their use is really necessary, of planning the work to maximize the information obtained and to minimize the number of animals required, and of providing the best possible care and attention for them.[11]

Experimentation based on *in vitro* methods is both ethically and economically attractive, but before 'alternative' methods can replace conventional procedures it is necessary to be certain that the information they provide is of equal quality and scope in protecting the health of humans and other animals. Critical assessment will show that the so-called 'alternative' methods would be better described as 'complementary', because they are not yet sufficiently well proven or robust to replace the procedures used today. There is growing interest in non-animal techniques, and their future development seems likely to be rapid provided that they are shown to give valid information for predicting harm.[12,13]

Which species to use is a difficult matter. Scientific points in favour of a particular species are that it is known to respond to analogous compounds in a way similar to humans (something improbable in the development of a new drug), that a sufficient number of healthy animals are available, that they can be properly handled (i.e. considerations of ferocity, size, ability to make clinical observations and to obtain samples for laboratory tests), and that there is adequate background experience of their toxicological and pathological responses to permit interpretation of the findings. The ability to detect and measure the pharmacodynamic response desired in humans can be a strong factor in favouring one species over another, as it would permit ready comparison of the therapeutic and toxic doses.

In practice almost all conventional toxicity testing is carried out in a rodent and a non-rodent species, in the expectation that such a wide range would suggest what is likely to occur in humans. Regulations are usually framed in a general manner, but testing is conventionally carried out in the rat and dog. The mouse and the golden (Syrian) hamster are alternative rodents, and a primate is sometimes used instead of the dog, commonly the baboon (*Papio* spp), cynomolgus (*M. fascicularis*) or rhesus (*M. mulatta*) monkey. For topical studies the rabbit is the standard species for tests on the eye because it is reasonably docile and has large eyes, which facilitates biomicroscopy and in which the medicament can readily be retained. For work on the skin both the rabbit and guinea pig are commonly used, with the ordinary or mini-pig as less tractable alternatives. The rat and mouse or hamster are the standard species for carcinogenicity tests.

In reproductive toxicity experiments it is customary to use the rat and the rabbit. The former is chosen because of its convenience (size, availability and wealth of background knowledge), and because other extensive toxicological and metabolic studies will have been carried out on it. The latter is used because it is one of the few species that responds to the embryotoxic and teratogenic effects of thalidomide. Occasionally a foetal toxicity study may be carried out on the dog, pig or primate, but although the last two may sometimes be closer to humans in certain respects, their practical disadvantages far outweigh any but very special pharmacodynamic or pharmacokinetic considerations.

Good Laboratory Practice regulations

All formal toxicity studies on pharmaceuticals, and many pharmacokinetic and metabolic studies also, are expected to conform to the Good Laboratory Practice (GLP) regulations.[14] These are a complex set of rules to demonstrate the validity of the data produced in toxicity experiments; they require written protocols and amendments, permanent recording and storage of data and a provision for checking conformity by internal and external (Department of Health) inspectors. It is necessary for all relevant procedures to follow written Standard Operating Procedures (SOPs).

Work carried out according to the GLP codes will be internationally acceptable, which is now essential in the development of a new medicine.

The GLP system has made toxicity testing more formal and cumbersome, but it should not affect the scientific responsibility of the toxicologist to design and perform whatever investigations may be necessary to reveal and understand the toxic effects of a compound. Investigative flexibility can be retained – at the cost of more forethought and more records.

Acute, subacute and chronic toxicity tests

Acute tests

Acute toxicity tests are now used to establish an approximate lethal dose of a compound in different species by different routes of administration, as it is agreed that there is usually no value in making a precise LD_{50} determination (the dose which would be lethal to 50 per cent of a population), which would require many animals. The tests are carried out by giving progressively increasing doses of the compound to small groups of animals until an end-point, usually death, is reached, or until an arbitrary large limit has been reached.

All animals must be carefully observed during the tests and at autopsy for any effects apparently associated with administration of the compound. Limiting pharmacological effects may be manifest; these may give an indication of the target organs for toxic effects, and the result may give some guidance about the choice of doses for subsequent repeat-dose toxicity studies (for a general review see Boyd[15]). In a non-rodent species one or two animals may be given a few increasing doses whilst being monitored very closely. The intention is not to find a lethal dose but to gain information about the relation between high doses and observable actions.

Acute studies should be carried out using at least those species and those routes of administration intended for use in repeat-dose toxicity studies. The intravenous route should usually be used in any event since it gives the best estimate of 'intrinsic' acute toxicity, uncomplicated by such factors as absorption from the gut or other sites of administration.

The numbers of animals used in acute studies is changing. Previously, LD_{50} values have been estimated in groups of small animals, usually rats and mice, and the approximate lethal dose, which requires use of far fewer animals, has been estimated in short-term experiments of a pharmacological type in larger species, including the dog. Nowadays, the approximate or a fixed dose procedure is employed.[16]

Subacute and chronic tests

The distinction between subacute and chronic toxicity tests is arbitrary and the term repeated-dose tests may be preferable. However, in shorter term tests of up to, say, 3 months' duration the aim must be to push the dose as high as possible to determine end-organ toxicity.

In such studies the daily doses may be adjusted in the course of the test if they appear to be too high or too low. In tests of longer than 3 months' duration it is less usual to adjust doses, which should have been established in the shorter term test. The common aim is for the highest dose to produce some minimal adverse effect (e.g. reduction of up to 10 per cent in the rate of body weight gain) without causing the death of so many animals that an examination cannot be made at the termination of the test.

Certain general principles govern the conduct of repeated-dose toxicity tests; for details of numbers of animals, biochemical and haematological investigations, lists of tissues to be taken for histology, etc. reference should be made to the Association of the British Pharmaceutical Industry (ABPI) Guidelines for Preclinical and Clinical Testing of New Medical Products (1977),[17] and to the guidelines issued by regulatory authorities.[7,8] It is instructive also to compare the experiments carried out to detect the hazards of a candidate medicine with those applied to a new food additive or other household product destined for widespread use by man.[18,19]

The basic features common to all repeated-dose toxicity studies are:

1. It is necessary to examine a range of doses so that any likely effect will be produced and the dose–response relationship be examined. The high dose is generally selected as one that causes no more than slight (say not more than 10 per cent) reduction in weight gain during treatment, probably as determined in a preliminary trial. Alternatively, in the case of a non-toxic compound, the dose may be chosen as not exceeding 100x to 200x the anticipated human dose, or may be related to a readily detectable pharmacodynamic action or to a blood level. The low dose would normally be a low multiple of the anticipated human dose and the middle dose would be the geometric mean of the other two.

2. The route of administration should be that intended for humans, as far as possible. It may be constrained by the non-specific effects of the stress caused by certain procedures, but oral treatment by gavage once or even twice daily is conventional, as is once or twice daily injection or topical application, and exposure to an aerosol is feasible albeit more difficult. For a topically applied agent absorbed from topical sites, appropriate tests should be carried out with systemically administered compound, as well as topical studies.

3. Two mammalian species, a rodent and a non-rodent, are normally used, commonly the rat and the dog. Dosing should start while the animals are immature. Ideally, the pharmacodynamic, pharmacokinetic and metabolic profile of the compound should be similar in the chosen species and in humans. This ideal may be difficult to achieve, partly because much work will already have

been carried out in animals before work in humans can begin. Nevertheless, if the profile of the compound being tested turns out to be significantly different in humans from either of the chosen species, there may be concern about the validity of extrapolation from the toxicity studies. Similarly, if absorption is limited in the test species, that, too, will jeopardize the value of the experiments. It is important in toxicity testing to demonstrate the overall validity of studies by a pharmacokinetic comparison with other laboratory species and with humans.

4.   The studies should be designed to determine whether any detected adverse effects are reversible, i.e. a recovery group should be included.

5.   It is very important to measure the plasma concentration of compound in animals in repeated-dose toxicity studies, and sometimes to monitor a key metabolite as well. This has a number of advantages. It is possible to check that animals have been dosed on any given day of the study, and there will be an indication of whether there is a build-up of compound in the blood with repeated dosing. Perhaps most important of all, the plasma concentration of a compound is a more relevant parameter than the administered dose. An indication will also be obtained of non-linear kinetics at any given dose level i.e. saturation of a normal metabolic process leading to cumulation of a drug or its metabolites. The ratio between the respective plasma concentrations associated with a given toxic phenomenon and with a therapeutic effect is likely to give a better indication of therapeutic ratio than just the relation between the toxic and effective doses.

The requirement for a plasma assay method necessitates early development of an analytical method or it may become a rate-limiting step in the development of a drug.

6.   The duration of administration of a new drug in toxicity studies governs the period for which the drug can be administered to humans in clinical testing. Recommendations acceptable to many regulatory agencies are given in the EC Guidelines.[7] One point worth noting is that in shorter term tests the dosing period is relatively short compared with the total time from instigation of the study to issue of the report. The number of tissues to be processed and slides to be examined are the same irrespective of the duration of the study. Thus it may be false economy to carry out, say, a 2-week rather than a 1-month test, as the latter will allow more protracted continuous studies in humans.

Reproductive toxicity testing

The search for a possible effect of a new medicine on reproduction is complex, because of the diversity of processes to be considered: production of gametes; fertilization; implantation; intrauterine development of the zygote into an embryo; birth; and postnatal growth to maturity. Several distinct types of preclinical test procedure have been developed for separate investigation of the principal stages in the overall process of reproduction, representing both empirically based scientific procedures and the precedent of past findings, most notably the consequences of administration of thalidomide to humans. (General accounts of reproductive studies and references to more specialized investigations are given by Wilson and Warkany,[20] Neubert *et al.*[21] and Snell;[22] regulatory requirements in the UK have been published by the Department of Health and Social Security (DHSS),[23] and they remain extant in the EC.[7])

Types of tests

The aim is to employ procedures which will generally reveal any potential adverse effect during the production and fertilization of gametes (so-called 'Fertility' or 'Segment 1' test), during embryogenesis ('Foetal Toxicity', 'Teratology' or Segment II test), or during birth and subsequent development ('Peri- and Postnatal' or Segment III test). The extent to which these stages are separated in practice and the nature of the detailed examinations conducted in each may differ from country to country because of local regulatory preference.

Overall regulatory requirements in the UK (ABPI) Guidelines[8,17] conform to those in the EC[7] (see Chapters 7 and 8). The pattern of the procedures is for the fertility test to comprise morphological examination in late pregnancy of dams dosed before and during embryogenesis after mating with males dosed for 70 days prior to mating, as well as behavioural and anatomical tests on offspring, some of which are allowed to develop for several weeks after birth; for the teratology test to cover morphological study of foetuses from dams treated during the sensitive period of organogenesis, and sometimes their subsequent maturation; and for the peri- and postnatal test to comprise extensive behavioural and autopsy investigations of pups from mothers treated during the latter part of pregnancy and lactation. A principal variant of this scheme, which is common in the USA, it to extend the fertility test to include dosing of the dams before and throughout gestation and to examine the breeding performance of randomly chosen pups ('two-generation test') in the hope that this procedure will cover all three phases of reproductive toxicity testing. The approach in Japan[8] differs in that dosing in the three types of study is strictly limited to the periods prior to fertilization, during embryogenesis and during late pre- and postnatal development.

Selection of doses and route of administration

The same principles apply to reproductive studies as to general toxicity tests (see above). Non-specific stress due to the general toxicity of an excessively high dose should be avoided, as it may itself affect the ability of animals to provide viable sperm, to ovulate or to copulate, and it may harm the viability and growth of the developing foetus, even to the extent of producing morphological abnormalities, which may sometimes be confused with a specific harmful action of the test compound.

Choice of species

Current practice is to carry out fertility tests in the rat, using any of the conventional random-bred strains. Foetal toxicity studies are also carried out in the rat and in the rabbit. The latter is required because it is the only convenient laboratory species that responds to thalidomide. Peri- and postnatal testing is carried out in the rat.

The advantages of the rat include the considerable amount of background knowledge of its responses, the data likely to be available about the pharmacodynamic and pharmacokinetic properties of the substance in it, the ready availability of healthy, defined stocks, the relative ease of handling adequate numbers of rats in the laboratory and the relative rapidity of its maturation and gestation.

It is not often necessary to do tests in other species. There may sometimes be good scientific reason for considering alternatives, for example in investigation of the predictive significance of the mechanism of an induced abnormality, particularly if a compound is thought to be likely to affect the processes of implantation and placentation, which differ in humans and the rat and rabbit. If an alternative species is to be considered the choice may be made from amongst:

Mouse	Very well studied but small size detracts from examination techniques.
Syrian hamster	Unusual placentation; not easy to dose.
Dog	Large size; limited number of pups; mating tedious.
Pig	Resembles humans in many respects; large and difficult to handle, prolonged gestation.
Primate	Resembles humans in many respects; less well studied than other species; handling and husbandry more difficult; prolonged gestation.

Whatever animals are used, their husbandry must be of the highest quality to maintain their health, to prevent stress and other non-specific disturbing factors and to ensure that environmental factors, such as lighting, pheromones, etc. are standardized, thus ensuring endocrine factors controlling reproductive activity and performance are held constant.

Outline features of tests

Fertility test

In principle, the processes that might be affected comprise the production of gametes, mating and fertilization to produce the zygote. The nature of the test is partly determined by the period of about 6 weeks for gametogenesis in the male rat. Although the ovum in the female completes its major development prenatally, final maturation and ovulation occur in mid-oestrus cycle, after which the oocyte remains viable for only a limited period unless fertilized. The test procedure must permit detection of effects on the complex physiological processes of spermatogenesis, ovulation and fertilization.

In the rat, groups of about 20 young males (usually selected immediately after weaning) are treated with the test substance for 60 days to cover a full cycle of spermatogenesis, including storage and final maturation of spermatozoa in the epididymis. Identical-sized groups of females are treated for 14 days to exclude any action on ovulation, which is assessed by regular examination of vaginal smears. The animals are then allowed to mate naturally, on a 1:1 basis, and the females are examined regularly for a vaginal plug as evidence of successful copulation. The mated females are dosed until day 7 of gestation (time of implantation) and are then followed until day 18 of gestation, i.e. until just before the time of natural birth, regular observations being made of their health, behaviour and weight gain. About two-thirds are then killed and autopsied.

The numbers of corpora lutea are counted as a measure of ovulation, the numbers of viable and dead embryos and implants are compared (to reveal intrauterine deaths) and the weights and sexes of the foetuses are recorded. In turn, the foetuses are examined for abnormalities of external form (e.g. cleft palate and limb lesions), a proportion is dissected to study the viscera, others are X-rayed or more often cleared in alkali and the bones stained with alizarin to reveal skeletal lesions, and others may be examined by the Wilson (coronal) slicing technique to show abnormalities in the head. Of the animals permitted to litter normally, the numbers of live and dead pups and their sex are recorded, the subsequent weight change and behaviour of the dams are observed, and the pups are followed to 42 days of age with periodic assessment of growth and physical and behavioural development.

As mentioned above, the females are dosed until day 7 of gestation, as it is considered that treatment until that time may also reveal any effect on transport of the zygote and formation and implantation of the blastocyte. In one variant of the test, dosing of the mothers is stopped on the day of mating to reveal any effect until that stage, without risking obscuration by an action postfertilization. In another, the offspring of dosed parents are mated and subsequent development of their foetuses is followed.

The data are analysed statistically to show any differences related to treatment in reproductive ability, in the weight gain of the dams and the pups, in ovulation and implantation, in intrauterine survival and growth, in the incidence and nature of foetal abnormalities, and in postnatal development assessed as survival, growth and maturation of external appendages and behaviour.

Although not intended to be a study in pharmacokinetics, it is valuable to check the plasma level of the drug from time to time, particularly in males of the parental generation during their prolonged exposure.

This experimental design is economical, particularly as animals with persistent infertility can be withdrawn for further investigation, i.e. mated with an untreated partner of the opposite sex to check one possible source of the infertility, autopsied or left without treatment for a period to permit recovery from a drug effect before a test mating. In a more rigorous type of experiment treated animals would only be mated with an untreated partner, but this would double the number of animals required *ab initio*. It appears more efficient first to seek an effect and then to devise experiments to investigate its specific cause, e.g. by functional, endocrinological or other means.

Foetal toxicity test

As the processes of organogenesis are the focus of this type of investigation, the dams alone are treated in the sensitive period. Morphological study of the foetuses, and sometimes assessment of the growth and functional development of pups, then follows.

In a typical test in the rat, groups of 20 to 30 adult females are followed by daily vaginal smears for at least two oestrus cycles to confirm that ovulation is occurring normally. They are then mated with adult males, the morning on which a vaginal plug is found being counted as day 0 of day 16. On day 18 or 19 (dependent on the strain, i.e. just before natural parturition with its risk of loss of abnormal foetuses by cannibalism etc.) up to 20 dams are killed and dissected to show the numbers of corpora lutea, live and dead implants, and the numbers, sexes and sizes of the foetuses. The latter are examined externally, and then one-third of each are used for dissection, study of Wilson slices and skeletal preparations. Similar statistical analyses are made as before of quantal and quantitative data.

The test is often extended by permitting up to an additional 10 females per group to litter, counting the numbers of live pups and, if necessary, equalizing them to eight per group (four males and four females). Physical growth of the young is followed until virtual maturity at 42 days of age, together with periodic assessment of developmental milestones such as opening of the eyes and ears and the acquisition of motor and other skills, e.g. nest seeking, balance, etc. The intention is to compare the overall rate of bodily growth and of functional maturation of the nervous system across the treatment groups.

A foetal toxicity study in the rabbit is comparable to the basic test in the rat. It is more reliable, however, to use primiparous does, brought into controlled ovulation by prior injection of a gonadotrophin, and to employ artificial insemination by a proven donor buck. Dosing of pregnant females runs from days 8 to 18 of pregnancy and they are necropsied on day 28.

A valuable addition, best carried out in a parallel foetal toxicity experiment and particularly in the rat, is to assay drug in the maternal plasma, in amniotic fluid and in foetal tissue once or twice during the test. Proof of placental transfer of the active agent is important additional confirmation of the value of the experiment

Peri- and postnatal test

Neither of the two previous studies permits adequate exploration of any possible drug action on late intrauterine growth, parturition and postnatal maturation.

These areas can best be explored in a further investigation, normally carried out in the rat. Pregnant females, 20 per group, are treated from day 15 of gestation until day 21 postpartum, when the young are weaned. The latter are followed without further treatment until day 42, when they are autopsied.

The growth and behaviour of the pregnant dams are assessed and so are the numbers of young born alive or dead, their sex and, as before, the physical growth and functional maturation of the pups.

Drug level in milk from lactating rats should be measured.

Carcinogenicity testing

This is best regarded as a special type of chronic toxicity testing, carried out mainly to show whether a compound has any potential to produce benign or malignant tumours.

There is some interest also in knowing whether it influences the normal background incidence of spontaneous neoplasms in laboratory animals, accelerating or retarding their time of appearance or changing the relative frequency of different types of growth, because that may reflect changes in endocrine status during the test.

There is general agreement that a candidate medicine should undergo carcinogenicity testing if:

1. It is to be administered to humans for a prolonged period. This is because carcinogenic activity requires prolonged and repeated exposure to a chemical.
2. Its chemical structure resembles that of a known carcinogen. Although unusual, there are examples of medicines of similar structure, e.g. to derivatives of hydrazines and steroids, proven to be carcinogenic in animals.
3. It is mutagenic under circumstances relevant to human treatment and in tests of established validity.
4. Other factors are sometimes advanced to justify carcinogenicity testing, but are of less general applicability:
    – if the compound is cytotoxic in low concentration;
    – if it has marked endocrine effects, causing direct or secondary hormonal stimulation of a target organ.

Certain substances are not themselves carcinogenic but they may promote the actions of other natural or administered carcinogens or act as co-carcinogens. The significance of these phenomena in causing cancer in humans is uncertain, so the use of special procedures to demonstrate 'promoting' activity is of doubtful value in defining the safety of a pharmaceutical.

The general technique of carcinogenicity testing is to administer the compound to rats and mice for the major part of their life span, e.g. for 24 months to the rat and 18 months to the mouse. Three dose levels and an untreated control group are employed, the highest dose level being chosen to cause minimal toxicity, e.g. 10 per cent reduction in weight gain. At least 50 animals of each sex are required for each treated group and 100 of each sex as the controls. The large numbers are necessary to permit adequate statistical power in the final analysis of the results, which is based on actuarial comparison of the incidence of the different types of tumours found in life and after death. The blood level of the compound or a major metabolite should be checked at intervals during the study to confirm the adequacy of dosing and to exclude excessive cumulation due to age, disease or non-linear kinetics. Expert statistical advice is required to design the experiment so as to obtain proper randomization and to avoid sources of bias.

For general details of carcinogenicity testing see the ABPI Guidelines,[17] and the Department of Health (DoH);[24] for critical discussions of various aspects see Dayan and Brimblecombe,[25] and Grice and Ciminera.[26]

The animals must be kept under optimal conditions to ensure adequate survival. They should normally be dosed by the route intended for humans. Repeated, careful clinical examinations are carried out, particularly to detect neoplasms, followed by detailed autopsy and an extensive histopathological survey of major tissues.

Problems may arise in analysis of carcinogenicity tests because of the high but variable incidence of spontaneous degenerative and neoplastic lesions in aged animals,[27] which may prevent adequate statistical evaluation of the findings either because of an excess of premature death or, more often, because of an excessively high incidence of tumours in the controls. A further complicating factor is realization that the incidence of spontaneous and induced tumours is dependent on the quantity and composition of the diet eaten by rodents, and that even slight undernutrition, whether due to restriction of the quantity of food available or failure to eat it, may dramatically change the incidence of neoplasms.[24]

Although the rat and mouse are conventionally used in carcinogenicity testing, there are significant objections to them under certain circumstances, in particular if metabolism of the compound is known to be quite different in humans, possibly leading to misleading results in the rodent, e.g. griseofulvin and phenobarbital, like some other medicines, are hepato-carcinogens in the mouse.[2] It may then be necessary to consider the hamster (Syrian) as an alternative.

Carcinogenicity testing is difficult, expensive and tedious. It should probably not be commenced too early in development of a drug because there will then be too many major uncertainties that may affect the nature of the experiment, but it must not be left too late because its duration may then delay marketing. Its timing depends on a calculated balance between the probability of success of development of the candidate drug and the cost and speed of its progress to a product licence application.

Mutagenicity testing

More than any other area of toxicity testing, detection of the mutagenic potential of a compound and interpretation of its significance is subject to uncertainty. Knowledge of a range of techniques and understanding of their possible significance is important because the ability to produce mutagenic damage implies that the substance has somehow affected DNA or its replication or some other aspect of cell division. A compound with that property, depending on the nature of the effect and the circumstances under which it occurs, might be able to produce transmissible genetic damage. There is also a strong although imperfect correlation for many compounds between the ability to produce mutation in somatic cells and to be carcinogenic in animal experiments, and so probably to carry a risk of tumour production in humans, at least under certain circumstances.

In general, a genotoxic compound is unlikely to be developed as a medicine because of the serious risk that it will be a carcinogen. The main exception to this is the development of cytotoxic anticancer agents. A non-genotoxic carcinogen may be developed if there are data to show that the mechanism of its oncogenic effects is unlikely to operate in humans, or if the human dose is well below the threshold that such compounds are considered to exhibit.

Testing for mutagenic potential is a relatively new science and there is still much to learn about optimizing procedures and about interpretation of the results.

Experience has shown the overall value of a battery of procedures, exploring different mechanisms of mutation, some done *in vivo* and others *in vitro*, and then always in the presence and absence of induced rat hepatic S-9 microsomes, as a surrogate for metabolic activation in the live animal.[28]

The principles of the methods are to test for point mutations in bacteria (the eponymous Ames' test) and mammalian cells *in vitro*, as their genetic organization is different from that in prokaryotic organisms. The production of chromosomal damage in mammalian cells *in vitro* and in bone marrow cells *in vivo* (metaphase analysis or a micronucleus test) is also sought as evidence of genetic damage of a different type. It is also possible to test selectively for genetic damage in germ cells by carrying out a Dominant Lethal test, which involves timed mating of dosed males and untreated females and assessment of the numbers of viable conceptuses.

Many other procedures have been devised and promoted, but they tend to be less well founded or validated, or more specialized. Amongst the more common are direct measurement of DNA binding and sister chromatid exchange. (Full technical details and a critical analysis of the interpretation of results are given in the UK Environmental Mutagen Society (UKEMS) handbooks,[29] which should be read in conjunction with the description of the scientific strategy in the DoH Guidelines.[28])

Key factors are the need to carry out experiments at high concentrations or doses, which risk activating aberrant metabolic or even chemical reactions irrelevant to humans (but the irrelevance must be proven by appropriate analyses) as well as sometimes permitting specific biological mechanisms or trace impurities to give misleading false positives.

A 'positive' in a genotoxicity test, even when confirmed in the essential replicate experiment, need not require abandonment of the compound, but it is an important signal of the need for much work before humans (except perhaps the terminally ill) should be exposed to the compound.

The tests will not be described here in detail (see UKEMS[29] for full information). The principles involved are:

1. *Point (gene) mutation tests*
   (a) Bacteria (Ames' test). Selected mutant strains of *S. typhimurium* are exposed to the test substance in the presence and absence of the S-9 microsomal metabolic activating system, and mutant reversion to the wild type is detected by seeking growth in a special histidine-free medium.
   (b) Mammalian cell. Special lines of V79 (Chinese hamster ovary) or L5178Y (mouse lymphoma) cells, selected for heterozygosity at the allele for a vital enzyme in nucleotide synthesis, are grown in a medium containing a nucleotide antimetabolite. Only null mutants are able to grow.
2. *Chromosome tests*
   (a) In cultured animal cells, or using human lymphocytes *in vitro*, metaphase spreads are prepared after incubation with the test substance and in the presence and absence of S-9 microsomes. Damage is shown by breaks in chromosomes, abnormal morphology or even aneuploidy.
   (b) Micronucleus test. In the mouse, clastogenic agents given orally or parenterally will cause lagging of chromosomes during a late stage in the maturation of erythroblasts in the bone marrow. The result is the appearance of one or even more DNA fragments in normoblasts ('micronuclei').

All these and most of the other procedures are essentially qualitative screening techniques. It is conventional[28] to have carried out all four types of test on a new medicine by the time of product license application.

Topical toxicity testing

Whether a preparation can cause local irritation, for example of the skin or the eye, is tested by application of the formulated product to the same site in a suitable species, commonly the rabbit, for up to 21–28 days. The importance of preexisting skin damage was formerly assessed by experimental treatment of abraded skin but this is not now regarded as giving useful additional information. Absorption from a local application should be measured, and if measurable plasma concentrations are achieved they should have been exceeded in other toxicity studies. If not, conventional tests to detect possible systemic toxicity should also be employed.

Certain materials result in adverse clinical reactions due to sensitization. The propensity of a substance to produce delayed hypersensitivity can be investigated with reasonable confidence by experimentation in guinea pigs, usually by giving one or more priming exposures (e.g. one injection with Freund's adjuvant, or multiple intradermal injections, followed by a simple patch test or a simple injection). The Magnusson–Kligman procedure is the best known sensitization test.

Medicines for ophthalmic use must be tested, usually in rabbits, for local irritant effects when instilled into the eye. In addition, it is necessary to check whether they are absorbed into the eyeball or general circulation. If so, the same comments apply as to compounds absorbed from the skin.

Medicines to be administered by inhalation must be subjected to toxicity studies by that route. The same guidelines relating to duration of exposure, choice of species, etc. apply as to systemic tests. Absorption from the respiratory tract is often considerable. Many techniques have been described for applying compounds to the lungs of rats and dogs.

If other routes are to be used in humans, then local irritancy must be checked, even if the systemic toxicity is well known.

Pharmacological safety studies

Tests designed to establish the pharmacological profile of a new drug with respect to its efficacy will have been carried out early in its development. These tests will usually have concentrated on the particular organs or systems involved in the therapeutic response to the drug. For example, effects on the cardiovascular system will have been studied in detail for antihypertensive drugs and on the central nervous system for psychotropic drugs.

It is necessary as part of the safety evaluation to establish whether effects, which may be considered to be adverse, originate in systems other than that involved in the therapeutic response.

Careful observation of animals in the acute and longer term toxicity studies may provide some indication but for a more detailed analysis pharmacological techniques should be used. Many techniques are available and suitable for this purpose. (For a detailed account see Zbinden and Gross.[30]) A few examples will suffice to indicate the types of test which can be employed.

Central nervous system
Observational techniques, such as that described by Irwin,[31] should indicate gross effects on the central nervous system – depression, stimulation, convulsions, etc. Such effects of compounds can be categorized further by, for example, ascertaining whether they modify barbiturate sleeping-time, the threshold for chemically or electrically induced convulsions, spontaneous motor activity, etc. All these procedures are, however, essentially descriptive. To obtain more information concerning the site and mode of action in the brain, complex electrophysiological procedures are often required. Even with these, extrapolation of results of animal studies to humans is very difficult. The subjective nature of many human behavioural responses to chemicals means that they are difficult, if not impossible, to reproduce in laboratory animals. Distribution studies (see below) are important. If a drug penetrates into the central nervous system, and especially if it is concentrated or localized there, it is reasonable to suspect that it may be capable of producing central effects,

even if they are not detectable in routine animal studies.

Cardiovascular system and autonomic nervous system

Anaesthetized dogs and/or cats are commonly used. Parameters measured to monitor cardiovascular function are likely to include the rate and force of contraction of the heart, cardiac output and arterial blood pressure; an ECG should also be recorded. Effects of any of these can be analysed in detail in further experiments.

Simple tests,[32] including responses to carotid occlusion, vagal stimulation, stimulation of preganglionic sympathetic nerves and to vasoactive substances (tyramine, isoprenaline, noradrenaline and acetycholine), can be used in the same animals to assess autonomic function.

It should be noted that the use of anaesthetized animals alone can give rise to misleading results. Anaesthetics can modify or prevent responses of the cardiovascular system to chemical agents. It is desirable, therefore, that basic studies, at least on heart rate and blood pressure, should be carried out in unanaesthetized animals, probably dogs.

Respiratory system

Effects on the rate and depth of respiration can be recorded from the same animals as are used to study cardiovascular parameters. Investigations on smooth muscle from the guinea pig respiratory tract are useful since responses of this muscle to active agents are usually similar to those of human respiratory muscle.

Biochemical studies

As indicated above, the early availability of an assay method for measuring concentration of drug in body fluids and tissues is becoming increasingly critical in the development of a new drug. Ideally, this should be a 'cold' method, but important information can be obtained using the radio-labelled drug, with which metabolic pathways can be detected and investigated before a non-isotope method specific to each compound has been devised.

Any risk of general systemic passage of the isotope should be minimized by placing the radio-label in the molecule where it is unlikely to be detached during metabolism.

The aim of early biochemical studies of drug metabolism should be to investigate the absorption, distribution, overall metabolism and excretion of the drug in animals, preferably in the species to be used in toxicity tests. This information is valuable in its own right, as it will characterize the behaviour of the drug and indicate whether interspecies differences are likely to exist. The information will also be useful for comparison with similar data obtained from humans when these become available.

Absorption and excretion can be studied by measuring the concentration of drug in blood, urine and faeces after administration by the chosen route and by comparing the results with the concentrations achieved after intravenous administration. Consideration should be given to carrying out such studies in pregnant and aged animals to ascertain whether the pharmacokinetics have been modified.

Distribution can be studied in a semiquantitative manner using whole body autoradiography. More quantitative results can be obtained by administering radio-labelled substance to groups of animals which are subsequently killed after various times. Selected organs and tissues are removed and levels of radioactivity measured.

Metabolic studies should ideally reveal the degree and nature of metabolism, ultimately including identification of metabolites. This is rarely possible in the early stages of development of a drug. It is sufficient to have an indication of the pattern of metabolism so that reasonable comparisons can be made between species, including humans.

Other biochemical studies likely to be carried out before embarking on extensive studies in humans are those designed to measure degree of binding to plasma proteins and to check whether there is induction or inhibition of liver microsomal enzymes. All this information is important in the context of possible interactions with other drugs.

Products of biotechnology

Biologicals, which are best defined as therapeutic substances of such molecular complexity that they cannot be adequately defined by conventional physico-chemical analysis, have become of increasing medical interest. There are the 'old fashioned' vaccines and polyclonal antibodies, new, chemically or biologically defined immunogens and monoclonal antibodies, and all the products of DNA technology, such as hormones, cytokines and growth factors.

Their toxicity testing is often limited by the difficulty of finding a responsive species, so that the high-dose pharmacological effects can be investigated, and their considerable antigenicity as foreign proteins.

The result is that repeated administration to a foreign species may lead to antibody production, which will terminate the activities that should be studied and perhaps replace them by irrelevant but dangerous immune complex formation.

The toxicity testing of such products is still evolving, but at present it is based on empirical assessment of the nature and properties of each substance, followed by relevant studies, if possible in a responsive species, for as long as the lack of an immune response permits.[10,33]

Conclusions

We have attempted in this chapter to review the non-clinical safety studies that are carried out in the process of development of a new medicine. Some must be completed before the first administration to humans, and others will be carried on concurrently with the clinical programme but will have been completed prior to submission for approval for marketing. The sequence of testing is, to some extent, governed by regulatory requirements, but it can also vary with the attitudes and practices of the particular pharmaceutical company and with the degree of enthusiasm for the potential medicine. With a novel compound showing a high probability of achieving clinical utility in an important disease there is justification for carrying out many of the tests listed here in parallel rather than in series. This entails risk and the commitment of significant resources but will shorten the development period. A more cautious approach may be indicated if the clinical utility is not immediately apparent and first requires confirmation in humans.

Although toxicity testing is only part of the essential preclinical development of a new chemical entity, it is costly in human and other resources, and in the time required; some approximate figures are given in Table 2.1 Although certain studies can be run concurrently rather than sequentially, and some may even be run at the same time as clinical experience of the compound is being gathered, toxicity experiments remain a costly burden and delay the progress of every new medicine.

Table 2.1   Specimen costs of toxicity tests

Test	Cost* (£ sterling)	Time to report (months)
Acute toxicity		
rat	1000	1.5–2
mouse	1000	1.5–2
Subacute toxicity		
rat	30 000	4 (1-month test)
dog	45 000	4 (1-month test)
Chronic toxicity		
rat	65 000	10 (6-month test)
dog	80 000	10 (6-month test)
Carcinogenicity		
rat	300 000	36
mouse	300 000	30
Fertility		
rat	85 000	12
Foetal toxicity		
rat	20 000	4
rabbit	18 000	4
Peri- and postnatal		
rat	20 000	6
Mutagenicity		
Ames'	1500	1
Cytogenetics *in vitro*	15 000	4
Miscellaneous	12 000	4

The figures refer solely to the cost of toxicological experiments in 1990 and the periods required to complete and report them. They are presented only as guidelines and individual experience may well differ in particular instances. The tests are assumed to be carried out on a stable substance for oral administration, according to Good Laboratory Practices, and to follow generally applicable procedures.

Many of the procedures described here are standard and have been used for years. There is now a healthy tendency for their value in predicting adverse effects in humans to be examined critically, but relevant data are not easily obtained and significant departures from these tests are not to be anticipated in the short term. Changes can occur however. The LD_{50} test is now unlikely to be used, and new techniques, e.g. mutagenicity testing, have been introduced over the past few years. For the future, pressures to use alternatives to whole animals will increase and, if they can be validated and shown to afford the same degree of protection to humans, *in vitro* techniques may play a greater role than at present.

Throughout the programme of non-clinical experimentation it should be realized that the purpose of the work is to indicate any *possible* hazard to humans. The decision whether they should be exposed to the predicted risk depends on the likelihood that the toxic action may occur (i.e. consideration of species differences, and difference of metabolic pathways, the relationship between dose and response, etc.) and an essentially clinical judgement comparing the severity of the reaction with the harmful effects of the disease to be treated. On their own, neither the detection nor the absence of a toxic response in laboratory experiments can clear a candidate medicine for use in humans; they are only part of the information necessary in assessing its potential therapeutic value.

References

1. Fletcher AP (1978). Drug safety tests and subsequent clinical experience. *Journal of the Royal Society of Medicine* **71**: 693.
2. Tardiff RG, Rodricks JV (1987). *Toxic Substances and Human Risk: Principles of Data Interpretation*. New York: Plenum.
3. Lumley CE, Walker SR (1990). *Animal Toxicity Studies. Their Relevance to Man*. Lancaster: Quay Press.
4. d'Arcy PF, Harron DWG (1992). *Proceedings of the First International Conference on Harmonisation*. Belfast: Queen's University of Belfast.
5. Barnes JM, Denz FA (1954). Experimental methods used in determining chronic toxicity. *Pharmacological Reviews* **54**: 191.
6. Paget GE (ed.) (1970). *Methods in Toxicology*. Oxford: Blackwell.
7. Committee on Proprietary Medicinal Products of the European Community (1989). *Rules Governing Medicinal Products in the European Community*. Brussels: CEC.
8. Alder S, Zbinden G (1988). *National and International Drug Safety Guidelines*. Zollikon, Switzerland: MTC Verlag.
9. Dayan AD (1990). The toxicological background. In O'Grady JF, Linet O (eds.) *Early Phase Drug Evaluation in Man*. London: MacMillan: 39–62.
10. Dayan AD (1992). Toxicity testing of rDNA products. In Cromelin D (ed.) *From Clone to Clinic*. Dordrecht: Kluwer
11. UFAW (1989). *UFAW Handbook of Laboratory Animal Management*, 3rd edn. London: UFAW.
12. Balls M, Riddell R, Worden A (1983). *Animals and Alternatives in Toxicity Testing*. London: Academic Press.

13. Office of Technology Assessment (1984). *Alternatives to Animal Use in Research, Testing and Education*. Washington: US Government Printing Office.
14. DoH (1989). *Good Laboratory Practice. The United Kindgom Compliance Programme*. London: Department of Health.
15. Boyd EM (1972). *Predictive Toxicometrics*. Bristol: Scientechnica.
16. van den Heuvel MJ, Clark D, Fielder R *et al*. (1990). The international validation of a fixed-dose procedure as an alternative to the classical LD_{50} test. *Food and Chemical Toxicology* **28**: 469–82.
17. ABPI (1977). *Guidelines for Preclinical and Clinical Testing of New Medicinal Products. Part 1 – Laboratory Investigations*. London: ABPI.
18. Committee on Toxicity of Chemicals in Food, Consumer Products and the Environment (1982). *Guidelines for the Testing of Chemicals for Toxicity*. DHSS Report on Health and Social Subjects, No. 27. London: HMSO.
19. International Programme on Chemical Safety (1988). *Environmental Health Criteria No. 70. Principles for the Safety Assessment of Food Additives and Contaminants in Food*. Geneva: WHO.
20. Wilson J, Warkany J (1965). *Teratology Principles and Techniques*. Chicago: University of Chicago Press.
21. Neubert D, Merker HJ, Kwasigroch TE (eds.) (1977). *Methods in Prenatal Toxicology*. Stuttgart: Georg Thieme Verlag.
22. Snell K (ed.) (1982). *Development Toxicology*. London: Croom Helm.
23. DHSS (1978). *MAL 36. Notes for Guidance on Reproduction Studies*. London: DHSS Medicines Division.
24. DoH Committee on Carcinogenicity (in press). *Guidelines for the Testing of Chemicals for Carcinogenicity*. London: HMSO.
25. Dayan AD, Brimblecombe RW (eds.) (1978). *Carcinogenicity Testing: Principles and Problems*. Lancaster: MTP Press.
26. Grice H, Ciminera JL (eds.) (1988). *Carcinogenicity Testing*. Berlin: Springer Verlag.
27. Cotchin E, Roe FJC (1967). *Pathology of Laboratory Rats and Mice*. Oxford: Blackwell.
28. DoH (1989). *Guidelines for the Testing of Chemicals for Genotoxicity*. Report on Health and Social Subjects No. 35. London: HMSO.
29. UKEMS (1990). *Basic Mutagenicity Tests: UKEMS Recommended Procedures*. Cambridge: CUP.
30. Zbinden G, Gross F (eds.) (1979). *Pharmacological Methods in Toxicology*. Oxford: Pergamon Press.
31. Irwin S (1964). Drug screening and evaluation of new compounds in animals. In Nodine JH, Siegler PH (eds.) *Animal and Clinical Pharmacologic Techiniques in Drug Evaluation*. Chicago: Yearbook Medical Publishers: 36–54.
32. Green AF, Armstrong JM, Farmer JB *et al*. (1979). Autonomic pharmacology: report of the main working party. In Zbinden G, Gross F (eds.) *Pharmacological Methods in Toxicology*. Oxford: Pergamon Press: 9–48.
33. Dayan AD (1990). *Toxicity Testing of DNA Products*. In Cromelin D (ed.) *From Clone to Clinic*. Dordrecht: Kluwer.

3

Making drugs into medicines
John M. Padfield

The process of pharmaceutical research and development (R & D) is complex, involving interactions not only between the 'laboratory' disciplines but also with Registration, Medical, Production and Marketing Departments. Effective interactions are vital if appropriate research objectives are to be set and targets achieved in bringing forward new products in the minimum time commensurate with sound science and acceptable economic return.

The 'research' phase of this process, described in Chapter 1, should have clear objectives in terms of therapeutic targets but the mixture of logical experimentation, creativity and serendipity does not always follow an exact time scale. The 'development' phase, on the other hand, has a much more clearly defined set of objectives, many of which (e.g. long-term toxicology studies, stability studies, etc.) have defined time targets.

Thus, the title of this chapter describes in simplistic but accurate terms the essential elements of the R & D contributions. For our purposes 'drugs' are the raw materials emanating from research programmes that have been shown to have activity in animals when administered in solution or as simple suspensions. Drugs are also those materials manufactured by Chemical Development groups in the R & D phase and by Primary Production factories in the manufacturing/selling phase. 'Medicines', on the other hand, comprise the dosage forms that are administered to patients, together with the delivery system/package, and they emanate from development programmes. The dosage forms are a mixture of the drug with other materials (usually called 'excipients') presented in a form suitable for use by the patient, e.g. tablet, cream, aerosol, etc. The package may simply be a container (bottle, vial) or it may also be the delivery system (e.g. cream tube, aerosol inhaler, prefilled syringe). More attention is now being given to the presentation used to administer the drug since it is possible, by inappropriate selection of excipients, manufacturing conditions, packages etc., to modify, reduce or even destroy the inherent activity of the drug. In addition, more emphasis is also being placed on 'controlled-release' presentations of drugs to reduce side effects and increase dosing intervals.

The development phase

The exact point of transition between 'research' and 'development' varies from one company to another but, in general, a drug is regarded as being a research candidate until its animal activity has been confirmed in human volunteers when, if acceptable, it becomes a development candidate.

The primary objectives of medicine development therefore are:

1. To ensure that the efficacy of the drug demonstrated during the research phase is maintained by appropriate choice of dosage form and formulation.
2. To encourage patient compliance by appropriate choice of the above and of packaging where appropriate.
3. To demonstrate long-term safety and efficacy through the conduct of appropriate non-clinical and clinical studies.
4. To develop suitable manufacturing processes to ensure consistent quality and to provide a robust, economical, mass-production process.

These objectives can only be met satisfactorily through detailed multidisciplinary project groups, each discipline recognizing the contribution and constraints of the others. The exact nature and scale of these interactions often depends on the relative locations of the groups. For example, some local laboratories of foreign multinational companies may have little input during the 'research' phase or in the type of presentation to be developed. They will, however, make vital contributions to the local requirements for packaging and process development, and generate data to satisfy regulatory authority requirements.

The laboratories of a home-based R & D pharmaceutical company will, however, be totally involved in all phases of the R & D process as illustrated in Fig. 3.1.

Like Ptolemy we all consider ourselves the centre of the universe, but it is true to say that the pharmaceutical and analytical sciences play a key role in the transition from drug to medicine. The relative proportions of analytical scientists to pharmaceutical scientists is also critical since the pharmaceutical scientist frequently cannot make progress until analytical data is provided. Indeed it has been light-heartedly suggested that a pharmaceutical scientist working for an afternoon can keep an analytical scientist busy for 2 weeks!

Typically a Pharmaceutical Science group will be involved in:

Advice to the research groups on suitable salt forms of a drug, their impact on drug availability and preliminary assessments of the drug's stability.

Provision of materials, to Good Laboratory Practice Standards, for toxicology studies, both in the research and the development phases.

Discussions with Chemical Development and Primary Production groups on the chemical, but more particularly the physical (e.g. crystal size, crystal habit, polymorphism), properties of the drug so that a

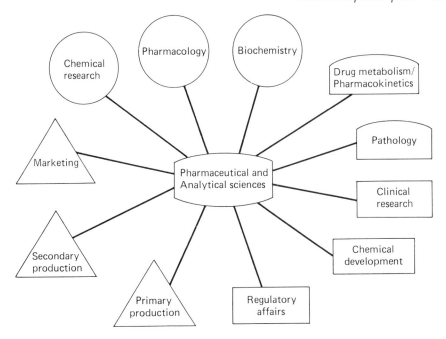

Fig. 3.1 Inter-relationships between research (○), development (□) and operating (△) arms of a pharmaceutical research and development company.

satisfactory manufacturing process for the medicine can eventually be established. Some types of manufacturing process are critically dependent on the physical properties of the drug and, if any changes to those properties occur during the drug manufacture, e.g. change in particle size, change of crystal form to plates from needles or vice versa, then Secondary Production may be severely affected.

Conducting stability studies on the drug to define any special handling requirements of bulk (e.g. tonne) quantities, suitable bulk packs for storage and transport, and a shelf life (expiry date) for the drug.

Discussions with Marketing to confirm the type of presentation wanted. For example, if for oral use, is a solid (tablet or capsule) or a liquid (syrup or perhaps soluble tablet) dosage form wanted? If a tablet, what size, shape or colour is desirable? Do the marketing groups have unlimited freedom in the type of packaging available for use (e.g. plastic blister packs, aluminium foil strips, plastic or glass bottles) or are the properties of the drug/medicine such that it must be protected from moisture, oxygen or light?

Discussions with Secondary Production to confirm that the type of dosage form, its manufacturing process and the packaging operation is feasible not only in large sophisticated factories but also in smaller, less sophisticated ones. In general, one international manufacturing process is desirable in order to ensure uniform quality and also to avoid duplication of process development costs, varieties of equipment, validation, stability testing, etc.

Discussions with Registration so that the standards set for the drug are likely to be acceptable to all registration authorities, that all excipients selected for use are approved internationally (both by regulatory e.g. DHSS, FDA and by pharmacopoeial e.g. BP, USP bodies) and that the formula, process and stability data to be generated will meet the needs of the most demanding authorities. It is usual to work to the 'highest common denominator' (often the USA and Japan) in terms of registration requirements although not all of the information is required by all authorities.

Discussions with Medical groups over the provision of materials for human volunteer and clinical trials. Most Pharmaceutical Science groups use the manufacture of clinical trial supplies, which usually escalate dramatically as the development phase proceeds, as part of the 'scaling-up' process to provide information on the manufacturing process to be proposed eventually to Secondary Production. The provision of clinical trial materials is discussed later in this chapter.

Formulation and process development activities related to provision of a manufacturable, marketable medicine. This involves generation of all the stability data necessary for registration authorities in order to define storage conditions and shelf life together with any special conditions necessary for transport. As indicated previously, this requires close collaboration with the analytical scientists who also set the standards (specifications) for the medicine.

Before these activities are examined in detail, Table 3.1 summarizes the very wide variety of dosage forms and associated packs available for use in administering drugs. Of course, not all are suitable for all drugs.

Pharmaceutical development of a medicine

There are essentially four stages to the pharmaceutical development of a medicine, as shown in Fig. 3.2. These are:

- Preformulation
- Formulation development
- Process development
- Scale-up

While it is not appropriate to discuss here the pharmaceutical science in detail, it is important that the reader should understand the principles involved.

Table 3.1 Types of medicines, by route of administration

Route	Dosage forms	Packs
Intravenous	Aqueous solutions, dry powders for reconstitution	Glass ampoules, glass vials closed with rubber plugs or disc seals, prefilled syringes
Intramuscular	Oily solutions and suspensions; aqueous solutions and suspensions	Unit-dose sterile packs
Subcutaneous	Aqueous solutions and suspensions, implants	Plastic and metal tubes; unit-dose plastic packs
Cutaneous	Lotions, creams, ointments, pastes, gels, modified-release creams and ointments; transdermal systems	Glass and plastic bottles and droppers; plastic and metal tubes; unit-dose plastic packs
Ocular	Drops; ointments; controlled-release polymers	Glass and plastic bottles and droppers; plastic bottles with atomiser; glass and plastic bottles with pumps
Nasal	Drops; squeeze sprays, metered sprays	Glass and plastic bottles; blister and foil unit-dose packs
Buccal	Rapid dissolution tablets; controlled-release (bioadhesive) tablets; gargles	Metal cans and glass bottles with valve and actuator; plastic devices with capsules; glass bottles; plastic and glass unit-dose ampoules
Inhaled	Solution and suspension pressurized metered aerosols; powder inhalers; nebulizer respirator solutions and suspensions	
Oral	Tablets, soluble tablets, effervescent tablets, dispersible tablets, enteric-coated tablets, layer tablets, controlled-release tablets; capsules, enteric coated capsules, controlled-release pellets, matrices, osmotic systems; syrups, elixirs, suspensions	Glass and plastic bottles; blister and foil unit-dose packs
Rectal	Fat-based suppositories, water-miscible suppositories, osmotic systems	
Vaginal	Vaginal tablets; pessaries; polymeric systems	Unit-dose packs
Intra-uterine	Controlled-release polymeric systems	

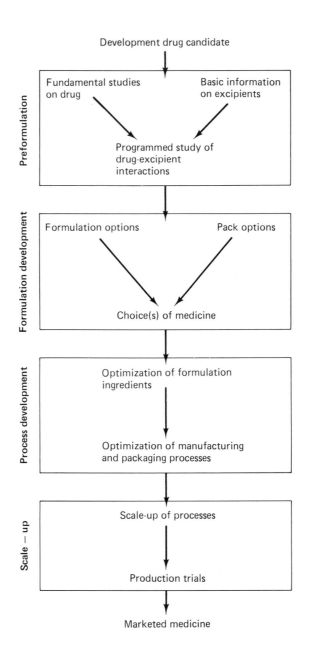

Fig. 3.2   The four main stages in pharmaceutical development.

Preformulation

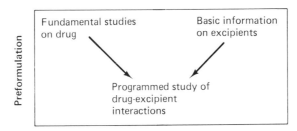

During this stage fundamental studies are conducted on the drug prior to formulating dosage forms. This is often the first opportunity that the pharmaceutical scientist has of examining such properties of the drug as those listed below

Physicochemical properties

Assay (potency) reproducibility

It is of paramount importance that the development scientist is aware of what variations might occur in the potency of the drug since, during the R & D phase, greater purity is often achieved than during continuous large-scale manufacture. Normally a drug specification will limit the drug assay to 97 per cent of theoretical to allow for such variations, although in the development phase purities of 98–99 per cent may be achieved. It is important to know whether the variation is due to increased amounts of known manufacturing impurities or to degradation occurring during manufacture. Both could have implications for the long-term stability of the drug and medicine.

Impurities and degradation products

Implicit in the above is a knowledge of the impurities that could occur during manufacture of the drug, and the degradation products that could arise. Manufacturing impurities may be intermediates used to synthesize the drug, catalysts used in the chemical reaction, by-products of incomplete synthesis or alternative routes of synthesis, alternative isomers if the synthetic route involves isolation of an optically active isomer or solvents.

Degradation products arise from some instability of the drug once it has been formed during synthesis. It is important to identify and quantify the impurities and degradation products since toxicology studies undertaken with 100 per cent pure drug may not be considered relevant to large-scale manufactured drug containing, say, a total of 5 per cent impurities or degradation products. Hence, at the preformulation stage a specification for the drug outlining limits of drug potency, impurities and degradation products is developed.

Stability

At the preformulation stage only a limited evaluation of stability can be undertaken because drug is usually in short supply and must be channelled into priority groups such as Toxicology. However, an early appreciation of the conditions of temperature, pH, moisture, etc. likely to affect the drug adversely are important so as:

1. To ensure that the bulk drug is stored under conditions likely to maintain its quality.
2. To ensure that early formulations used for animal studies are of adequate quality.
3. To provide some indication of what formulations, presentations and packages are possible for the medicine.

For example, a liquid presentation of a drug unstable in water due to hydrolysis (e.g. penicillins, cephalosporins, aspirin) may not be a feasible objective except in a granular/powder form suitable for reconstitution by the pharmacist. Furthermore, a drug that is highly hygroscopic would not be ideally suited to presentation in a hard gelatin capsule (as it may remove a significant quantity of water from the capsule shell and make it very brittle) or even as a tablet packed in a polyvinyl chloride (PVC) blister pack (as the moisture ingress through PVC packs is sufficient to cause physical changes such as swelling, loss of hardness, in the tablet). The stability of drugs and medicines is so fundamental to the development process that a separate section is devoted to the subject later in this chapter.

Solubility

This is an important parameter for any drug, and is usually determined over a wide range of temperature (e.g. 5°C to 50°C) and pH (2 to 8) to cover formulation and biopharmaceutical considerations. The formulator of an injection, for example, needs to know the limits of concentration and pH within which he can work to allow for optimum injection volume, stability and to ensure no changes occur during transport. Solubility–temperature relations are particularly important with regard to storage and transport since it is not unknown for medicines to be exposed to temperatures below 0°C. Freezing and thawing studies may be required if the likely concentration of the drug in the medicine is close to its solubililty at 5°C. This is to ensure that, if the drug did come out of solution at low temperatures, it would rapidly redissolve. Failure to do so could result in incorrect dosage. Similar considerations occur when drugs are formulated as suspensions since a finite, albeit small, amount of the drug will be present in solution, and this may crystallize out of solution at low temperatures and then undergo crystal growth as the temperature is raised, with potential consequences for poor suspension stability.

Polymorphism

Some drugs can exist in more than one crystalline form. Often there is only one stable polymorph as other forms are thermodynamically meta-stable and revert to the stable form. However, phenobarbitone, for example, exists in several stable polymorphic forms only one of which may be therapeutically active. In such cases it is vital to ensure that the formulation or process does not produce reversion to a potentially less active polymorph.

Hygroscopicity

This was mentioned earlier in relation to stability but it is an important factor to be noted separately. The degree of moisture uptake and its consequences both need to be considered. The consequences may not only be physical changes (e.g. swelling of tablets) but may produce a greater risk of microbial spoilage or may promote chemical instability. In Fig. 3.3 four hypothetical cases are considered. Drug A would produce no problems in any formulation or package. A slight concern might arise if it was a drug considered for administration by inhalation since the relative humidity (RH) of the respiratory tract is greater than 99 per cent at 37°C. Under such conditions rapid crystal growth can occur that may affect efficacy depending on the area of the lung it is desired to reach. Hiller *et al.*[1] have demonstrated that some increase in particle size occurs in aerosol inhalation products at high humidity but that the magnitude of the increase (1–2 μm) is unlikely to influence efficacy. Dry powder inhalers (e.g. Rotahaler* and Spinhaler**) may be more at risk if a hygroscopic drug is to be used but there is little that can be done without producing other concerns about the lung being exposed to additional excipients (e.g. membrane-coating materials). Drug B represents a good profile for a drug to be used in temperate (less than 55 per cent RH) climates (e.g. Europe) when any type of pack could possibly be used. However, in tropical (greater than 75 per cent RH) climates (e.g. Far East, parts of the USA, parts of Australia), permeable containers (e.g. PVC blister packs) are probably not appropriate and a foil-strip pack is probably the only alternative. For Drugs C and D a foil-strip pack would be the only type suitable for all markets, the difference between the two drugs being that D would also require very stringent manufacturing conditions (less than 10 per cent RH). This places considerable constraints upon Secondary Production operations and of course may significantly influence the unit cost of the medicine.

Physicomechanical properties

Particle (crystal) size and shape

The mean size and the size distribution of a drug can be important. For a drug to be administered as an aerosol to the lung, size can determine penetration into the airways; for a suspension medicine it will influence the physical stability and sedimentation properties; for a tablet it can determine dissolution rate and bioavailability. Together with other properties such as shape, flow and compressibility, size can influence the type of tablet to be developed and the quality of the Secondary Production process.

Frequently drugs are 'micronized' to produce the majority of particles

*Trade mark of the Glaxo Group of Companies
**Trade mark of Fisons Ltd.

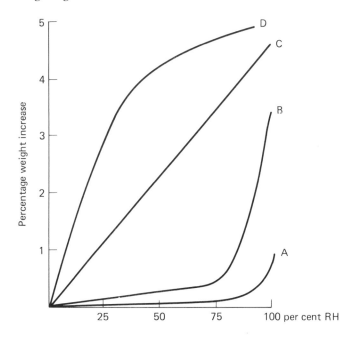

Fig. 3.3 Four hypothetical profiles demonstrating degrees of hygroscopicity. RH, relative humidity.

in a size range less than 10 μm and micronized drug is often the form used in suspensions (since small particles, being lighter, settle less readily than large ones) and in aerosols, dry powder inhalers, etc.

Particle shape is less frequently determined, but it can affect tablet size (through effects on bulk density), flow on a tablet machine, suspension sedimentation and other features. The most common shapes resulting from the crystallization of drugs in Primary Production are flat plates, which can adhere together and cause poor flow, and needles which, depending on their length and breadth, can have variable influences.

Bulk density
This is the volume occupied by a given mass of powder and is a determining factor in many medicines where the drug is not present in solution. While there is no ideal value for bulk density (usually quoted as grams per cubic centimetre), a drug of low bulk density will occupy a large volume and therefore would produce a larger tablet or would require a larger hard gelatin capsule shell than a drug having a high bulk density and occupying a small volume (Fig. 3.4). Of more importance is the range of bulk density between batches of drug from a given Primary Production process since, if wide, it will cause variations in tablet size and in the fill of manufacturing equipment. Since one of the primary objectives of medicine development, outlined at the beginning of this chapter, is to produce a product of consistent quality using economical, mass-production processes, such variations must be minimized.

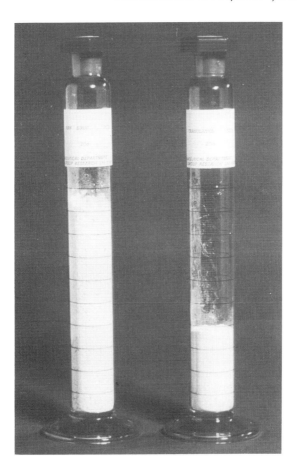

Fig. 3.4 Bulk density of solids. The container on the left contains material low bulk density (0.2 g/cc) and that on the right material of high bulk density (0.6 g/cc). Both cylinders contain identical weights of drug.

Flow

Solid-dose formulations (tablets, capsules) account for the vast majority of medicines in use and require high-speed manufacturing equipment. Many tablet machines produce 4000 tablets/min, i.e. approximately 2 000 000 tablets in an 8-hour working day. As the process involves powder flowing from a hopper into a small hole (the die) prior to compression between an upper and lower metal punch, it is imperative that the powder flows almost like a liquid to avoid variations in fill weight and hence tablet thickness. In this type of equipment the die has to fill with powder to within ±2 per cent of the target weight within milliseconds. Determination of the inherent flow properties of the drug at the preformulation stage is thus a prerequisite for deciding what type(s) of medicine can be developed, what additional processing will be necessary and what type of excipients will need to be added to the drug to make it flow more readily if it has poor inherent flow. As indicated earlier, size and shape can have profound effects on powder flow.

Compressibility
In order to make a tablet it is necessary to make the drug particles bind together to form a hard compact. Certain drugs have an inherent brittle nature such that on compression they fracture but may not bind together to form a tablet. In such cases it is necessary to add excipients of a plastic nature which will deform upon compression and bind together the fractured drug particles. On the other hand, some drugs are of a plastic nature and may not require plastic excipients as they would not form hard compacts. In such cases brittle excipients could be used.

Biopharmaceutical properties

Partition coefficient
The relative affinity of a drug for oily or aqueous phases influences transport across biological membranes. Lipid solubility favours drug absorption, cerebral transfer, etc.

pK_a
Many drugs are weak electrolytes and are partially ionized in solution. pK_a is the pH at which the compound is 50 per cent ionized. Acids are more highly ionized in alkaline solution and vice versa. The significance is that the ionized fraction is not appreciably lipid soluble and is poorly absorbed. However, the two fractions are in equilibrium and in practice it is found that acids with a pK_a above 3 and bases with a pK_a below 8 are absorbed satisfactorily.

Dissolution rate
With solid dosage forms it has often been found that the dissolution rather than the diffusion rate is the rate-limiting step in the absorptive process. The dissolution rate is therefore a most important factor influencing bioavailability – the extent and time course of entry of a drug into the circulation. Bioavailability differences have been shown between formulations of numerous common drugs, especially those with low water solubility. They are only likely to be clinically important with drugs that have a steep dose–response curve and a narrow therapeutic ratio, particularly if they are used in serious illnesses.[2] All these apply to digoxin, and the incident of 1972 provided a classic example of how formulation and processing can affect clinical efficacy.[3]

However, there are numerous other examples where such pharmaceutical factors have no influence on efficacy. It is therefore of the utmost importance to examine critically the need for bioavailability testing in the light of the data on a particular drug. Most companies now perform dissolution tests routinely in development programmes. The data are included increasingly in pharmacopoeias and regulatory submissions and the US Food and Drug Administration (FDA) requires dissolution testing in the specifications of all newly registered solid dosage products, regardless of the relevance of the data for clinical use. However, most companies still regard such testing as an 'in house' rather than a registration requirement.

It is clear that prior knowledge of the many properties of a drug before formulation is undertaken allows selection of suitable excipients to satisfy the objectives of medicine development as listed previously. For example,

> An appreciation of the pH-stability profile of the drug for use in a liquid formulation enables one to set up accelerated stability studies of the drug in the presence of a variety of suitable buffer salts before choosing some for formulation development. Antibacterial and antifungal preservatives, active at the pH selected, may be chosen at this stage for compatibility studies including confirmation of microbiological efficacy in the presence of the buffer salts, drug, etc.
>
> An appreciation of the flow and compression properties of the drug enables one to select suitable flow/compression excipients for incorporation into the tablet or capsule before accelerated stability testing in conjunction with other materials such as disintegrants (to aid the tablet or capsule to break up in the gastrointestinal tract, maximizing the surface area for drug release), lubricants (to facilitate ejection of the compressed tablet from the die), flavours, colours, etc.

Of course, not all factors are determined for all drugs. For example, physicomechanical properties are unimportant for a drug to be presented solely as an injection or a syrup.

Whatever presentation is to be developed, the final outcome of the preformulation stage is a programmed study of binary, tertiary, etc. mixtures of the drug with suitable excipients in order to provide a basis for formulation development.

Formulation development

One function of the pharmaceutical scientist is to create options for the Marketing groups. As a result of the preformulation programme, therefore, the available options have to be declared. For example, the aqueous solubility of the drug may make solid oral dosage forms or suspensions the only options. The taste of the drug may require substantial taste-masking

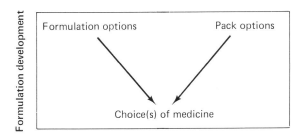

work or use of a capsule. If the drug is substantially degraded at low pH values (less than 4), then enteric coating of the tablet or capsule may be required. Alternatively, the solid-state stability of the drug in the presence of moisture or oxygen may be such that careful selection of excipients and packages must be made.

Knowledge of the preformulation properties also allows initial consideration of the package options, which may again preclude certain formulation options. Many different packaging materials exist for a given presentation, as shown in Table 3.1.

The resistance of containers to moisture may be assessed by filling them with dry calcium chloride and following the weight uptake (corresponding to ingress of moisture) at 37°C/75 per cent RH as a function of time. Typical data shown in Fig. 3.5 demonstrate that plastic blister packs do not provide a barrier to moisture and that their utility depends on the susceptibility of the formulation to moisture.

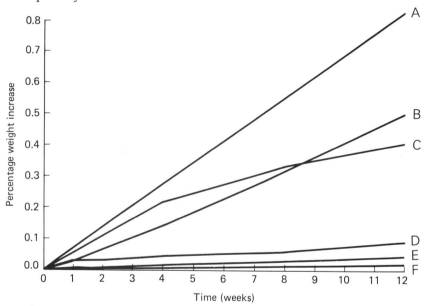

Fig. 3.5 Influence of pack-type on moisture ingress: A, polyvinyl chloride blister; B, Securitainer; C, Aclar blister pack; D, high-density polyethylene container with Clic Loc lid containing foil-faced liner; E, glass vial with polythene snap-on lid; F, aluminimum foil strip pack.

Fig. 3.6 shows the different delivery patterns that emerge from different nasal presentations. Selection of one will depend on the potency of the drug, its site of action and the accuracy of dosage required.

It is not possible to describe in detail the formulation development process for all products but, by way of example, the thought process behind the development of a tablet will be described.

Consideration has to be given as to whether the tablet will be manufactured by 'wet granulation' or by 'direct compression'. Wet granulation

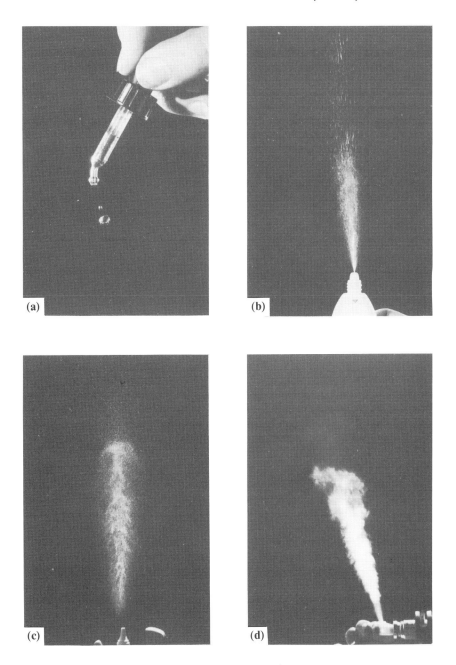

Fig. 3.6 Delivery patterns of different nasal presentations: (a) nasal dropper; (b) nasal squeeze bottle; (c) nasal metered pump spray; (d) nasal metered aerosol.

involves mixing the drug with suitable excipients such as starches or celluloses that will bind together the mixed mass when wetted. The wet mass is manipulated to produce granules (somewhat like instant coffee granules although more dense) which have good flow properties when dried. No water is included in the direct compression process, which simply involves mixing together the drug and excipients prior to compression. This is preferred for drugs susceptible to moisture but, if the drug represents a significant proportion (greater than 40 per cent) of the final tablet weight, its physicomechanical properties are critical. Wet granulation is more widely used than direct compression as it is more 'forgiving' in terms of variations in the physicomechanical properties of the drug. However, with a drug of high water solubility, very strong binding can occur with consequent poor drug availability.

Consider two drugs A and B with properties assessed by preformulation studies as shown in Table 3.2. Both have adequate chemical properties and their degradation pathways are known. Neither drug is likely to have any bioavailability problems (unless there is a narrow window for absorption) as solubility is good at all pH values likely to be encountered in the gastrointestinal tract and the rate of dissolution from simple formulations is also good. The essential differences between the way the drugs would be treated lie in their physicomechanical properties, their relative stability to moisture in the solid state and the dose to be contained within a single tablet.

Table 3.2   Properties of two hypothetical drugs

	Drug A	Drug B
Assay	> 98%	> 98%
Impurities	Trace catalysts, solvents	Trace catalysts, solvents
Degradation products	Two known hydrolysis products	One known main hydrolysis product
Stability	Solution stability fair	Solution stability good
	Solid-state stability in contact with water very poor; when dry excellent	Solid-state stability excellent
Solubility	> 10% w/v water	> 50% w/v water
Polymorphism	Two forms known	One form known
Hygroscopicity	Moisture uptake at RH > 60%	Moisture uptake at RH > 90%
Size	Mean size $200 \times 20 \ \mu m$	Mean size $70 \times 20 \ \mu m$
Shape	Long needles	Micro-needles
Density	< 0.25 g/cc	< 0.6 g/cc
Flow	Poor	Fair
Compression	Good	Poor
pK_a	8.4	4.5
Log P*	2.6	2.74
Dissolution Rate	Rapid	Rapid
Dose	200 mg	1 mg

* The logarithm (to base 10) of the partition coefficient. RH, relative humidity.

Drug A is moderately hygroscopic and the moisture it takes up leads to hydrolysis in the solid state, thus giving an unstable product. For this reason the obvious choice of manufacturing method is direct compression but the physicomechanical properties are less than ideal for such a process. Thus the pharmaceutical scientist can either select wet granulation, keeping the contact time with water as short as possible and drying out the tablets prior to packaging, or he can work on the physicomechanical properties in an attempt to make the direct-compression formulation work since, in the long term, that is likely to give a more stable product with a longer shelf life.

Let us assume that the pharmaceutical scientist chooses the latter course; he has to raise the bulk density by at least two-fold in order to produce a tablet of reasonable size. With poor flow properties it is not likely that the final tablet weight will be less than 400 mg (i.e. a 50 per cent drug content) and with a bulk density of less than 0.25 g/cc a large tablet would result. The low bulk density (and consequent high occupied volume) is a result of the long needle crystals which also cause the poor flow by interlocking. If a means could be found, therefore, of reducing the size of the needles somewhat without making them too small then perhaps flow could be improved.

Grinding the drug in a mill would not be appropriate since too much fine powder would probably be formed, but the good compressibility of Drug A makes two other options possible – 'slugging' or 'compaction'. Slugging involves compressing very large tablets of the drug alone, at slow speed where flow properties are less important; the slugs are subsequently broken down to give granules of high bulk density and good flow. The compaction process involves feeding the drug between two large rollers which compact the drug between them and produce a long 'flake' (or sheet) of drug. This is subsequently broken down to give dense granules. The granules could have a mean size of some 150 μm and a bulk density of 0.6 g/cc.

Having thus achieved the objective of improving the physicomechanical properties, one important physicochemical check is necessary. Drug A is known to exist as two polymorphs and, since it is known that physical processing can bring about polymorphic change, it is essential to confirm that the slugging or compaction of Drug A has not brought about an adverse change. This is normally done by infra-red spectrometry but it may be necessary to conduct X-ray diffraction studies.

Assuming that all is well, excipients have to be chosen either to add bulk to the tablet or to aid flow or assist compression. Many materials are available, e.g. starches, lactose, maltose, celluloses. The best ones would be selected by observing the mixing and tableting processes, ensuring equal distribution of drug throughout the mix and evaluating the tablet for weight uniformity, size, hardness (resistance to crushing), friability (resistance to abrasion), disintegration time (rate of tablet break-up) and assay uniformity (confirmation of no de-mixing during tableting).

Whilst de-mixing is always a possibility in any heterogeneous system its significance will be less important where the drug represents a large proportion of the tablet weight. In the case of Drug A the slugging process produced granules with such good flow properties that it was possible to provide a tablet weighing 300 mg in total. This represents a 66.67 per cent content of Drug A per tablet and tablet weight and thickness could be monitored as reliable indicators of drug content uniformity, together with analysis of a sample taken from 10 or 20 tablets that have been powdered and mixed together.

Once several options had been identified, accelerated stability studies would be performed to investigate chemical degradation. As Drug A is sensitive to moisture, challenge to high humidity conditions is essential at this stage to provide an indication of likely packaging needs (probably a foil-strip pack) and probable shelf life and storage requirements.

Turning to Drug B, which has no apparent solid-state stability problems in the presence of moisture, the unit dose would allow a very small tablet, say 50 mg (2 per cent drug content), to be developed. However, as the drug does not have inherently good flow and compressibility properties a larger tablet, say 200 mg (0.5 per cent drug content), could be preferred for direct compression in order to 'dilute out' such properties. In such cases the potential for segregation of drug from excipients both at the mixing and tableting stages is great and, if such a process was selected, considerable analytical work would be essential to check that this did not occur. Excipients that would 'bind' the drug to them, perhaps in imperfections (crevices) in their surface, would be the most suitable.

Alternatively, the pharmaceutical scientist could choose the wet granulation approach for Drug B where, because of the intimate mixing of the drug and excipients in a damp mass, dosage uniformity is more reliably attained. With a drug of such high solubility it is possible that very strong binding between drug and excipients could occur so that the tablet fails to disintegrate readily. Thus, adequate amounts of disintegrants (e.g. starches) must be included in the granules to break them down *in vivo* and release the drug for dissolution and absorption. Whatever formulation is chosen, a unit content of only 1 mg will necessitate chemical analysis of 10 individual tablets to check for content uniformity. In such a case the British Pharmacopoeia (BP) would require each tablet to contain 80–120 per cent of the stated content except that one tablet can be between 75 and 125 per cent.

The final outcome of the formulation development stage should be the Marketing groups giving an idea of what presentations they would like to develop and the pharmaceutical scientist saying which formulations in which packs are practical. When the preference of the Marketing group is known, the pharmaceutical scientist can make his choice of formulation ingredients. More than one option for any given presentation will have been developed by the pharmaceutical scientist in case one proves unsuitable at a later stage, e.g. stability or processing failures. However, as the work will now increase dramatically, full resources can only be allocated to one formulation option per presentation.

Process development and scale-up

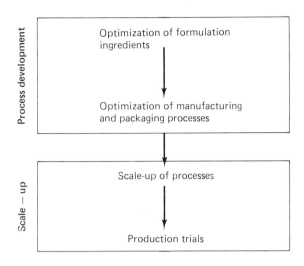

The objective of the process development stage is to begin to translate the laboratory developed formulation into one that can be manufactured on a large scale in Secondary Production. Thus the pharmaceutical scientist has to know where the medicine will be manufactured, the equipment available at those sites, any particular restrictions on the availability of the desired excipients and environmental restrictions such as a discharge of solvents into the atmosphere etc. Most pharmaceutical companies aim for a common formula and process throughout the world and the pharmaceutical scientist has therefore to balance the ideal against the attainable. A scientifically perfect medicine that creates production difficulties is less desirable than a compromise that is scientifically sound but capable of manufacture under all expected conditions.

Consideration also has to be given to the regulatory status of the excipients; are they materials approved in the pharmacopoeia (an official book of standards) of each country, are they readily available at reasonable cost, are their qualities (e.g. purity, moisture content, particle size, microbial content) equivalent to those of the material studied during formulation development? Frequently pharmacopoeial standards relate only to chemical properties of the excipient while, for a robust product, consistent physical properties are often more important. For example, magnesium stearate is widely used as a tablet lubricant but many grades exist, all of which would meet pharmacopoeial standards. Many studies have shown that minor differences in quality and processing methods can considerably influence its utility. White soft paraffin, a major diluent of creams and ointments, has many quality variations which can affect its ability to form a suitable medicine. The most notable variation is in its rheological (flow) properties which influence whether or not the drug remains suitably dispersed or whether the medicine 'bleeds' giving liquid separation.

If a particular particle size range of an excipient is required, steps have to be taken at this stage to identify the limits that are acceptable and to set appropriate specifications that can be adhered to. As an example of such a requirement, the lactose used as a carrier for the drug in dry powder inhalation products has to be suitably coarse (>50 μm) to prevent inhalation into the lung and yet of a size to allow good mixing with the drug within the capsule.

Similar considerations apply to packaging components. If the package contributes significantly to the stability of the medicine (e.g. as a moisture barrier for a tablet, for maintenance of sterility for an injection, for dosage uniformity of an aerosol) confirmation that suitable packaging materials are available at all manufacturing sites must be obtained.

Once suitable excipients have been chosen and tentative specifications set, experimental work continues on a gradually increasing scale to determine the processing parameters for each stage of the process. Returning to the wet granulation of Drug B, this would include optimization of the time required for dry mixing of the ingredients of the formulation, the volume of granulating fluid to be used, review of the characteristics of the granules produced, the time required for further mixing with extragranular excipients such as disintegrants and lubricants, followed by optimization of compression characteristics on the tablet machine. If the tablet is to be coated, for taste-masking, colour or other reasons, the film-coating process too has to be optimized.

The scale of the process development work relates directly to the likely batch size of the production process. Furthermore, as by this stage in the development of the medicine extensive clinical trials will be proceeding, manufacture of clinical trial supplies will be performed on an increasing scale so providing valuable information on the process. As an example, a tablet of say 300 mg weight might be manufactured on a 300 kg scale, i.e. 1 million tablets per batch. The formulation development work would probably be undertaken on a 1–5 kg scale, gradually working up through 10–30 kg batches at the process development/clinical trial stage.

As unforeseen problems can occur during scaling up, for example non-equivalence of different size manufacturing vessels, differences in stirring conditions, temperature changes due to the longer time bulk quantities take to heat up/cool down than small quantities, the objective at the scale-up stage is to proceed stepwise and only to commit large quantities of drug, still likely to be in limited supply prior to manufacture of production quantities, when reasonable confidence exists of a successful outcome. The above example would be scaled up through 100 kg batches eventually to 300 kg batches as full production trials. Usually a minimum of three production trials will be undertaken with production staff learning about the process and probably taking sole charge of the final batch. These production trials may form the launch stocks of the new medicine and therefore it is important that all steps are taken to guarantee the quality of those batches through thorough adherence to the principles of Good Manufacturing Practice (GMP). These are regulations designed to assure the quality of products through in-built controls in the production process. It is now accepted that one 'builds' quality into a product from the outset as described here rather than simply 'controlling' quality by analysis of a limited sample after manufacture.

The successful outcome of the process development and scale-up stages is the marketed medicine. The formulation will have been soundly developed, the package secure, the process optimized for robustness, economy and quality, and if all goes well the pharmaceutical scientist will never be called in to Secondary Production as no problems will arise. But then we have been dealing with hypothetical situations!

Stability testing and shelf life determination

Reference has already been made to aspects of evaluating the stability of drugs and medicines in order to assure maintenance of quality throughout their intended life. The meaning of 'quality' is discussed later, but stability evaluations are important to the industry, to regulatory authorities, to pharmacists and ultimately to patients. The tests should provide data that will give confidence that the medicine is stable under the conditions under which it is manufactured, transported, stored, sold and used.

Because of the importance attached to the evaluation of stability and the determination of shelf life (expiration dating in the USA), the industry expends considerable resources on stability testing and is constantly seeking new predictive methods for assessing at the earliest possible point whether or not a medicine will be stable. No time is available for lifetime (say 2, 3 or even 5 years) stability studies at the recommended storage conditions prior to seeking regulatory approval, and the accelerated stress tests which are used must therefore confidently reflect what is likely to happen under less stressful conditions at some point in the future. It is the function of the regulatory authorities to assess whether or not the stability data presented, usually of limited duration (say 6–12 months), provide sufficient confidence that the quality of the medicine will be maintained throughout the shelf life being claimed by the applicant.

Manufacture and distribution of medicines
Before considering the types of stability testing to be performed one should be aware of the potential conditions to which the medicine could be exposed during manufacture, distribution, storage or use.

Manufacture
Obviously there are considerable variations in both temperature and RH between different countries throughout the world and also within countries in different seasons. Moreover, some countries (e.g. USA, Australia) have considerable regional differences in climate. Without adequate environmental control (e.g. air conditioning) it is possible, during manufacture, for a product to be exposed to temperatures around the world between 59°F(15°C) and 90°F(32°C) and RHs between 20 per cent

and 99 per cent. Sensitive products may thus require control of some aspect of the environment, and it is the function of the stability testing programmes to determine suitable limits of temperature and/or relative humidity that are attainable and economic.

Some sort of stress may well be encountered by the drug and medicine during manufacturing, processing or packaging. Examples are discussed below.

Temperature
For injections, sterilizing by autoclaving requires a minimum exposure of 121°C for 15 minutes. For creams, temperatures up to 60/70°C for an hour or so are not unusual. For tablets, temperatures up to 50/60°C for 15 hours or so can be attained during drying of wet granules.

Humidity
Aqueous injection solutions, syrups, suspensions, etc. have to be resistant to hydrolysis. Creams, lotions, etc. may experience condensation of water vapour during a cooling phase in manufacture and microbiological growth could occur.

Oxygen
All products will include atmospheric oxygen unless steps are taken to exclude it; for example, nitrogen can be used to displace dissolved oxygen present in solution in the product and also oxygen present in the head-space above the solution. Not all the oxygen can be removed in this way.

Mechanical stress
Creams, ointments, syrups and suspensions are all pumped from vessel to vessel and from vessel to package during manufacture and may be subjected to shearing forces. Tablets must have considerable strength to withstand compression at high speeds followed by bulk handling and further stress during packaging.

As soon as the product is manufactured it starts to age; i.e. degradation begins and continues at a rate that is a function of the environment to which the medicine is exposed.

Distribution
After manufacture the medicine passes to a warehouse and it is at this point that the manufacturer starts to lose control of what happens to it. As distribution proceeds, the medicine becomes gradually more vulnerable as protective components are gradually removed. For example, a manufacturer may send to his warehouse 20 wooden pallets each having 128 cardboard outer cartons containing 10 cardboard packs each of 10 glass ampoules. Each pallet will be overwrapped with plastic shrink-wrapping. The warehouse may send a number of individual outer cartons to a wholesaler who may break these open to send five packs of ampoules to a hospital pharmacy. The pharmacy may send one pack to a ward whereupon the nurse or clinician may remove one or more ampoules from

a plastic tray within the pack, discarding the pack in the process. Thus, not only is the medicine now exposed to light, which may be a problem for a light-sensitive medicine, it is also exposed to a greater risk of breakage; furthermore, the storage instructions and expiry date have been discarded with the pack.

Distribution, therefore, involves a complicated sequence of different challenges of ill-defined magnitude and duration. Manufacturers have major problems in designing studies that will cover all eventualities but there must at least be an awareness of the potential stresses:

- Environmental: temperature; moisture; radiation; oxygen; pressure.
- Mechanical: vibration; inversion; deformation
- Contamination: chemical adulteration; microbiological; infestation

Table 3.3 illustrates that these stresses are not equally encountered during all stages of the distribution process. The most dangerous stresses are not the catastrophic ones, but those that can lead to medicines of poor quality passing undetected to the patient.

Table 3.3 Major stresses during distribution and use

	Environmental	Mechanical	Contamination
Warehouse	−	+	−
Transport	+ +	+ +	−
Wholesaler	+	+ +	+
Pharmacy	+	+	+ +
Patient	+ + +	+ + +	+ + +

Let us briefly consider what would happen to a pallet of goods transported from London to Singapore. The stresses will differ depending upon whether air or sea is chosen, but let us examine the former. The most damaging mechanical shocks are experienced during loading and unloading, and the major airlines specify that the pack to be transported (e.g. the pallet) must be capable of 'withstanding a 1.2 m test drop on to solid concrete in the position most likely to cause damage'. Assuming that this stage is successfully accomplished, loading will take place at ambient London conditions – 59°F(15°C), 60 per cent RH, 1000 mb atmospheric pressure – and, if the doors are closed and the aircraft is grounded for some time, solar heat gain may cause a significant increase in temperature and corresponding decrease in RH (Fig. 3.7). During take off and ascent, a rapid fall in pressure may occur along with a more gradual decrease in temperature, with corresponding changes in RH, until a cruising altitude is reached. These conditions will be maintained for hours, possibly interrupted by a stop in the Middle East, until the aircraft descends towards Singapore. The earlier changes are then reversed, although more rapidly since the ambient conditions are higher – 86°F(30°C), 90 per cent RH, 950 mb atmospheric pressure. If the aircraft is opened immediately, the cold goods are exposed to the warm, humid atmosphere and condensation will immediately occur. Recent information from British Airways indicated

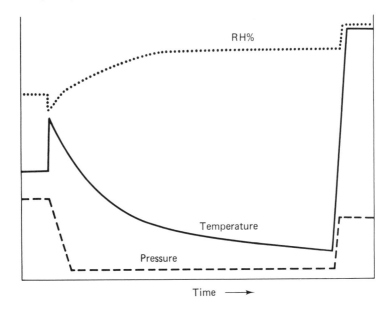

Fig. 3.7 Environmental changes to which a medicine could be exposed during air transportation from London to Singapore, RH, relative humidity.

that the manufacturer also has to be aware that hold temperatures vary in different aircraft.

Use
The product is often most vulnerable when it is in the patient's hands as:

The pack is opened and thus the product is exposed to the environment.
The patient frequently receives medicines from the pharmacist in packs different from those in which the manufacturer has undertaken stability studies.
The patient may mix several solid-dose medicines within one container.
Microbiological contamination may occur.

The onus is thus on the manufacturer to attempt to minimize the risk of a medicine deteriorating by, for example, including antimicrobial preservatives or, for medicines critically affected by environmental factors, using packs that will go directly to the patient.

Stability testing
Armed with this knowledge of the stresses that the medicine may encounter, how does the scientist study its stability profile?
The first essential is a 'stability indicating analytical method' which may

have been developed during preformulation studies but now is essential before stability studies can start. This method should be capable of high precision for the drug and must be capable of separating the drug from its impurities and degradation products. It therefore follows that the analytical scientist must have thoroughly considered the potential routes of degradation, possibly isolated some degradation products and checked them back as a discriminating test of the analytical method.

The next stage depends upon the type of medicine to be tested, as shown in Table 3.4. Some tests (e.g. assay of solutions at high temperature) are amenable to quantitative accelerated testing (e.g. Arrhenius testing – see below) whereas others (e.g. assay of tablets at high temperatures) may be, provided that the results are treated with some caution. Other tests (e.g. tablet hardness, medicine appearance, odour, etc.) are interpreted in the light of experience.

The reasons why some tests are amenable to quantitative acceleration while others are not lies in the nature of the reaction involved. Simply,

Table 3.4   Typical stability evaluations for some medicines

Medicine	Typical tests conducted
Tablet	Assay
	Levels of degradation products
	Moisture content
	Appearance and dimensions
	Hardness
	Friability
	Disintegration time
	Dissolution rate
	Pack condition
Syrup	Assay
	Levels of degradation products
	Appearance, taste and odour
	Viscosity
	pH
	Preservative assay
	Antimicrobial effectiveness
	Pack condition
Multidose injection vial	Assay
	Levels of degradation products
	Appearance and clarity
	pH
	Preservative assay
	Antimicrobial effectiveness
	Sterility test (initially and at end of life only)
	Tonicity agent assay
	Pack condition, including physical tests on rubber plugs

most reactions occur by one molecule interacting with another; for example, water interacting with a water-labile drug produces hydrolysis of the drug. The chance of such interactions occurring depends on the relative proportions of each molecular species and their positioning one to another. In a non-viscous liquid, molecular motion is unrestrained, large numbers of water molecules are available for interaction and the degree of hydrolysis that occurs depends on the lability of the drug. A number of factors can influence such molecular interactions but temperature would clearly play a large part. Increases in temperature will increase molecular motion and will therefore increase the degree of degradation. Similarly, decreases in temperature will bring about a decrease in degradation as will an increase in viscosity since in both cases molecular motion is diminished.

As most drugs degrade in solution by a reaction process which obeys first order chemical kinetics (i.e. the higher the concentration the greater the rate), a stability test that determines the concentration of drug (e.g. mg per 5 ml) over a given time interval will provide a straight line on a graph if plotted logarithmically as shown in Fig. 3.8. By study at a number of temperatures a family of lines can be drawn, the slope of each being the reaction rate constant for a given temperature and starting concentration. As a rule of thumb it can be considered *very generally* that the reaction rate doubles for each 10°C rise in temperature. However, extrapolations must be treated with caution since some reactions change very rapidly with temperature and others show discontinuities throughout the temperature range.

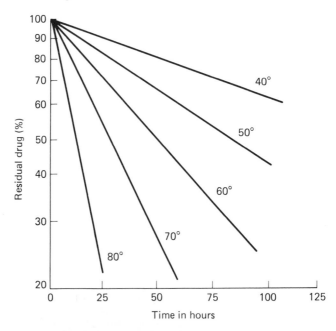

Fig. 3.8 Influence of temperature on the degradation of a medicine following first order chemical kinetics.

It is more usual, therefore, to apply the data from Fig. 3.8 to the Arrhenius equation which says that the reaction rate constant is inversely proportional to the absolute temperature (°K). Plotted logarithmically (Fig. 3.9) this provides a clear indication of any discontinuities and enables the 'activation energy' for the reaction to be determined from the slope of the line. Higher values of activation energy indicate that the temperature dependency of the degradation process is greater. If the Arrhenius plot is linear it can be extrapolated to lower temperatures (Fig. 3.9) and hence an estimate can be made of the reaction rate at potential storage temperatures (e.g. 30°C, 25°C, 4°C, etc.). As reaction rates have units of time^{-1}, an estimate of the shelf life in days/months/years can be reached.

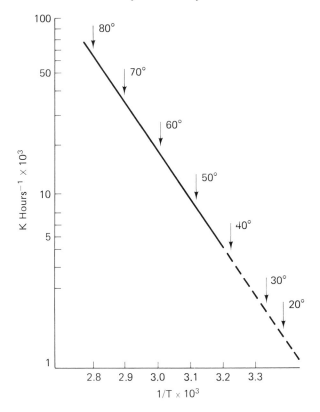

Fig. 3.9 Arrhenius plot showing the linear relationship between the degradation rate constant (obtained from each line in Fig. 3.8) and the inverse of absolute temperature to enable the shelf life to be determined.

Such test results are somewhat of an ideal in the complex medicines available and Arrhenius testing principles can only be applied in a limited way for solid dosage forms, e.g. tablets. The reasons are fairly straight-forward and relate primarily to considerably restricted molecular motion and non-ideal homogeneity (i.e. the drug will be distributed throughout the tablet but in discrete 'pockets') providing variations in concentration throughout the tablet. Moreover, if the drug in the tablet degrades by hydrolysis, the moisture content of the tablet at normal storage temperatures will be critical and the only function of high temperature studies will be to drive out the moisture from the tablet producing artificially good results. Thus, accelerated testing has its place with tablets and capsules, but rarely are temperatures above 65°C used for tablets and 40°C for capsules, and then care is exercised in interpreting the data obtained.

Such testing is only one component of a stability test profile as all factors being studied must be satisfactory before a medicine can be marketed. For example, a tablet with good chemical stability yet that readily takes up water vapour leading perhaps to decreased hardness or split tablets is unacceptable. Equally an erythrosine (red) coloured, strawberry flavoured syrup packed in a clear plastic bottle is of little value if it loses its flavour by volatilization through the plastic and its colour due to light. This would have to be rectified by use of a glass bottle, probably amber, and may require an outer carton for light protection.

Thus typical stability protocols such as that shown in Table 3.5 are often constructed providing high temperature, early warning, predictive data up to 6 months followed by longer term confirmatory testing. For a new drug being registered for the first time it would be unusual to provide less than 12 months data on the medicine in the marketed pack at the Product Licence/New Drug Application stage. Longer term confirmatory studies on earlier packs may be included in the application if it helps the case for the requested shelf life. It is, however, required that the stability programme, incompletely reported in the application, be continued and the results eventually reported to the regulatory authorities to support the shelf life given or even to extend it. Moreover, it is now increasingly becoming accepted that regular stability monitoring of production batches of the medicine is desirable in order to confirm that the process is remaining under control. Such testing is usually undertaken to a less demanding protocol.

Table 3.5   Typical programme for evaluation of drug stability

Storage conditions (°C)	Time (months)						
	1	3	6	12	18	24	36
4	{√}	{√}	{√}	{√}	{√}	{√}	
20				√	{√}	√	√
20/75%RH				√		√	√
30			√	√	√	√	√
30/75%RH			√	√		√	
40		√	√				
50	√	√	{√}				
60	√	√					

RH, relative humidity.

The meaning of quality

The Oxford English Dictionary defines quality as 'a particular grade of excellence . . . possessed by something'. For a medicine that excellence will depend partly on who is considering the quality.

1. A production manager will consider the medicine of suitable quality if no difficulties are experienced during manufacture and targets of specification and delivery can be met.
2. A quality control analytical chemist will consider the medicine of good quality if the results of the tests performed match a specification that has been set. Such a specification may include chemical, physical and microbiological tests.
3. A pharmacopoeial/regulatory person, however, will be more concerned that the tests performed agree with those considered acceptable for that type of product and which appear in pharmacopoeial monographs, e.g. that the correct strains of micro-organism and technique are used in antimicrobial effectiveness tests.
4. A clinician will, in all likelihood, not be concerned with any of the above – after all he relies on the manufacturer's reputation and the regulatory authorities to monitor that – but will judge quality by efficacy and safety. Thus he will be aware of the research work that was undertaken and will wish to see consistent clinical performance batch to batch, month to month, etc.

Quality standards are constantly under review to see whether they are appropriate to current practice. If problems arise indicating weakness in standards, new tests are adopted or existing ones tightened, as happened with digoxin where a dissolution test standard was adopted.[3] The old concept of 'quality control' is now invalid and we now more frequently use the term 'quality assurance'. At all stages in the development, manufacture and distribution of the medicine, assurance must be available that a product will be and will remain of good quality. Quality cannot be controlled into products. Increasingly, regulatory authorities are taking a position where they are expecting proof at the first approval that the quality links between product development and manufacturing are secure enough to provide assurance that product made in a decade's time will have the same safety and efficacy as when developed.

The supply of clinical trial materials

The supply of clinical trial material is often the greatest area of contact between clinical and pharmaceutical staff within the industry. However, despite the importance of the contact it is not necessarily the closest, often due to misunderstanding of the features involved in both the clinical and pharmaceutical aspects associated with setting up clinical trials.

The clinician is responsible for the patient and the trial design and, therefore, he wishes to ensure that, if a double-blind trial is required, the compromised by poor patient compliance associated with having to take multiple dosage forms.

The pharmaceutical and analytical scientists thus have to be aware of the trial design and be in a position to offer alternative presentations to conduct the trial optimally. Thus the pharmaceutical scientist has responsibility for:

Identifying suitable dosage forms

Developing appropriate manufacturing procedures and documentation to meet regulatory GMP requirements

Ensuring use of suitable packaging materials to provide stability and, if necessary, double-blind protection

If a competitor's medicine is manipulated, ensuring that it is bio-equivalent with the marketed medicine

The analytical scientist has responsibility for:

The purity of the drug included in the dosage form

Quality assurance on the manufactured medicine

Ensuring, where placebos are used, some means of identifying the active from the placebo medicine, and ensuring that the placebo is free from contamination by any of the drugs under study

Methods of producing double-blind supplies

Most trials are of a double-blind nature and the level of work involved for the pharmaceutical scientist depends upon whether the trial:

Has simple placebo controls

Has matching competitor medicines

Has non-matching competitor medicines and placebo controls to both the drug under study and the competitor medicine

Placebo controls

The supply of placebo medicines to one's own active medicine is relatively straightforward. Thus, when the active medicine is a white or coloured tablet, a clear or coloured syrup, etc. the degree of difficulty is not too great. Difficulties arise when trials are undertaken against a marketed medicine which will almost always bear some form of identification. It is ethically unjustifiable to put such identification on placebos and so unmarked active medicines will require manufacture.

The factors to be taken into account when matching placebo to active medicines are: shape, size, marking, colour (external and internal), texture (external and internal), weight, taste and after taste, and smell.

Matching competitor products

It is usually necessary either to request the competitor company to provide their drug in a form to match your medicine, or for you to manipulate products are suitably matched. Furthermore for a double-blind, double-dummy study the clinician has to be sure that the study will not be their medicine in some way. As delays are frequent in obtaining the competitor drug in an alternative form, if it can be obtained at all, it is more usual to manipulate the competitor medicine. Table 3.6 illustrates some of the techniques available for matching competitor products. Clearly if your product cannot be matched, it too will require manipulation.

Table 3.6   Some techniques for producing matching tablets

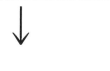

Increasing
complexity,
time and
cost

Small tablets placed in capsules
Tablets placed in (coloured?) rice paper cachets
Ground tablets placed in capsules
Film or sugar coat for normally uncoated tablets or tablets
  having coats of different colours
Formulate new tablets from basic ingredients

The factors to be taken into account when matching the competitor medicine to your own are, in addition to those listed for placebos:

- disintegration time
- dissolution rate
- bioequivalence

These factors do not need to be identical for your medicine and the competitor medicine but the 'availability', assessed by the above criteria, of the competitor product as marketed must not be impaired by the manipulation employed.

Non-matching competitor products
If it is not possible to match your medicine against the competitor – e.g. a tablet to be compared with an aerosol, a layered, controlled-release tablet to be compared with controlled-release pellets in a capsule, etc. – then placebos to each form must be made available so that the placebo of one active form can be included alongside the active of the other and vice versa (the double-dummy technique). The factors to be taken into account are identical to those listed above.

All of the above work takes time, not only to manufacture, pack and supply, but also, where development work is involved, to provide a medicine that satisfies the criteria specified. It may be necessary to perform some stability testing to ensure that the manipulation has not affected the long-term quality of the medicine. Thus, early discussions between clinical and pharmaceutical personnel are vital if satisfactory material is to be provided in good time.

Conclusions

It was stated at the outset that making drugs into medicines was a complex problem involving interactions between many people in a variety of disciplines. It has only been possible to scratch the surface of the detail involved but it is hoped that the reader, whatever their sphere, will have found that it helps interactions with others involved in the process.

References

1. Hiller, FC, Mazumer MK, Smith GM *et al.* (1980). Physical properties, hygroscopicity and estimated pulmonary retention of various therapeutic aerosols. *Chest* **775:** 318S.
2. Report of a WHO Scientific Study Group (1974). *Bioavailability of Drugs: Principles and Problems*. World Health Organisation Technical Report Series 536. Geneva: WHO.
3. Shaw TRD (1974). Non-equivalence of digoxin tablets in the UK and its clinical implications. *Postgraduate Medical Journal* **50 (suppl 6):** 24.

4

Clinical trials

Denis M. Burley and Louis Lasagna

A significant milestone in the development of a new drug is its first administration to humans. It is an important and difficult decision but less onerous than might be thought since it is usually taken by a team of medical and non-medical scientists in the light of accumulating preclinical data. Most drugs are first studied in non-patient volunteers. Limited studies are then undertaken in patients with the disease for which the drug is being developed. After this, clinical trials involving a much larger number of patients are completed. Further trials may be required after marketing. Following American practice these stages have become known as Phases I–IV. In detail and scale they represent a more or less continual progression from depth to breadth. Although the scientific principles and underlying philosophy of clinical trials are the same throughout the process, there are important practical differences between the phases, so it will be convenient first to describe them in more detail.

Although others can make an important contribution to the clinical evaluation of a new medicine, trials must remain under the control of able and well trained physicians. Only about 10 per cent of new chemical entities reaching humans are eventually marketed. Most of the remainder fail early in the trial programme. Knowing when to abandon a project is just as important as deciding when to continue it.

Phase I studies

Initial studies in humans are normally carried out in healthy volunteers, but it is probably better to refer to these as non-patient volunteers since inevitably those drawn from a healthy population will include some who are allergic, anxious, have undetected disease or who have minor abnormalities. Ideally the aim of these early studies should be to investigate pharmacodynamic and pharmacokinetic properties. However, many drugs do not have pharmacological effects in healthy people; for example, anti-inflammatory drugs and antibiotics. There are two essential objectives in initial Phase I studies. The first is to assess tolerability as well as safety of gradually increasing doses. The second is to obtain basic pharmacokinetic information. These are critical studies, and observations made during this stage will influence the design of later phases. Of course, the finding of unacceptable adverse effects may preclude any further development. The protocol for Phase I investigation is therefore vitally important.

Exceptions to the use of non-patient volunteers as first subjects are studies with anticancer drugs or drugs for the management of AIDS.

Design of a Phase I investigation

The design of the initial human evaluation will largely depend on the potential use of the drug; for instance, whether it is going to be used in the psychiatric, respiratory or cardiovascular field. It is thus only possible to make generalizations about the design. Some of the more important factors influencing the design are set out below:

1. The likely mechanism of action. If it has been possible to gain such information from the animal studies it is important to check whether the same conclusions apply to humans. If the mechanism of action is known, one may be able to predict more accurately where and when the drug will be of clinical use, and possibly to predict and avoid adverse reactions. Also, the design of the investigation becomes much simpler.
2. The predicted effect is likely to occur only in diseased subjects. If no pharmacodynamic effects are expected in non-patient volunteers, then it is essential to know the extent to which the drug has been absorbed from the gastrointestinal tract. In addition, checks can be made to find out whether what is presumed to be an adequate drug concentration is achieved in blood and urine, or at other appropriate sites.
3. Where a pharmacodynamic effect is expected, it often does not occur after a single dose. Repeated administration may be necessary and this may be more appropriate in Phase II when relevant patients are exposed.

Selection of investigators and site

The first administration of a novel compound to humans should be performed at a site where there are staff and facilities able to deal with any emergency situation. Some pharmaceutical companies have well equipped units on their own premises, but they do not always have staff who are familiar with resuscitation procedures or all the specialist fields in which the company may be interested. Increasingly, Phase I studies are being contracted out to commercial organizations or hospitals who specialize in conducting this type of work to the highest standards of Good Clinical Practice (GCP). In the UK there is an organization called the Association of Independent Clinical Research Contractors who arrange biennial inspections of members who carry out both non-patient and patient volunteer studies.

The clinical investigator has to be both a physician and a pharmacologist. He must have a good understanding of the details of the animal pharmacology and toxicology and be able to assess the validity and level of confidence with which the prehuman pharmacological conclusions have been drawn. This is necessary to understand the risk to which the volunteers are being subjected. Fortunately, experience has shown that in capable hands the early studies of drugs in humans are remarkably safe.

The planning of Phase I studies is shared between the company sponsoring the study and the unit carrying out the study, using the pooled knowledge from the sponsor, who is familiar with all the preclinical history of the candidate drug, and the experience of the investigator group, so as to minimize risk to volunteers and maximize the information obtained through studies of absorption, distribution, metabolism and excretion (ADME) of the drugs. It is therefore essential for the pharmaceutical physician to establish good working relations with academic or other specialist colleagues involved in such work. Active 'hands on' participation is valuable to obtain and maintain the commitment of others to the successful completion of the investigations.

Selection and care of subjects

Most Phase I studies are initiated in fit male volunteers who may be recruited through various teaching institutions or medical schools. Advertising through local newspapers, health care organizations, clubs, etc. is often employed. Increasingly, studies are being required in volunteers over the age of 65 and independent contract organizations and hospitals have set up panels of volunteers to meet this need. Since volunteers are usually paid for their time and the inconvenience of Phase I investigations which may involve overnight stays (or longer term residence in multiple dose studies), it is undesirable that the financial element should be the major factor in persuading subjects to volunteer. The danger is that they may too readily consent to the procedures proposed or may attempt to enter studies at too frequent intervals. Ideally 4 months should elapse between successive studies and no volunteer should ever knowingly be put in two studies at the same time. The dangers are obvious. Some units only recruit volunteers in stable occupations so that the financial arrangements are not of primary concern. Fortunately, volunteers can see the value of helping with medical research which does not directly benefit them, but which may well be of value later and particularly to their children or others in the family.

No volunteer should be in a position of subservience to the investigator or sponsor. This is one of the reasons why volunteers taken from the sponsoring companies are used much less now than in the past. All volunteers should be informed about the procedures to be carried out and must give their agreement, preferably in writing. They need to be told that they are participating in research that usually will be of no direct benefit to them. An explanation about the nature of the drug they may be taking should be given, with attendant risks so far as they are known as well as details of all the procedures to be adopted, such as blood sampling and urine collection. The fact that this may be the first administration of a drug to humans should be understood by the volunteers since it carries with it the implication that its handling in the body is under investigation and that safety can only be judged at this stage from previous animal studies.

There is advantage in bringing potential volunteers together at a meeting when a clinical investigator can address them and answer questions. Also, at least a week should be given for reflection or to enable a volunteer to discuss the matter with a friend or family before giving written consent. Once a subject has volunteered it is essential that they give a complete medical history, and that clinical examination and appropriate screening tests are carried out and interpreted by a doctor with a sound clinical background. Screening tests should include chest X-ray, ECG, full blood count and tests of hepatic and renal function. If the preclinical information indicates that the compound may have some effect on a specific organ, for example the thyroid gland, specific baseline tests such as testing of thyroid function should be carried out. Volunteers should be screened for hepatitis B, and in some European countries HIV screening is also required. In any event, history-taking should allow volunteers to be rejected if there is any likelihood that they could have acquired HIV.

If the subject is volunteering for the first time it is wise to inform the subject's general practitioner, as they may have pertinent information about the subject. Also, the subject's usual medical attendant should be informed of their participation in a study and a report given at the end of the study. This is easy to achieve in the UK, where people are normally registered with a local practitioner, but in many countries the medical arrangements are different and volunteers are frequently recruited without a previous medical history being available or indeed without the volunteer having a regular medical attendant. It is essential that the subjects and investigator be covered by adequate insurance. The ethics are fully dealt with elsewhere but, as with clinical studies in patients, the protocol for a Phase I study should be approved by a properly constituted Ethics Committee, or Institutional Review Board in the USA.

In most Phase I studies subjects are usually aged between 18 and 60. Furthermore, they are usually male. This is not male chauvinism; it is due to the fact that there is an increasing trend for companies to delay full teratology studies until the Phase I studies have been successfully completed. In addition, many potential female volunteers are on the contraceptive pill, which in some instances may affect the pharmacokinetics of the study drug. A drawback of restricting Phase I studies entirely to men, however, is that women may handle the drug somewhat differently, and this could be clinically important. Unless the disease for which the drug is intended is exclusive to males, it would seem sensible to find out whether the drug is teratogenic or not at an early stage, although the cost of such studies is considerable. It seems reasonable, at the earliest stage of clinical investigation, to restrict the age range, but if the drug is intended to be used in elderly patients or in children a full pharmacokinetic and pharmaco-dynamic investigation should be undertaken as soon as this becomes possible, bearing in mind the ethical problems that arise with studies in children. Indeed, in most countries including the USA it is only possible to give new drugs to children at much later stages in their development.

Drug administration

In the UK permission from the licensing authority is not required for the administration of a drug to non-patient volunteers. For this purpose a non-patient volunteer would be defined as a subject who is not expected to obtain therapeutic benefit. However, in the USA permission has to be obtained from Food and Drug Administration (FDA) before such studies can be carried out. As the predictive value of animal toxicity testing is often questionable, guidelines on the amount of animal toxicity testing required before initial drug administration to humans are necessarily empiric.[1]

In UK it is now regarded as satisfactory for many compounds if the drug is administered to two species, one of which is non-rodent, for 2 weeks (Table 4.1). This permits a single dose or a single short series of doses to be given to humans. Guidelines for initial dosage and subsequent increments are empiric, but many investigators start with the equivalent of about 2 per cent of the dose that is effective in animals and double this until either the expected dose is reached or the therapeutic effect or some toxic effect occurs. The route of administration must be the same in animals and humans. Although it is important to note that a minute dose of a radio-labelled drug will be all that is required for initial pharmacokinetic data, it is always better to correlate pharmacodynamic with pharmacokinetic changes. This can only be achieved with an effective dose in subjects capable of showing the pharmacodynamic effects. Wherever possible the dose of a drug should be titrated against its effect and, depending on the nature of the drug, this may have to be done in Phase II. Such dose titration studies will give more information than a single fixed dose study.

Repeated dosing in man must be preceded by longer toxicity testing in animals. The guidelines agreed to by the UK Department of Health and Social Security (DHSS) and the Association of the British Pharmaceutical Industry (ABPI) are set out in Table 4.1. Animal toxicity testing should give indications as to which organ systems to monitor, since no drug can be completely non-toxic.

The physician will want to ensure that, subject to the pharmacological properties of the drug, a high enough dose has been given to the animals.

Table 4.1 DHSS and ABPI guidelines for toxicity testing

Administration to humans	Toxicity programme
1–3 single doses	14 days in two species
Up to 7 days treatment	28 days in two species
7–28 days treatment	3 months in two species
1–3 months treatment	6 months in two species

The route or routes chosen for the animal study must be the ones intended for clinical adminstration of the drug. Variation in the route can result in important pharmacokinetic and pharmacodynamic differences.

Measurements

These will depend mainly on the drug and the disease for which it was developed. It is important to be open-minded and not only to check whether the same properties are found in humans as in animals but also to investigate whether there are novel ones not detected in the animal experiments. Especially important are the tests that are difficult or impossible to perform in animals, e.g. psychological testing. However, it is important not to make the study too complicated. Well validated, simple measurements are more useful than complex ones which may often be found to be unreliable. In appropriate circumstances electrocardiography, electroencephalography and the use of radio-isotopes can provide a great deal of information. The key to safety lies in good experimental design, using techniques and facilities with which the investigators are familiar and in which they have confidence.

In single-dose studies, if the compound is being given orally, it is essential to know whether the compound has been absorbed. At this stage of the drug's development an assay method sensitive enough to detect predicted low levels of the compound or its metabolite may not have been developed. In such circumstances the administration of a small dose of compound labelled with a radio-isotope should be incorporated into the investigation. In acute studies estimation of plasma concentration provides an indication of whether a drug or metabolite is responsible for the pharmacological effect. It will also reveal whether the drug obeys first or zero order kinetics. Volume of distribution and clearance will be obtained for most drugs. Pharmacokinetic data obtained from repeated administration are necessary to check on initial impressions obtained from acute administration data. Clearly, if the dynamic data correlate well with the kinetic data for the parent compound then this is strong presumptive evidence that the drug itself rather than a metabolite is responsible for the pharmacological effect. Sometimes a metabolite which is more pharmacologically active is identified, raising the possibility of developing that compound instead.

In both single- and repeated-dose studies volunteers should be monitored closely, with full blood counts and hepatic and renal tests which are repeated at appropriate times. If a serious untoward event occurs (which may or may not be due to the drug) it is essential to investigate the circumstances as promptly and as thoroughly as possible. If this is not done future volunteers or even patients may be put at risk unnecessarily, or a potentially useful drug may be withdrawn. Important adverse drug reactions can be looked for in Phase I studies, but these are usually identified at a late stage after a good deal of patient information has been obtained.

Phase II studies

The primary object of these studies is to determine whether a drug shows promise in one or more clinical indications. Patients rather than healthy volunteers are used as subjects. Early studies in Phase II are among the safest since they start with one or a few low doses of the new drug in a limited number of patients who are very closely monitored. Progression to multiple-dose studies or expansion of patient numbers is embarked upon after initial reassuring experience with the new drug.

It is quite legitimate for many of these early investigations to be uncontrolled and, provided they are properly conducted, they can contribute valuable data. They are best carried out by investigators who have a special interest in the treatment of the disease for which the drug is intended.

The trials should identify the most suitable dosage schedule; give an estimate of clinical efficacy in relation to concentration of the drug and its metabolites in body fluids and tissues, and provide information on adverse effects. They should if possible give enough information to allow a preliminary assessment of benefit/risk ratio. The pharmacokinetics of a drug should be investigated in patients because they may handle the drug differently from healthy people, either as an effect of their disease or because patients with the disease in question may be much older or much younger than the healthy volunteers studied in Phase I. Vigilant observation by an open-minded investigator may indicate even at this early stage some unforeseen property, beneficial or otherwise.

Phase III studies

Phase III trials are undertaken when there is evidence that:

1. An adequate degree of efficacy exists.
2. The risk profile of adverse reactions appears to be acceptable in terms of demonstrated efficacy.

Primary responsibility for this decision is obviously that of the clinical research department of the pharmaceutical company. However, it is very important that the opinions of the various hospital investigators involved in the Phase II studies are taken into account. Also, in most countries including the UK and the USA the requirements of the regulatory authority must be met. In the USA it is quite common for an 'end of Phase II' conference to be convened at which medical and scientific personnel from FDA participate.

In Phase III studies the number of patients is gradually increased as confidence in the drug grows. Several different types of trial design may be used and these will be discussed later. The objective of a Phase III clinical trial programme is not merely to obtain the approval of the government authorities so that a drug can be marketed. It is to generate information that enables the practising doctor to utilize the drug effectively, safely and put it to optimal use. Indications for use of the drug must be confirmed. Firm recommendations for dosage must be established. Those circumstances under which a different dosage is to be used should be clearly defined to ensure that as precise prescribing information as possible is available.

Phase IV studies

These are trials undertaken after obtaining a marketing licence. Phase II and III studies suffer from three major limitations:

1. Restricted patient populations.
2. Limited duration of patient exposure.
3. Limited patient numbers.

Consequently Phase IV trials should be constructed to show:

1. Drug efficacy in prolonged use where perhaps the natural course of a disease may be modified over a period of several months or years.
2. Adverse reactions which only occur with long term use or which occur only very rarely.
3. Comparative data with standard drugs.
4. A detailed examination of non-responders.
5. An assessment of overdosage and misuse or abuse liability.
6. New dosage forms.
7. New indications.
8. Drug interactions.

With regard to drug interactions it should always be borne in mind that drug metabolism can either be increased or decreased by the coadministration of another drug. Similarly, the excretion or absorption of a drug may be affected by another drug. Competitive antagonism at receptor sites may affect the efficacy of one or both drugs.

For most drugs which are given orally over long periods of time Phase IV trials will be often organized with the cooperation of general practitioners, although the situation is different in many other countries including the USA. In the UK there are now firm guidelines for the conduct of trials of licensed medicinal products in general practice.[2] These guidelines have been carefully drawn up to ensure ethical and scientific validity. Needless to say it still remains the ultimate responsibility of the pharmaceutical physician to ensure that these trials do meet the guidelines.

The experimental nature of clinical trials

Sir George Pickering in his Presidential Address to the Section of Experimental Medicine and Therapeutics of the Royal Society of Medicine said in 1949: 'Therapeutics is the branch of medicine that, by its very nature, should be experimental'. This statement crystallizes the view that scientific method is the proper way to evaluate therapeutic intervention in sick people and places a 'seal of approval' on the controlled clinical trial, which could be regarded as the centrepiece of pharmaceutical medicine.

There are of course examples of controlled trials dating back for centuries,[3] the most familiar being James Lind's classic trial in 1747 in 12 sailors suffering from scurvy, two being given vitriol as a dietary supplement, two cider, two vinegar, two oranges and lemons and two a mixture prepared by the surgeon. This experiment established the value of oranges and lemons as a cure for scurvy. Earlier in this century (1931) the Medical Research Council (MRC) created a Therapeutic Trials Committee which has been emulated more recently by the British Thoracic and Tuberculosis Association (now the British Thoracic Society) and for examples of well constructed, randomized, controlled clinical trials the early antituberculous chemotherapy studies with streptomycin, para-amino-salicylic acid (PAS) and isoniazid are well worth studying.[4-6]

Sir Austin Bradford Hill, through his classic work '*Principles of Medical Statistics*', which has run into numerous editions, set out the fundamental principles of clinical trials in his definition: '. . . the clinical trial is a carefully and ethically designed experiment with the aim of answering some precisely framed question'.[7] Sir Austin can properly be regarded as the Father of the medical branch of statistics and his contributions to the literature on clinical trial design have ranged over such subjects as the use of controls, the allocation of treatments, the measurement and reporting of results and the ethical problems that have to be faced when a patient consents to take part in a clinical trial or is randomized to a placebo treatment.

During the last 40 years the technique of the randomized controlled clinical trial has become accepted as the proper method for evaluating new therapeutic interventions and this has led to many valuable contributions to the literature on clinical trial design, the proper application of statistical methods, clarity in the presentation of data and appropriate decision making. Clinical judgment and experience have been supported by the proper use of scientific method and the pitfalls of relying solely on the former have been clearly demonstrated.

Some demonstrations of therapeutic activity have been so dramatic that clinical experience and scientific assessment would clearly have led to the same conclusions. The transformation of tuberculous meningitis from a fatal to a non-fatal disease by the advent of streptomycin and isoniazid, the truncation of the classic phases of pneumococcal pneumonia by the advent of penicillin and the cure of subacute bacterial endocarditis are familiar examples. But most therapeutic progress is brought about through a series of much smaller steps, or much less dramatic manifestations. It is in these situations that experience may be fallacious and judgment faulty or prejudiced, so that the discipline of scientific method must be invoked if one is not to be led along false trails or into blind alleys.

We are fortunate that since the Second World War there has been so much progress in the medicinal therapeutic field and that there are few medical conditions which are not at least partially amenable to drug therapy. This in itself has created ethical problems in recent years over such issues as consent to randomization and the use of placebos.[8] By their nature randomized trials tend to serve a collective ethic rather than an individual ethic, and as a result of 'experience' a practitioner must at least have some view as to the 'best' existing treatment. Hence it is argued that randomization which relegates the individual to the whim of the random number generator is unjustifiable and that the use of a placebo is a denial of treatment.[9]

If these sentiments were to lead us to retrace our steps away from scientific method and back along the path of unsupported belief the prospect would be appalling for both doctor and patient. However, in as much as our ethical anxieties have led us towards considering new methods of using controls through adaptive designs[10] or reconsidering old methods,[11] they have served a valuable function, and recognition of the importance of the individual through proper consent procedures has reduced the feeling that taking part in a clinical trial is simply a lottery.

Clearly in the future there will be much more discussion by informed laity and the legal profession (to say nothing of the media and various pressure groups) about medicinal treatment in general and the role of scientists and doctors. Some of our present views will need to be modified in the light of changing public opinion as to the role of the individual in society and the rights of the sick individual in relation to his medical attendant. In the USA certain AIDS advocacy groups have been very effective in pushing regulatory authorities and industry to involve them in protocol design and other matters. Ethical principles are not written on tablets of stone.

Organizing a clinical trial

The essence of good clinical trial design is careful planning, and the aim should be to maximize the benefit/cost ratio of any study, cost being measured not only in conventional terms but also in the use of patients. An inefficient trial utilizing human and technical resources which by its very design can provide no information to guide future therapeutic decisions is unethical from its inception.

The pressures engendered by the need to produce results from multiple Phase III clinical studies to satisfy health authorities and obtain marketing consent tend to lead to stereotyped thinking. The words of Bradford Hill when discussing the ethics of clinical trials,[12] ' . . . that one can make no generalization. One can lay down no general conditions. The problem must be faced afresh with every proposed trial', is equally true of clinical trial design. But guidelines are valuable and these we will try and set out.

The Protocol
The clinical trial protocol describes the procedure for carrying out a clinical trial starting with its aims and justification and ending with what

is often forgotten; how the trial should be terminated. It is therefore useful to have a schedule or check list to ensure that nothing has been forgotten. Detailed check lists have been published[13] but the main headings are as follows:

Aims:	questions to be answered; justification
Material:	patients selected – exclusions; consent
Trial Design:	group comparisons, crossovers; numbers required
Treatments:	allocation to patients – placebos
Measurements:	validity
Record keeping:	clerk and computer
Drug supplies:	matching, labelling; code
Handling adverse	
reaction:	reporting; code breaking
Report writing:	results; statistical considerations; conclusions
Closing the Trial	

The Team

The protocol must be written by a team[14] who collectively will have at their fingertips or in their cerebral computers all the accumulated information that will enable them to formulate a useful question (or questions) to be answered by the clinical trial and to decide whether that question can be answered with the resources and patients available. The protocol writing team will therefore include:

A *Physician* who is responsible for the care and welfare of the patients taking part in the trial.

A *Recorder* who is responsible for making patient observations and recording measurements.

A *Pharmaceutical Physician* who is the repository of the pedigree of the drug or drugs being used in the trial, their effects and side effects and their procurement.

A *Statistician* to advise on type I and type II error in relation to the hypothesis to be tested and the number of patients available.

A *Pharmacist* who will be responsible for the proper dispensing of drugs, often using a randomized procedure.

A *Monitor* who will be responsible for the logistics of the trial; the completion of records, the continuity of drug supplies and availability of finance.

In addition, the cooperation of a number of others who will inevitably become involved in various aspects of the trial is vital to avoid obstruction and frustration. The ward or outpatient Sister (charge nurse in the USA) and her staff should be brought into the discussions, together with departments of biochemistry, haematology, radiology, etc. who may be burdened with increased workload and can often provide valuable advice on measurements, methodology and recording. All should be quite clear about the extent of their involvement.

In outpatient studies the family practitioner should be notified that their patient is taking part in a trial and cooperation actively sought. They should also be notified when the trial has ended and the patient has been returned to their care, together with advice on future management which the trial results may have suggested.

The Physician
The Physician (or other clinician) responsible for the trial does not necessarily have to take an active part in the interviewing of patients and in recording observations, but the trial is their responsibility and they have to satisfy themselves regarding the credentials of the other members of the team, that patients are being managed in an ethical manner and conventionally according to the Declaration of Helsinki, and that they have given valid consent to any procedure being carried out.

The Recorder
The Recorder or Recorders are responsible for the proper collection of the measurement data (objective and subjective) that will form the basis of decision making when the trial is complete. They need to be aware of the problems associated with measurement such as bias, digit preference, intra- and interobserver error and the inconvenience associated with missing data.

The Pharmaceutical Physician
The Pharmaceutical Physician should regard it as their responsibility to be familiar with the literature not only of the drug in the trial, but the methodology and results of trials previously carried out with drugs of the same class. A literature search is an essential preliminary to any piece of scientific work and the physician should ask himself the following questions:

> Is the question worth answering?
> Has it already been answered?
> Can it be answered by the proposed trial?

and perhaps most important,

> Can the investigator answer it with the resources available?

It takes courage to shut down a trial when you *know* it will not yield useful information, let alone when you only *suspect* that it won't.

The Statistician
The role of the Statistician is covered in detail in the succeeding chapter. Suffice it to emphasize at this point the essential contribution that they can make in the planning stage of any trial. They are not just there to make sense out of nonsense at the end of the trial.

The Pharmacist

The Pharmacist of the past often became aware that the patient was participating in a clinical trial when they appeared with an empty bottle bearing the label 'the trial tablets – take one every morning'. This is no longer permissible and it is essential for all hospital drug supplies to be dispensed from the pharmacy according to a prepared randomization list. A randomization code should also be kept there in case it needs to be broken. In fact many hospitals have now appointed a pharmacist with special responsibility for clinical trial supplies.

The Monitor

The Monitor has to some extent been a response on the part of the pharmaceutical industry to the legal requirement that a pharmaceutical physician should be responsible (under signature) for the authenticity and accuracy of data submitted to health authorities. Such requirements are more stringent in the USA whose health authority (FDA) appears to have experienced a disturbing degree of dishonesty in the reporting of clinical trials data for new drug applications (NDAs). Nevertheless, many firms in the UK now employ clinical research assistants who are responsible for monitoring data collection and ensuring that data transferred for computer processing is not given a spurious authenticity by being printed in standard format. There is no substitute for the careful inspection of the original handwritten data on the original record form. If all the records are in the same handwriting with the same biro there are grounds for suspicion. It is most important that the record be accepted or rejected for analysis *before* the code is broken.

Trial aims

It is important not to attempt too much or to try to answer too many questions in a single trial. The number of patients available, the time constraints, the continued interest and dedication of the investigator, will all argue in favour of answering a few questions at a time and ensuring that they are answered well, whether negatively or positively.

It is assumed that a comparative study will be carried out, although other forms of study do have a place and will be considered later. Early on it is necessary to decide whether the comparison will be against a positive control (usually the 'best' of the other treatments available) or a negative control (placebo), or against both. With serious or life-threatening conditions comparisons will have to be against a conventional treatment if one exists, but for investigations involving simple illness or the management of symptoms placebo controls may be more appropriate.

Difficulties arise with trials in conditions such as hypertension or depression. It may be permissible to postpone effective treatment in order to carry out placebo-controlled studies in patients with mild forms of the illness, but patients with severe hypertension could be at risk from stroke or severe depressives at risk from suicide if effective treatment is withheld for a period. The problem with positive controls is that a finding of no difference between the new and standard treatments can be explained either by the fact that both are effective or by the fact that both are ineffective, and one needs to be sure that the standard treatment has been shown for that particular group in the past to be consistently superior to a placebo in order to dispense with the need for a negative control.[15]

Having decided on the nature of the comparison, the next consideration is what outcome measure is going to provide the best test of treatment effectiveness. The simplest objective measure, and one not likely to give rise to dispute, is mortality, but most Phase III trials do not have this as a likely outcome. Even here some major outcome studies of secondary prevention of myocardial infarction have led to disputes about the inclusion of some of the mortality data. All other measures, objective or subjective, will present problems which are considered later and in the next chapter. It seems logical to place strong emphasis on the patient's judgment concerning the benefit of treatment, particularly in conditions such as angina pectoris or rheumatoid arthritis. In the latter condition it may be tempting to judge a response by measuring erythrocyte sedimentation rate (ESR) or the titre of rheumatoid factor, but in practice the patient's experience of morning stiffness, joint tenderness and ability to carry out daily tasks is a much better guide to treatment response.

Finally, all treatments will involve a balance between risk and benefit, so it is necessary to evaluate carefully the adverse effects of new and comparative treatments. A single trial involving relatively small numbers of patients will not reveal uncommon hazards. Subsequent trials will add information and special examinations of body systems will be required if there are any pointers from previous studies (human or animal) of damage to important target organs such as the liver, the kidney and the blood-forming organs.

It is important in setting out the aims of the trial to indicate the nature of the hypothesis to be tested (usually the Null Hypothesis) together with the statistical limits for rejection and the power of the trial. Conventionally the Null Hypothesis is rejected when the probability of a demonstrated difference being due to chance (type I error or α) is 5 per cent ($P = 0.05$) or in some trials 1 per cent ($P = 0.01$). The danger of not finding a difference which is present is called the type II error or β. The power of a study $(1-\beta)$ is its ability to demonstrate the difference. β is often set at between 10 and 20 per cent and therefore the power is between 90 and 80 per cent. This is why expert statistical advice is so important; consideration of the likely sources of error and the minimum useful treatment benefit one hopes to detect govern the number of patients that must be entered into the trial (see also Chapter 5).

The patients

Since it is impossible to treat a whole population of patients with a given condition it is necessary to treat a typical sample, and herein lies a classic dilemma. Does one select a narrow homogeneous group who fulfil certain well defined criteria, or does one accept a wide range of patients under a given diagnostic umbrella? The disadvantage of the first method is that it may be hard to find sufficient numbers of patients because of the numerous exclusions, and the results of the trial may only be applicable to the chosen subgroup. On the other hand, by the choice of a wide range of patients positive results in an important subgroup may be so diluted that they are undetectable or do not reach statistical significance. It is perhaps best in most cases to choose a sample that is as broadly based as possible, yet define those patient characteristics that are most likely to affect response to treatment. By suitable randomization and a realistic choice of numbers it may be possible to have the best of both worlds and to detect not only overall benefit but also benefit confined to certain subgroups, provided always that the objectives are set out in advance. However, no trial sample is ever a random sample of any population and one should always be cautious when extrapolating data from the findings of a trial to the universe of patients with the disease under study.

The factors most commonly affecting response to treatment are:

- Age
- Gender
- Severity of disease
- Duration of disease
- Previous or current therapy

These will form the basis for choosing response categories, but others may be important in particular conditions; for instance the presence or absence of cavitation in tuberculosis trials.

The criteria for patient inclusion and exclusion must be defined in the protocol in unambiguous terms and it may be desirable to provide a checklist to ensure that ineligible patients are not included (Fig. 4.1). It goes without saying that if more than one centre is involved there must be agreement between investigators on both the validity and determination of diagnostic categories.

Conventional exclusions are:

- Children
- Women of child-bearing age
- Seriously ill or moribund patients
- Those with other diagnoses
- Those who are unlikely to cooperate with the trial regimen

In the past elderly patients were often excluded from studies, but since it has been demonstrated with many drugs that elderly patients respond differently and may need dose modifications it is now usual to carry out specific studies in elderly subgroups: a licence may not be granted to cover patients over the age of 65 unless such studies have been carried

---

Eligibility form*

Patient's name. . . . .

Hospital No. . . . .   Today's date . . . .

tick appropriate box

		Yes	No
Is he	Male?	☐	☐
	Between ages of 35 and 60 years (inclusive)?	☐	☐
Is there	A clinical history of myocardial infarct 2/12 or more ago?	☐	☐
	Either (a) 2 ECG's available showing typical infarct changes? Or (b) if only left bundle branch changes are there also SGOT, CPK or HDB results showing an infarct pattern?	☐	☐
Have you excluded	Cardiogenic shock?	☐	☐
	Serious dysrrhythmias?	☐	☐
	Heart failure?	☐	☐
	Other cardiac, renal, respiratory or CNS abnormalities, making the patient unsuitable for the study?	☐	☐
	Diabetes?	☐	☐
	A history of bronchospastic disease (i.e. asthma, chronic bronchitis etc.) contraindicating beta-blockage?	☐	☐
Can you confirm that	(a) he is not on, or needing, anti-hypertensive drugs?	☐	☐
	(b) he is not taking a tricyclic anti-depressant drug?	☐	☐
	(c) if he is on beta-blockers already, these have not been taken for longer than one month?	☐	☐
	(d) he is fit to return to previous employment, or light work if previously heavy manual labour?	☐	☐

*If the answers to all the questions listed above are 'YES', then the patient may be eligible for the trial and you should now proceed to fill in the Initial Assessment Form (Form II).
If one of the answers to the questions above is 'NO', then the patient must be excluded from the trial.

Fig. 4.1 An eligibility form.

out. In addition, some studies in fecund women may be carried out if adequate birth control techniques are being used, or in women who are sexually inactive or lesbians.

Although some exclusions are usually prudent, one has to take care not to extrapolate uncritically the results of the trial to such excluded patients at a later date. In addition patients will need to be excluded if the new treatment under examination may cause a particular hazard; for example, to patients with heart failure, bradycardia or asthma in trials of β-adrenergic blockers.

Study design

If the clinical trial is the centrepiece of pharmaceutical medicine, then the randomized comparative group study is the centrepiece of clinical trials and has become accepted generally as the method of choice for the study of therapeutic remedies. The comparative group study is therefore taken as the basis for considering the problems of design and the numbers of patients to be recruited, followed by considerations of other common types of design and more recent ideas that have been put forward to meet some ethical objections.

If we do not know which of two treatments is best and we randomize administration between two groups, then so far as we can judge on the evidence available they are going to be equally efficacious. This state of ignorance is represented by the Null Hypothesis (there is no difference between the treatments). The aim of our study is to test this hypothesis and utilize a statistical test of significance to suggest whether we should accept or reject it. It is very much a clinical decision, however, as to what level of significance is chosen. Equally, it is very much a clinical decision as to what additional benefit is worth seeking and detecting, for clearly it is going to take a lot more work and a lot more patients if we wish to detect small differences in outcome rather than quite large ones.

To return to statistical significance, we first have to decide how sure we want to be that any difference we do detect has not arisen by chance. In the nature of things randomization imbalance and inherent variability in measurements of biological variables will throw up chance results that are misleading. How frequently are we prepared to be misled? As mentioned previously it is customary to choose a 0.05 (5 per cent) risk, but since it is really a clinical decision the level of significance should be set flexibly. It would seem sensible to accept a smaller per cent risk of obtaining a false positive result when current treatment is satisfactory and acceptable than when it is unsatisfactory or hazardous. Whatever you choose will again affect the numbers in the study. The smaller the probability (P) of obtaining a false positive result the larger the numbers. We have seen therefore that numbers are affected by:

1. The size of the difference the clinical trial is hoping to detect.
2. The P value.

There is, however, a third factor which is perhaps less easily understood and which often escapes consideration in clinical trials, both in design and in reporting:

3.   Power.

The power of the study is its ability to detect the worthwhile difference between treatments that you are hoping for. In other words, it is no use looking for a 25 per cent improvement in clinical effectiveness, asking for a 95 per cent probability that a positive result is the correct one (5 per cent due to chance) and randomizing 50 or 60 patients to the two treatments under study, if with these numbers there is only a faint chance of picking up the positive result. Yet this is how so many studies are set up. The literature abounds with examples.[16,17]

The cynic might say that when pharmaceutical companies are testing a new remedy against a placebo they take more care to ensure the numbers are sufficient to pick up differences should they exist than when, for example, they are comparing their new antidepressant with a standard agent: it may be useful to show that your new antidepressant is as effective as say amitriptyline and this may well come about if the trial is not sufficiently powerful to pick up any difference one way or another, something which is clearly improper because one can never 'prove' no difference and one should not set up a trial with this objective. Temple has discussed these points in relation to clinical trial submissions in the USA.[15]

Tables[18] and nomograms[19] have been published to aid the calculation of numbers required in group comparative studies (see also Chapter 5).

Finally, the statistical test chosen has an influence on the power to detect differences that do exist. A familiar example would be the use of the conventional 't-test' with paired data when the 'paired t- test' is appropriate and more powerful.

Randomization

The purpose of randomization is to avoid bias, and to ensure that all patients have an equal chance of being allocated to either or any group.

It also provides a valid basis for statistical calculations after the data are collected. The clinical trial groups should therefore differ from each other only by chance. It does not of course eliminate imbalance but, since statistical tests are based on an estimate of random variation, it achieves its purpose. If one is seriously concerned that some factor or factors which influence response to treatment may by chance be allocated to one treatment group in an unbalanced way, this can be limited by stratification.

Stratification

Stratification is carried out by randomly allocating treatments to different classes of patients by the use of separate dispensing lists; for example, male list, female list. In addition, severity of disease may be deemed a factor of importance in determining response to treatment, in which case the patients may be divided up into: severe disease; moderate disease; mild disease. This would now entail six dispensing lists as follows:

1. Male: severe disease
2. Male: moderate disease
3. Male: mild disease

4. Female: severe disease
5. Female: moderate disease
6. Female: mild disease

If further factors are stratified the number of dispensing lists will grow as a multiple of the number of levels for each stratification factor and this could become very cumbersome administratively and put a strain on the dispensary. Another technique for achieving balance on any number of variables has been described by Taves,[20] using a 'minimization' technique.

Randomization itself is carried out *after* the patient has been admitted to the trial, and in order to avoid any selection bias the randomization code attached to the dispensing list is usually constructed from a table of random numbers and is kept in the dispensary. The doctor admitting patients to the trial has no knowledge of and cannot know in advance which patients have been allocated to each treatment. This is why randomization techniques involving the use of alternate patients, for example, or the final digit of the patient's hospital number should not be used since preknowledge or 'preguesses' as to the likely treatment allocation may cause the physician to selectively reject an eligible patient.

Although tables of random numbers are usually used if the aim is to produce a balanced randomization, another method of constructing a randomization list is simply to draw coloured balls from a bag, or marked pieces of paper from a hat, having put into the bag or hat originally an equal number of alternatives and a total representing the number of patients to be recruited. However, with stratification this is more difficult since one does not know at the outset how many patients in each subset are going, to arrive. In theory therefore one should have a dispensing list for each subset that is as long as the anticipated patient total (since all the patients recruited could fall into the same subgroup). A series of dispensing lists to cover the stratifications indicated above might start as follows:

Male: Severe disease

Name	Treatment Code
1.	X
2.	Y
3.	Y
4.	X
5.	etc.

Male: Moderate disease

Name	Treatment Code
1.	Y
2.	X
3.	X
4.	Y
5.	etc.

and similarly for groups 3–6.

It is a wise precaution to balance the treatments every four, six or eight subjects when relatively small numbers of patients are likely to fall in one or other stratification group, to avoid chance imbalance in treatment allocation. This has been done in the dispensing lists shown above after every four patients. If there are three treatments then the balance may be struck after six, nine or twelve subjects.

One other advantage of a stratified randomization is that it clearly indicates the patient subgroups which are going to be studied in the analysis and will help to ward off accusations of 'data dredging'.

Having achieved a predictable degree of balance through randomization, it is important not to introduce bias in the management of patients. Complete blindness of the patient and the investigator to treatment allocation is the best way of achieving this, but clearly blindness is not always possible, for example in dietary studies or comparisons of medical with surgical treatment. It is essential in such trials that management is standardized apart from the treatments under test. It is often difficult to ensure that this has been achieved. Breaking blindness can also occur as a consequence of adverse drug reactions (ADRs) or a dramatic beneficial effect.

Matched pairs

It might be though that prematching of patients for relevant factors (age, sex, severity of disease, etc.) might be the best way to overcome imbalance in small trials. Each pair of well matched patients could then have the two treatments randomly allocated. But this again begs the question that we will not know exactly what to match for and the more complicated we make the matching the greater will be the difficulty in securing a 'pair'. It tends to be a self-defeating exercise except if one uses a computer programme for the Taves scheme.[20]

Crossover trials

The attraction of crossover trials is that since all subjects receive both treatments during the study, the variance due to individual patient differences is thought to be cancelled out. However, the impact of time related differences is substituted and the patient is almost never the same in the second time period as in the first, and in addition treatment administered in the first time period may continue to influence responses in the second time period, unless it is possible to incorporate a 'wash-out' in between.

Crossover designs are necessarily restricted to those treatments that do not have a fundamental influence on the disease process as opposed to producing temporary relief of symptoms. An advantage is economy of numbers in that half the number of patients are required compared with a parallel group study. On the other hand, the duration of the trial may be prolonged, particularly if there are more than two elements to the crossover

Statisticians prefer to analyse parallel group studies because of the difficulty in disentangling carry-over effects from one treatment to another, even if balance is achieved between the patients receiving the drugs in the first treatment period and subsequent treatment periods. The problems inherent in the analysis of crossover designs, such as interaction between the treatments and periods, have been examined by Hills and Armitage[21] and by Cox.[22] An important conclusion reached by Hills and Armitage is that the choice of a crossover design takes a chance on the possibility of an interaction between treatments and the periods of administration and that, to be safe, a crossover trial should be of sufficient size so that it can be analysed as a parallel group study. This of course sacrifices the advantage of smaller numbers, but if numbers are limited then it is important to have evidence that the basic assumptions concerning interactions have been considered and are properly presented when the study is written up.

There are a number of balanced designs that are of great value for studies in other scientific fields, such as engineering and agriculture, which are occasionally useful in medicine.

Latin square design

Where a number of treatments are being evaluated in a crossover study, it may be important to ensure that equal numbers of patients receive the drugs in all possible orders, or at least an equal number receive them as first agent, second agent, third agent, etc. For instance, with three treatments, ABC, there are six possible orders:

    A B C
    A C B
    B A C
    B C A
    C A B
    C B A

Therefore by randomizing patients into six equal groups, a complete balance can be obtained. However, it is usually sufficient to construct a Latin Square as follows, using three groups:

    A B C
    B C A
    C A B

so that each treatment features as first treatment, second treatment and third treatment. For four treatments a Latin Square would be:

    A B C D
    B C D A
    C D A B
    D A B C

all the letters featuring equally in columns and rows. It is an easy matter to construct larger squares or consult Fisher and Yates.[23] To maintain balance in the analysis, drop-out patients would need to be replaced.

Factorial design

In this design we are concerned with evaluating more than one treatment. One example is a β-blocker and a diuretic in moderate hypertension in the elderly. Groups of patients could receive either no treatment, the diuretic, the β-blocker or both. This would permit a comparison of both treatments against control, as well as diuretic against no diuretic and β-blocker against no β-blocker. A classic experiment was reported by Mainland,[24] whereby a study of X-ray bone densitometry simultaneously investigated seven variables – two kilovoltages two positions, two processing methods, two strengths of developer, two fixation periods, two washing periods and two drying methods. This resulted in $2^7 = 128$ possibilities. Nevertheless, if one wished to study, say the effect of the two drying techniques, there would be 64 films using one and 64 films using the other.

Such designs give a full play to analysis of variance – a powerful parametric statistical technique by which the contributions of the individual factors can be assessed.

Long-term prevention studies

During the last 15 years a number of long-term studies have been performed with the aim of reducing morbidity and mortality from coronary artery disease; earlier studies involved the investigation of agents such as stilboesterol, thyroxine and nicotinic acid and more recently a variety of β-adrenergic receptor blockers, antithrombotic agents and diet. This has given rise to a spate of literature on what might be called the science of prevention studies.

First, a distinction has to be drawn between the 'explicative' and the 'pragmatic' approach.[25] The explicative approach tries to investigate mechanisms of drug action by determining whether the application of a particular preventive measure reduces mortality in those patients who accept and adhere to the regimen. The pragmatic approach is to adopt a policy in a clinic whereby the results of intervention in all patients are analysed whether they comply with treatment or not. Since in the practice of medicine it is usual to offer a treatment to any patient with a particular disease state, before being able to take into account compliance with the suggested treatment it would appear sound to analyse results in comparison with any other treatment policy using all the patients admitted, even if after admission they never received even one tablet of the therapy or made the slightest effort to stick to an allocated diet. This was originally discussed by Peto and colleagues[26] in relation to trials of anticancer drugs under the phrase 'intention to treat', and subsequently developed by Lovell[27] in respect of studies in coronary artery disease. Further contributions by Hampton[28,29] and Mitchell[30] made it almost mandatory to set out analyses of such prevention studies in a specific diagrammatic form (Fig. 4.2).

The great merit of this diagram is that it clearly shows where the patients were drawn from, how they were randomized, how they complied with treatment, what mortality results were obtained for each subgroup and the comparative mortality for each treatment on an 'intention to treat' basis.

Uncritical adherence to this formula has led to two side effects. First, a reluctance to accept any subgroup results, however significant and however clinically important (data dredging again!), and second, it has inhibited consideration of whether in fact treatment policies are applied uncritically in the clinic. In clinical trials selection bias has to be avoided, but in real life a physician may well withhold a treatment if he feels the patient will not comply properly, or alternatively he may take special steps to ensure that a critical treatment is administered regularly and correctly. Hence the results of prevention studies already published may well underestimate, through dilution with unsuitable or non-compliant patients, the value of certain agents in coronary prevention.

Clearly subset analyses are less reliable than the main total patient analysis, both for statistical reasons – the more you analyse the more likely you are to discover chance benefits – and logistical reasons – you are unlikely to be able to recruit enough patients overall to avoid

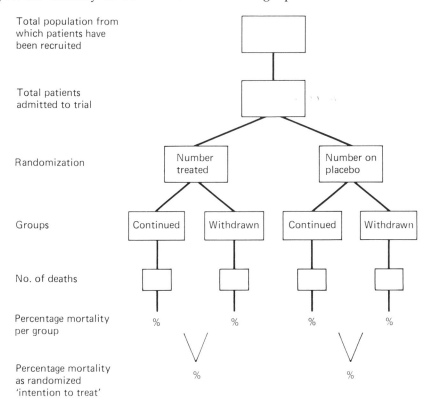

Fig. 4.2 'Hampton' scheme for data presentation in prevention studies.

gross reductions in your ability to detect real differences in subsets. Nevertheless subset analyses are valuable for generating hypotheses and occasionally the differences stick out like a sore thumb.

The enormous logistical problems attendant upon prevention studies are closely connected with the number of patients necessary to detect clinically important changes in mortality over quite long periods of time, when untreated mortality is itself quite low. Table 4.2 shows the total numbers required to demonstrate reductions of 10–50 per cent when the fatality rate in untreated patients during the trial period is either 5, 10 or 15 per cent. For this Table α is set at 0.05 and β at 0.129. If these frightening numbers are not obtained then there will be a sacrifice of power and a consequent reduction in the chance of detecting a worthwhile difference if one exists. Further allowance will have to be made for the diluting effects of substantial numbers of dropouts.

Table 4.2

Per cent reduction in events	Event rate in untreated patients during trial period		
	5%	10%	15%
10	76 000	36 000	8800
20	18 640	8600	5440
30	7600	3640	2300
40	4040	1840	1240
50	2420	1160	740

The organizational costs of such trials have run into several millions of dollars in some US studies, and even in the UK, after financial constraints and every effort to simplify procedures where possible, costs of up to a million pounds have been incurred. In one US study it is reported that Pinkerton's detective agency was employed to trace dropouts!

In addition there are ethical problems concerning the use of placebo control groups now that a range of trials with β-blockers has already demonstrated reductions in mortality. This ethical issue has given rise to strong emotions over the proposed placebo-controlled trial of vitamin supplements in pregnancy to investigate their effect on the incidence of spina bifida.[31,32] Since there is already evidence that vitamin supplements may reduce the incidence, it is hard to establish this through a properly conducted placebo-controlled study, especially as the hazards of giving vitamin supplements routinely to *all* pregnant women are probably small.

To overcome the objection that a potentially beneficial prevention treatment might be denied to a placebo group long after evidence of its value was available, it has become customary to examine the data at intervals (6 monthly or annually). If the results are deemed to be signficantly in favour of, or significantly adverse, to a treatment, the trial could be stopped and acted upon accordingly. This has substantial implications with regard to type I error and 'multiple looks' at the data have to be accompanied by a reduction in the *P* value attached to the decision making process.[33,34] It is also necessary to have an independent monitoring committee looking at the data at the appropriate intervals who do not communicate with the trialists unless a decision is reached which will mean an interruption of the trial. This happened with a recent β-blocker prevention study, where it was decided halfway through the trial that there was only a remote possibility of coming to a favourable conclusion with regard to drug therapy by the time all the patients had been recruited and carried through the trial; therefore further commitment of resources was unjustifiable.

It was concern over ethical issues of this kind that led to consideration of certain other adaptive trial designs.

Adaptive designs

The ultimate in 'multiple looks' is to examine the results as each patient completes their assessment and to make a decision to curtail the trial when certain statistical criteria have been satisfied. *Sequential charts* can be constructed to facilitate the recording of results and the most familiar are the closed designs shown in Fig. 4.3. In Fig. 4.3a patient results are obtained from matched pairs in a parallel group study or within patients in a crossover study. A preference for treatment A is recorded by placing a X vertically on the 'leggings' and for treatment B by placing a X in the next box horizontally. With this design it is possible to reach a decision that A is superior to B (or vice versa) after a minimum of eight patients or patient pairs, because the trial is closed immediately the next X crosses the boundary of the chart. With the closed design a 'no important difference' result is registered when a X enters the space between the two legs. It is to be noted that 'tied pairs' or patients unable to express a preference between A and B do not contribute information and cannot be entered on the chart. It is also to be noted that a X must enter a boundary after a certain maximum of preferences has been recorded (58 on this chart), which helps to limit the size of the trial unless there are a large number of tied pairs. With open designs[35,36] the trial can be prolonged indefinitely because it only terminates when one of the outside boundaries is crossed. In Fig. 4.3b, usually called a 'bat's wing', the result favouring treatment A is recorded as a line drawn as a north-east diagonal and a result favouring treatment B as a south-east diagonal. The construction of the charts will depend as usual on:

1. The magnitude of the difference between the treatments that you hope to detect (θ), e.g. 80:20.
2. The P value (α), e.g. 0.05.
3. The power (1−β), e.g. 95 per cent.

However, since the results are inspected after each entry the 5 per cent probability of a type 1 error ($P = 0.05$), will require more patient results than for non-sequential studies. In Fig. 4.3b a line must reach a boundary after 40 usable results if not before.

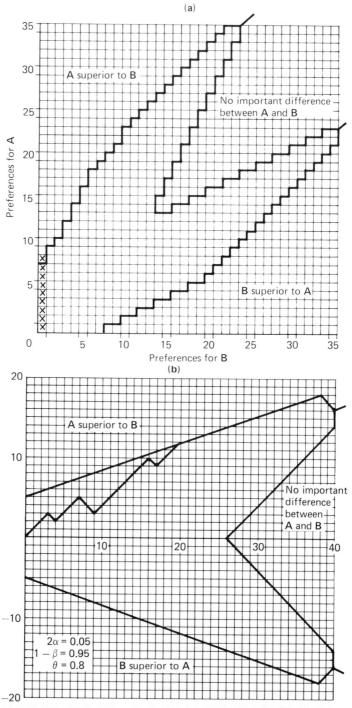

Fig. 4.3   (a) and (b) demonstrate two methods of constructing sequential analysis charts (closed designs).

Sequential studies help to overcome some of the ethical problems that arise with parallel group studies; for instance the fear that many patients may receive an inferior treatment after unexpectedly favourable results have occurred with a new treatment, or will continue to be put at hazard when the new treatment is unexpectedly dangerous. However, a limiting factor in sequential studies is that the preference (treatment A better than treatment B or vice versa) needs to be either global or dependent upon some single important measure of outcome and this may pose difficulties. Those interested in studying sequential trials and their modifications in more detail should consult Armitage.[37]

In other adaptive designs the proportion of patients allocated to treatments may be varied according to the results that have already accumulated. The first group of patients is allocated randomly on a 50:50 basis, but as results come in suggesting that one or other treatment is superior the proportion is altered, with the objective of reducing the number of patients being allocated to a treatment that shows a trend towards inferiority.[38] As with sequential trials it is important that the results should come in fairly quickly to maximize the benefit of these adaptive approaches and again it is necessary to have some single measure of outcome which is of overriding importance.

Finally there are a number of non-randomized designs whose aim is to maximize the expected benefit to the individual patient. Such designs have been proposed by Lellouch and Schwartz[39] and Zelen.[40]

Placebos and blindness

Placebos are composed of pharmacologically inactive substances that can be used for baseline comparisons against a new remedy provided there are no ethical objections. They are invariably made to resemble the active material so that both patient and investigator blindness can be preserved after randomization. Indeed, minimal specifications for the manufacture of matching materials have been set out by Joyce.[41] In addition, Hill *et al.*[42] have studied the qualities of matching samples and have made the additional point that active materials may age differently, the active white tablets becoming off-white after 6–12 months. The arguments for and against the use of placebos in clinical trials have been discussed previously by Joyce.[43]

Conventionally, a single-blind trial is one in which the patient is kept in ignorance of which treatment is being employed although the doctor knows. This technique is not often used and it is customary to try and preserve blindness both for the doctor and the patient, to avoid bias in the assessments – the 'double-blind' trial. In some countries drug regulatory authorities will only consider seriously such double-blind studies.

Problems when allocating patients to treatments
Preserving blindness when dispensing matching materials has already been mentioned but special difficulties arise if the treatments are dissimi-

lar (an injection and a tablet) or dosage increments are to be allowed. The 'double-dummy' technique allows each patient, as shown in Fig. 4.4, to receive a capsule plus a tablet, but for half the tablet is a dummy and for the other half the capsule is a dummy. Similarly, active and dummy injections can be used, although the use of a mock injection for half the patients could be regarded as unethical discomfort.

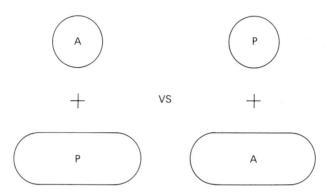

Fig. 4.4   The 'double dummy' technique.

Dosage increments can be organized by having the assessor blind to the drug dispensing. The assessor simply indicates that a dose needs to be increased (or decreased) and this is acted upon (or not) within the dose ranges allowed by the trial. It may be difficult to preserve blindness, however, since the patient may give away to the doctor what is happening to his treatment.

Another method is to have complex packaging of active and dummy tablets, as shown in Fig. 4.5.[44] Every patient takes three tablets three times daily and hence it is possible to organize anything from once daily treatment (using eight dummies) to a maximum of three treatment tablets three times daily (no dummies). As usual the increased complexity increases the danger of errors both in the preparation of the individual sachets and in the dispensing. Also, poor patient compliance with the full programme of nine tablets daily will have capricious effects on treatment response.

Seeing when blind
Double-blind trials may fail to achieve blindness for a number of reasons:

1. The 'matched' treatments may be distinguished easily through initial differences in colour, size, weight, etc.[41]
2. Well matched tablets may age differently. A white active preparation may become off-white after 6 months, whereas its matched placebo may remain pure white.[42]
3. Patients or doctors may make deliberate attempts to break the code

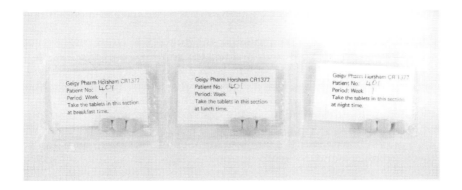

Fig. 4.5 Complex packaging of active and dummy tablets.

      (a sort of 'defeat the clinical trial' game). In a β-blocker trial patients bit into tablets which were supposed to be swallowed and found that some were sweet tasting and some were bitter tasting.

4.   One of the 'blind' treatments may produce a physiological response or side effect that the matching placebo or alternative treatment does not. Bradycardia and cold extremities with β-blockers or dry mouth with certain antidepressants are examples of this.

5.   One of the treatments may modify the course of the disease under assessment in such a way that outcome variables and end events are missed. For example a β-blocker may suppress the pain of a cardiac ischaemic episode so that electrocardiographic changes or enzymes are not measured.

Measurement in clinical trials

Since a decision about the value of a new treatment is going to depend on measuring changes in some variable or variables, the choice of a relevant indicator of improvement or deterioration is of the greatest importance.

      Measurements can be *subjective* depending on a doctor or patient's view of changes in symptoms (rheumatic stiffness, depression, headache, etc.) or through *objective* recording of parameters or events (blood pressure, haemoglobin, anginal attacks, death). It is generally considered that objective records are preferable where there is a choice, but this is not necessarily so. Treatment may well influence symptoms more than a disease process (e.g. rheumatoid arthritis) and from the patient's point of view his symptoms and survival often seem more important than clinical signs or the results of laboratory tests. Indeed, Scott and Huskisson[44] have suggested that the most relevant outcome variable may be the one the patient chooses as the best description (for them) of the progress of the disease. Hence, measures should not be chosen simply because they are fashionable, complicated, cheap, expensive, interesting, or any other adjective; they simply have to be relevant and to have been validated through previous use as reliable predictors of outcome.

Outcome has two main components; the immediate effect on wellbeing and the long-term prognosis. In a clinical trial it may only be possible to test one of these; indeed, if the aim is to postpone death in a β-blocker intervention trial there may be no immediate benefit noticed by any of the patients and for the great majority of them the trial will end, say 2 years later, without the patient or the doctor being able to judge whether treatment has had any benefit at all.

It is preferable to study a limited number of variables, both for the sake of simplicity and to avoid spuriously significant results which are inevitable if multiple estimations are made. In any event the statistician will need to calculate the trial numbers based on a clinically relevant change in just a few measurements, or even one.

Types of measurement

There are essentially three types:

1. *Interval*
   Made by a recording instrument on a scale (ruler, blood pressure machine) in which there is a mathematical relation between each observation.
2. *Ordinal*
   Where responses to treatment can be classified on a scale of response but not otherwise quantified, as in mild, moderate, severe pain levels.
3. *Nominal*
   Event recording.   Alive: Dead
   Better: Not better

Different statistical methods are applicable to these different types of measurement. *Parametric statistics* concern interval measurement and the most well known are Students 't'-test and analysis of variance. *Non-parametric statistics* handle ordinal and nominal data and the most familiar tests are the Wilcoxon rank tests and the Chi square tests.[45,46]

Rating scales

These were designed to give what some would say are spurious numerical values to subjective material. The Hamilton rating scales in depression were actually designed to help standardize the diagnosis of depression and to aid different skilled observers to reach a measure of agreement on the diagnosis and severity of depression. In order to use these scales properly observers need tuition and practice. These scales were not initially designed for comparative purposes in drug trials although they are now often used in this way. Large numbers of rating scales have now been devised particularly in the area of psychiatry, neurology, mental handicap, etc. Their use needs to be tempered with caution; have they been validated as a reliable and relevant measure of outcome?

The analogue scale is very popular and is a device for converting a subjective response to a number between 0 and 100. For example:

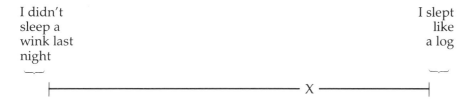

I didn't   I slept
sleep a   like
wink last   a log
night

The patient is invited to place a X which represents how well they slept last night between the extremes at each end of the 10 cm line. A ruler is then used to measure the position of the X in millimetres (67). This figure is then used as if it were an interval parametric measure. The hazards and inaccuracies attendant upon this approach have been investigated by Seldrup and Beaumont[47] and commented upon by Curson and Curson.[48] It is beyond the scope of this chapter to discuss the statistical hazards of converting subjective ordinal information to an interval scale and then employing a number to parametric statistical tests. In the past this has been defended by the insistence that the power of the test has not been illegally enhanced by rejecting non-parametric methods and that such methods if used lead to a similar P value.

Missing data and missing patients

Patients default from clinical trials for a number of reasons, but these can be grouped into those associated with the trial and those not associated with the trial. The former are often related to the side effects of therapy, but dislike of the hospital, the investigations or even the investigator are other possible reasons. Non-trial reasons might be moving from the district, or because they were killed by falling under a bus. It is possible, however, that patients leave an area to get away from the trial, or they fall under a bus because of a sedative effect of one of the drugs!

Every effort has to be made to trace defaulting patients and ascribe a reason. Clearly drug-related defaulters are highly relevant to the trial conclusions and must participate fully in the data analysis. The handling of incomplete data has been discussed by Chaput de Saintonge and Vere.[49]

Missing data from compliant patients are another matter and may be due to inadvertence, lost or broken samples and recording mistakes. If a small amount of data are missing in a random fashion this will probably not seriously affect the trial analysis. Alternatively good monitoring may enable missing data to be 'recovered', albeit a day or two late. This becomes progressively unsafe the longer the interval between patient attendance and the discovery that an important assessment was not performed or recorded. Sometimes a missing value may be estimated from other variables and tested to see if analysis gives similar results with and without it. However, if the amount of missing data are substantial the fact will have to be admitted and the conclusions of the study tempered with appropriate caution.

Finally, intermediate values are often not used in the analysis of trials, since the best comparisons are often the pretrial and end-trial results. In crossover studies, where carry-over drug responses are likely, the end of period value, after say 6 weeks, is likely to be more useful than values recorded immediately after the crossover. However, intermediate values can throw valuable light on the time course of drug action and will support the beginning and end comparisons if they show a steady trend to change. These issues have been discussed in more detail by Evans.[50]

Adverse reactions

The handling of adverse reactions in clinical studies is often deficient because the main aim of a study is to evaluate efficacy. Also the significance of isolated events in small numbers of patients is hard to establish. Nevertheless, in the finality the place of a new treatment in the therapeutic armamentarium is going to be assessed as a balance between efficacy and hazard. Across a number of clinical studies some impression of adverse effects is bound to emerge, hence careful recording of each event is vital, as is communication between one centre and another.

It is important to distinguish those reactions that are predictable from the pharmacology of the drug, such as dry mouth due to the anticholinergic effects of antidepressants, and those that are unexpected (idiosyncratic). Defaulting in clinical trials is often linked with adverse reactions and hence the need for provision in the protocol for following up patients who do not report at the expected time.

It cannot be expected that rarer adverse effects (and these are often the most serious) will be picked up in clinical trials. As a rule of thumb, a 1 per cent incidence is unlikely to occur in less than 300 patients, and a 0.1 per cent side effect in less than 3000 patients. Occurrence of such an event does not, however, prove cause-and-effect, since it is unusual for an adverse effect to be so uniquely drug-induced that one can rule out 'spontaneous' or disease-related adverse events. The rule of thumb described above cannot be used if one is trying to detect a drug-related event that occurs against a background of similar but unrelated adverse events. Some form of postmarketing surveillance (PMS) will be necessary to discover such uncommon happenings.

In clinical trials side effects are often classified as:

Trivial: Nuisance value only
Mild: Impairing patient function, but not leading to discontinuance of treatment
Serious: Leading to discontinuance of treatment

It is fairly easy to solicit a battery of trivial reactions in clinical trials by asking specific questions, e.g. have you had any headaches? Alternatively a patient may be asked to fill in a questionnaire about side effects at each visit. Such information may be useful to get an idea of 'background noise' before the trial starts, or when the patient is on a placebo, from which will emerge some reactions with a significantly higher incidence when the patient is on an active agent. The discovery of impotence on diuretic therapy in the MRC mild hypertension study is a good example of a significant reaction that is often not mentioned by the patient and that has a background incidence from other causes.[51] Serious reactions will clearly be classified as treatment failures in the analysis.

Finally, appropriate forms should be fully completed and sent to the health authority concerning all suspected adverse reactions in clinical trials (for more detailed discussion see Chapter 6).

Logistics

Since a clinical trial should be a 'carefully planned experiment', it is essential to have a coordinated plan and efficient documentation. Planning decisions range from simple local arrangements for recruiting small numbers of patients for a restricted pharmacodynamic study, to the almost military style operation required for an intervention trial on dietary changes or drugs (clofibrate or β-adrenergic blockers) on coronary artery disease mortality. The vast problems set by these latter studies have already been referred to but are really beyond the scope of this chapter and have been the subject of whole chapters or books in themselves.[52–54] Nevertheless, some of the elements required for these big studies are worth listing since they have more general application.

A main coordinating committee to decide and agree:
1. the disease definition of the patients to be included
2. the exclusion criteria
3. the trial design
4. the trial end-points and their definition
5. the method of allocation of treatments to patients
6. the measurements to be made and when
7. how side effects are to be handled
8. how drop outs are to be detected and followed up
9. how compliance with treatment is to be assessed
10. how the patients are to be informed about the trials and communication with the patient's family physician is to be effected
11. submission to and liaison with independent ethics committees

Monitoring subcommittees
These may be required to assess trial end-points independent of the trial organizers (e.g. assessing electrocardiograms for allocation to 'definite' or 'probable' myocardial infarction). They may also assess changes in

laboratory and other tests (e.g. reading X-rays blind for extent of disease or cavitation in tuberculosis trials).

A quality control group
This assesses by regular monitoring the completeness and reliability of the recorded data – particularly important before processing the results onto computer files which may give bad data an air of respectability. Also legal requirements may require a medical adviser to certify and take responsibility for the data package. When using foreign data to support drug licensing applications, good quality control arrangements are much more reassuring to health authority assessors.

Pharmacy drug monitoring group
Continuity and accurate dispensing of drug supplies is so important that major hospitals often employ clinical trial pharmacists. In addition they can advise on monitoring compliance. Although compliance with drug therapy is often better in clinical trials than in ordinary therapeutic practice there may be problems if any of the treatments are unpleasant, if the patient feels well and does not see the need to continue therapy, and if the trial is long term so that participants lose interest. Drug taking can be monitored by a variety of techniques: pill counting, direct drug assay in urine and blood, indirect assay using a marker.[55] Best of all is to fully supervise drug administration which has even been possible in some outpatient trials of antituberculous therapy.

Documentation

In times past the production of good record forms has been very much an individual matter enabling an investigator or pharmaceutical physician free rein for creativity.[14] Now nearly all the data will be transferred to a computer file so it is necessary to enter information on standard coded forms. However, many of the old principles still apply, particularly the need to maximize simplicity and convenience. Most doctors cannot record data accurately even if they measure it accurately and often disobey simple instructions – like putting a cross where a tick is required and confusion about the use of some American terms like the word 'check'. The time factor is also vital. For instance, if it takes 20 minutes to measure and record all the patient observations at each visit and 1000 patients are to be recruited for the trial with an initial attendance 2 weeks before trial entry and subsequent follow up at 0, 3, 6, 9 and 12 months, it will take one doctor working 8 hours a day, 5 days a week to complete the work when the patient entry is at its maximum, and he won't be able to take any holiday! The motto must be: don't collect data if it is irrelevant, can't be used, can't be analysed or will simply clog up the computer or the statistician's office.

Essentials to be considered are:
- A protocol
- An eligibility form

- An initial assessment form
- A form for each follow-up visit
- Forms for recording laboratory data
- End-point forms
- Patient questionnaires
- Instructions about treatment changes or use of non-trial drugs
- Side effect forms and reason for patient withdrawal
- Dispensing code and where it is held
- A concluding or exit form
- A timetable

Finally, an operating manual may be needed as a guide to the correct completion of the documentation, to remind physicians of the criteria being used for diagnosis, the diagnosis of an end-point and of the measurement of response variables. For very long trials regular newsletters have proved valuable to investigators, particularly in multicentre studies, both to highlight problems that have occurred and to sustain interest and camaraderie.

Termination of the trial

Patients usually get what they perceive to be better treatment when they are taking part in a clinical trial. Certainly they may be allocated more doctor or investigator time and have a larger number of investigations carried out upon them. This increased attention often has a favourable influence on the patient's condition and it has been frequently observed that the morbidity and mortality in the placebo group in prevention studies is lower than historical data would suggest. Indeed, this is one of the reasons why historical controls from routine clinics make poor comparative groups compared with those being treated contemporaneously.

When the trial is over the patient may feel neglected and deteriorate. If he has done well on a new therapy, which has not been shown to be superior to the control drug for the majority, he may find the treatment withdrawn or it become unobtainable. These issues have to be considered and patients must be eased out of a clinical trial in a humane and ethical manner. If they are returned to their general practitioner when they have been attending the hospital outpatient department for their assessments, it is essential to write a full letter to him about the future management of his patient and to offer further outpatient appointments if things are not going well. Also remember to thank everyone who contributed to the trial's success and where appropriate send them a copy of the report.

Obtaining patient cooperation

The help of patients is essential for clinical trials to be carried out at all. Fortunately most patients are extremely cooperative and in the UK often prefer to leave it to their medical attendant to look after their best interests.

This confidence must not be abused or undermined through discourtesy or neglect. Patients participating in clinical trials often like to know the answers to the following questions:

What is the purpose of the study?
Who can participate?
Why should I be involved?
What will happen during the study?
How much time will I have to spend at the hospital/away from work?
How long is the trial going on for?
What are the potential benefits for me?
How does the medicine work?
What are the dangers and side effects?

Finally, the patient complies with treatment and the trial better if they are told:

That their participation is much appreciated.
That it is important they cooperate with every aspect of the trial.
That they keep all appointments at the specified time (and you should see them then).
That if they change their address or are going on holiday they should notify you well in advance.
That if they take any medicines outside the trial medication they should tell you.

Disadvantages of controlled clinical trials

The two main problems for the clinician are that clinical trials are inflexible and restricted. To obtain balance and control a great deal of artificial rigidity has necessarily to be built in, which is at odds with normal clinical practice. The patients participating in the trial may only represent a small subgroup suffering from the disease requiring treatment; alternatively the results from a broad group of patients may not be sensitive enough to pick up certain kinds of patients who do benefit.

Nearly all clinical trials, however negative, usually throw up individual patients who appear to obtain considerable benefit and who are most reluctant to discontinue when the trial is over. But it is only rarely that one is able to spot some common factor in the 'responders' which would suggest a further trial to be performed in that subgroup.

From the economic point of view clinical trials can be costly, cumbersome and take up a great deal of time, particularly long-term studies. The cost benefit of the trial has therefore become an important item in the balance sheet.

A negative result ('it did not achieve statistical significance')
It is well worth quoting in full the final paragraph from Rose's paper on bias.[56] It goes as follows:

'The power of controlled clinical trials is less than is generally supposed and it is still regrettably common to equate a failure to demonstrate an effect with the positive verdict that the treatment is useless. This danger would be avoided if authors and editors made it a practice in any trial with a seemingly negative outcome to give a confidence interval for the estimated effects. If this embraces what would be regarded as a clinically important result, then the only valid conclusion is that the question remains open and a more powerful trial is needed.'

The inclusion of confidence interval data helps the reader to decide whether a result that is reported broadly as 'not statistically significant' could have a concealed clinically important result or whether, even allowing for the vagaries of chance, it is hardly likely that anything of importance has been missed. It might equally be said of significant results that a confidence interval helps one not to become 'overenthusiastic' when the lower end of the confidence interval embraces only a trivial improvement. In Fig. 4.6 A is 'not significant', but we might be missing a clinically important improvement that a larger and more powerful trial would have confirmed. B is 'statistically significant' but may not be as good as the median result suggests.

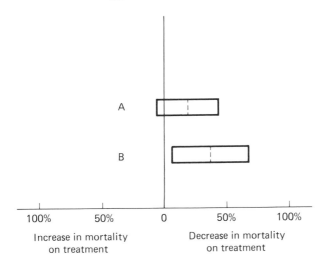

Fig. 4.6 Ninety-five per cent confidence intervals for mortality in two prevention trials with β-blockers.

Causes of failure
Some of the causes of failure in clinical trials could be listed as follows:

1. Lack of clarity of the questions to be asked with consequent incorrect trial designs being used. Trying to answer too many questions at once.

2. Failure to consult a statistician at an early enough stage.
3. Wrong investigator chosen; inadequate access to right patients, too busy and does not effectively delegate the work to competent assistants.
4. Inexperienced pharmaceutical physician working without adequate supervision.
5. Delays in getting approval of ethical committees and regulatory authorities leading to the loss of interest of the investigator.
6. Inadequate follow-up by the physician and the clinical trials team. The frequency of follow-up visits will depend on the nature of the trial which in our opinion should never be less frequent than once a month. Telephone contact should be made no less frequently than 2 weeks. Infrequent follow-up leads to a feeling of lack of commitment by the investigator.
7. Failure to produce the clinical trial materials on time leading to loss of interest by the investigator. Failure to keep up the supply of clinical trial materials leading to interruption or delay in recruitment.
8. Selecting the wrong patients; that is choosing patients with the wrong type of the disease, or those unable to comply with the requirements of the protocol.
9. Inadequate recruitment when the investigator seriously overestimated the number of patients who would be available and suitable.
10. Lack of compliance by the patients because of a badly formulated drug, for example too large a capsule or tablet.
11. Poorly designed record card leading to omission of important information. Lack of supervision by the clinical trials team to ensure that good record cards are completed fully.
12. Failure to achieve an effective method for collection of record cards and/or blood samples.

Although any of these faults can occur in a single centre trial they are far more likely to occur in a multicentre trial. *Multicentre trials* have the advantage of being able to provide larger numbers of patients in a given time. However, they require experienced and vigilant coordination in order to be successful and to avoid many of the pitfalls listed above. Multicentre trials, though, can be successful providing that all the investigators are involved at the earliest stage in the planning of the protocol and in working out the detailed mechanics of the study, particularly the standardization of diagnosis, recruitment and measurement. This can only be achieved by frequent meetings and commitment which not only produce scientifically valid results but also give a fine sense of achievement for all those concerned.

Uncontrolled studies

These are often in the nature of pilot studies with a new drug and can provide valuable information of practical importance for the later design of controlled trials. For example, such studies may enable one to determine suitable dosage and dosage intervals. Also, pilot studies may be used to test a protocol, rather like 'de-bugging' a computer programme.

Most uncontrolled Phase III and IV studies are performed in general practice, which after all is the scene for most uncontrolled drug administration. The artificiality of clinical trials and the emphasis on group results rather than individual response has already been commented upon. Knowledge of how the drug is handled in general practice and how well or badly it is working is valuable even if assessments cannot be controlled. Lasagna[57] has pointed out that our current methodology is deficient in estimating benefit and making sense of the cost/benefit equation. A drug's actual performance is what we care about, not what it ideally might do.

Clinical trials in general practice

The requirements for good clinical trial design are no different for studies under general practice conditions. Since 80 per cent of drug therapy is prescribed by family practitioners in the UK and some medical conditions are hardly ever seen in hospital clinics there are positive reasons for preferring general practitioner trials. The objectives and mechanisms for such trials are often different because of limited laboratory facilities and time constraints. Most trials have to be conducted using a large group practice, or across many practices with different doctors or assessors. Controlled studies using matching materials need an efficient organization and monitoring service. Nevertheless, the rewards for conducting good studies are substantial, both in terms of realism and patient numbers. Some company medical departments run very successful general practitioner clinical trial groups, providing opportunities for quite sophisticated studies and education in clinical trials methodology.

The monitoring of adverse reactions and a proper assessment of the balance between effectiveness and harm broadens the base of knowledge concerning drug activity. It may also help to accumulate information on the general acceptability of a new drug formulation and patient compliance. Difficulties arise with the use of placebos in control subjects simply because patients attending a general practitioner clinic expect to receive an accepted treatment and therefore comparative trials against existing therapy are more usual. This leads to a second difficulty in that a patient in a trial may need to have an effective treatment withdrawn if an alternative is to be substituted, and this may be unacceptable. For example, it would probably not be ethical to take a patient with well controlled hypertension and put him in a study with a new agent, unless there was substantial evidence that the new agent was at least as effective or might produce less adverse effects. It would also be imprudent to include a wash-out period during which blood pressure might return to baseline levels.

In recent years uncontrolled general practitioner trials have fallen into disrepute because they have been used as promotional exercises to obtain widespread usage; the science being secondary to the major aim of encouraging continued prescription after 'the study' is over. This has led in the UK to the publication of guidelines for general practitioner trials drawn up as a result of a joint agreement between the British Medical Association (BMA), the Royal College of General Practitioners (RCGP) and the ABPI[2].

References

1. CIOMS (1983). *Safety Requirements for the First Use of New Drugs and Diagnostic Agents in Man*. Geneva: The Council for International Organisations of Medical Sciences.
2. (1983). Code of Practice for the Clinical Assessment of Licensed Medicinal Products in General Practice. Joint agreement between BMA, RCGP, and ABPI. *British Medical Journal* **286**: 1295.
3. Bull JP (1959). The historical development of clinical therapeutic trials. *Journal of Chronic Diseases* **10**: 218.
4. (1948). Streptomycin treatment of pulmonary tuberculosis. A Medical Research Council investigation (1948). *British Medical Journal* **ii**: 769.
5. (1950). Treatment of pulmonary tuberculosis with streptomycin and para-amino-salicylic acid. A Medical Research Council investigation. *British Medical Journal* **ii**: 1073.
6. MRC (1953). Isoniazid in the treatment of pulmonary tuberculosis. *British Medical Journal* **ii**: 521.
7. Hill AB (1971). *Principles of Medical Statistics*, 9th edn. London: The Lancet
8. Clayton DG (1982). Ethically optimised designs. *British Journal of Clinical Pharmacology* **13**: 469.
9. Burkhardt R, Keinle G (1978). Controlled clinical trials and medical ethics. *Lancet* **ii**: 1356.
10. Weinstein MC (1974). Allocation of subjects in medical experiments. *New England Journal of Medicine* **291**: 1278.
11. Cranberg L (1979). Do retrospective controls make clinical trials inherently fallacious? *British Medical Journal* **ii**: 1265.
12. Bradford Hill A. (ed.) (1960). *Controlled Clinical Trials*. Oxford: Blackwell Scientific Publications.
13. (1977). Aide-memoire for preparing clinical trial protocols. *British Medical Journal* **2**: 1324.
14. Burley DM (1970). Preliminary design – the ideal clinical trial. In *The Principles and Practice of Clinical Trials*. Edinburgh and London: E & S Livingstone.
15. Temple R (1982). Government viewpoint of clinical trials. *Drug Information Journal*, **January/June**: 10.
16. Freiman, JA, Chalmers TC, Smith H *et al*. (1978). The importance of beta, the type II error and sample size in the design and interpretation of the randomised controlled trial. *New England Journal of Medicine* **299**: 690.
17. Ambroz A, Chalmers TC, Smith H *et al*. (1978). Deficiencies of randomised control trials. *Clinical Research* **26**: 280A.
18. Clarke CJ, Downie CC (1966). A method for the rapid determination of the number of patients to include in a controlled clinical trial. *Lancet* **2**: 1357.
19. Altman DG (1982). Statistics and ethics in medical research. In *Statistics in Practice: Articles published in the British Medical Journal*. London: British Medical Journal: 7.
20. Taves DR (1974). Minimisation: a new method of assigning patients to treatment and control groups. *Clinical Pharmacology and Therapeutics* **15**: 443.

21. Hills M, Armitage P (1979) The two-period cross-over clinical trial. *British Journal of Clinical Pharmacology* **8**: 7.
22. Cox KR, (1968). *Planning Clinical Experiments.* Springfield, IL: Charles C. Thomas USA.
23. Fisher RA, Yates F (1974). *Statistical Tables for Biological, Agricultural and Medical Research.* Edinburgh: Oliver and Boyd.
24. Mainland D (1956). Measurement of bone density. *Annals of Rheumatic Diseases* **15**: 115.
25. Schwartz D, Flamant R, Lellouch J (1980). In: *Clinical Trials*, translated by MJR Healey. London: Academic Press.
26. Peto R, Pike MC, Armitage P *et al.* (1976). Design and analysis of randomised clinical trials requiring prolonged observation of each patient. *British Journal of Cancer* **34**: 585.
27. Lovell RRH (1977). Problems of interpretation in secondary prevention trials in coronary heart disease. *Medical Journal of Australia* **i**: 224.
28. Hampton JR (1981). Presentation and analysis of the results of clinical trials in cardiovascular disease. *British Medical Journal* **282**: 1371.
29. Hampton JR (1981). The use of beta-blockers for the reduction of mortality after myocardial infarction. *European Heart Journal* **ii**: 259.
30. Mitchell JRA (1981). Timolol after myocardial infarction: an answer or a new set of questions? *British Medical Journal* **282**: 1565.
31. Wynn J (1982). Spinal bifida: trials ahead. *Nature* **299**: 198.
32. Leck I (1983). Spinal bifida and anencephaly: fewer patients, more problems. Editorial, *British Medical Journal* **286**: 1679.
33. McPherson K (1974). Statistics: the problems of examining accumulating data more than once. *New England Journal of Medicine* **290**: 501.
34. Pocock SJ (1978). The size of cancer clinical trials and stopping rules. *British Journal of Cancer* **38**: 757.
35. Bross I (1952). Sequential medical plans. *Biometrics* **8**: 188.
36. Bross I (1958). Sequential medical trials. *Journal of Chronic Diseases* **8**: 349.
37. Armitage P (1975). *Sequential Medical Trials.* Oxford: Blackwell Publications.
38. Day NE (1969). A comparison of some sequential designs. *Biometrika* **56**: 301.
39. Lellouch J, Schwartz D (1971). L'essai therapeutique: ethique, individuelle ou ethique collective? *Review of the Institute of International Statistics* **39**: 127.
40. Zelen M (1969). Play the winner rule and the controlled clinical trial. *Journal of the American Statistical Association* **64**: 131.
41. Joyce CRB (1968). *Psychopharmacology: Dimensions and Perspectives.* London: Tavistock Publications.
42. Hill LE, Nunn AJ, Fox W (1976). Matching quality of agents employed in double-blind controlled clinical trials. *Lancet* **i**: 352.
43. Joyce CRB (1982). Placebos and other comparative treatments. *British Journal of Clinical Pharmacology* **13**: 313.
44. Scott PJ, Huskisson EC (1979). Measurement of functional capacity with visual analogue scales. *Rheumatology and Rehabilitation* **16**: 257.
45. Siegel S (1965). *Non-parametric Statistics in the Behavioural Sciences.* New York: McGraw Hill.
46. Langley R (1970). *Practical Statistics for Non-mathematical People.* London: Pan Books Ltd.
47. Seldrup J, Beaumont G (1975). A methodological study of the visual analogue scale applied to normals. *Journal of Clinical Pharmacology* **11**: 46.
48. Curson DA, Curson VH, (1983). *Rating Scales in Clinical Research: Use and Misuse.* Washington: II World Conference on Clinical Pharmacology and Therapeutics.

49. Chaput de Saintonge DM, Vere DW (1982). Measurement in clinical trials. *British Journal of Clinical Pharmacology* **13**: 775.
50. Evans SJW (1982). What can we do with the data we throw away? *British Journal of Clinical Pharmacology* **14**: 653.
51. Medical Research Council Working Party on Mild to Moderate Hypertension (1981). Adverse reactions to bendrofluazide and propranolol for the treatment of mild hypertension. *Lancet* **ii**: 539.
52. Greenberg G (1982). Logistics and management of clinical trials. *British Journal of Clinical Pharmacology* **14**: 25.
53. Hampton JR (1981). Organisation of multicentre clinical trials. In Evered D, O'Connor M (eds.) *Collaboration in Medical Research in Europe.* London: Ciba Foundation/Pitman.
54. Klimt CR (1979). Principles of multicentre clinical studies. In Boissel JP, Klimt CR (eds.) *Multicentre Controlled Trials. Principles and Problems.* Paris: INSERM.
55. Ellard GA, Jenner PJ, Downs PA (1980). Evaluation of the potential of isoniazid, acetyl isoniazid, and isonicotonic acid for monitoring the self administration of drugs. *British Journal of Clinical Pharmacology* **10**: 369.
56. Rose G (1982). Bias. *British Journal of Clinical Pharmacology* **13**: 157.
57. Lasagna L (1974). A plea for the 'naturalistic' study of medicines. *European Journal of Clinical Pharmacology* **7**: 153.

5

Statistical considerations
Win M. Castle and Alan F. Ebbutt

This chapter is divided into three parts: (1) a revision section for those whose elementary statistical knowledge has gone rusty; (2) a discussion of statistical problems that are commonly encountered in the pharmaceutical industry; and (3) a reminder to the reader that there are problems, particularly in assessing drug safety, and so far there are no solutions. This last section is deliberately provocative.

Statistical revision notes

The areas revised are descriptive statistics, reliability, probability, significance tests and their conclusions. There are no apologies for oversimplification in these revision notes.

Description of data

Types of data
Non-numerical results that only allow allocation to groups are 'qualitative'. Examples are ethnic group, whether or not a subject has a particular disease, whether or not they are a protocol violator, etc. Some qualitative data have an implied order, e.g. severity may be classed as mild, moderate and severe.

'Quantitative' results are measurements, answering the question how much or how many. This numerical (quantitative) data may be discrete (measured in whole numbers, e.g. number of asthma attacks per year) or continuous, e.g. height or weight.

The difference between qualitative and quantitative data is important from the statistical point of view as they are illustrated, summarized and analysed differently.

Illustrating qualitative and quantitative data
To present qualitative data diagramatically; pie diagrams, pictograms, bar charts and proportional bar charts are used. They are intended to save words and make points clearer. They should each be fully labelled, simple and honest.

Before illustrating quantitative data measurements are grouped. The number in each class is called the frequency. The frequency in all the classes is called the frequency distribution. This grouping makes illustration easier, but the price is some loss of detail. Ideally, 10 to 25 different groups can be used. The frequency distribution is represented by a histogram or frequency polygon. When two or more frequency distributions are superimposed it is better to use two frequency polygons. Three dishonest tricks used with quantitative data are: suppressing the zero; inflating the scale; and extrapolation. Fortunately there are many less examples in promotional literature than there used to be.

Qualitative data
Qualitative data can be presented simply as counts or summarized as *ratios, proportions* (or percentage) and *rates*.

A ratio is $\dfrac{\text{number of sheep}}{\text{number of goats}}$

and a proportion is $\dfrac{\text{number of sheep}}{\text{number of sheep} + \text{number of goats}}$

The percentage is 100 times the proportion. It is wrong to state these indices without quoting the number involved. A rate is similar to a proportion but its denominator is a static measurement whereas the numerator is counted over a period of time.

The two most commonly used rates, the prevalence and the incidence, are often confused. The prevalence is larger. Basically the prevalence tells us how *common* is a situation (e.g. how many new prescriptions of a particular drug), whereas the incidence tells us how *often* the situation occurs (e.g. number having prescriptions). Consider the pregnancy rate for rabbits in 1992. The *incidence* rate is the number becoming pregnant during 1992 divided by the number of rabbits exposed to risk during that year. The *prevalence* rate has the same denominator but the numerator is all those rabbits who are pregnant during 1992 – unlike the incidence it includes those rabbits becoming pregnant during 1991 who delivered during 1992. Prevalence rates themselves can be pinpointed to answer the question how common is the situation at a particular moment in time (the 'point' prevalence) as opposed to the 'period' prevalence which includes all those in the given situation over a period of time.

Quantitative data (and the normal distribution)
Terms used to describe quantitative data must define both the middle and the amount of scatter.

The fact that many quantitative variables either follow the 'normal' distribution approximately or can easily be transformed to do so is very useful and helps statistical analyses. The normal distribution is symmetrical and bell-shaped and has two points of inflection (where the shape of the curve changes from being convex to concave).

The mean, median and mode

The three most useful measures of the middle are the mean, the median and the mode. The *mean*, or average, has the symbol $\bar{X}$ and is the most reliable measure. It is markedly affected by extreme values. The median and mode are calculated after the results are placed in order of size in an array. The *median* is the middle value in an array (or the average of the middle two values if *n* is even). It is usually used if we are particularly interested in whether cases fall in the upper or the lower half of the distribution. As 50 per cent of cases fall below the median in an array, the median could also be called the 50 percentile. The *mode* is easy to distinguish, being the most fashionable, the value which occurs most frequently. If a frequency distribution is bimodal it usually indicates that the group is not homogeneous and two very different groups are mixed together. In the normal distribution the mean, the median and the mode fall in the same place.

The variance, standard deviation and range

Measures of variation are used to indicate the spread of the curve. The *variance*, s^2, and its square root, the *standard deviation*, s, are the measures of choice; the range is occasionally used. The highest and lowest results often need to be quoted and *the range* of the results is easy to calculate but has the same disadvantage as the median and mode; that it is not a reliable measurement. It is used as a measure of variation when the median is used as a measure of the centre. The range is the difference between the highest and lowest values.

The formulae for calculating the variance (s^2) are:

$$\frac{\Sigma\,(X - \bar{X})^2}{n-1} \quad = \quad \frac{\Sigma\,(X^2) - (\Sigma\,X)^2}{n-1}$$

where $\bar{X}$ is the mean and Σ means add together.

The formulae are numerically identical (remember first work out the results in brackets). The standard deviation in the normal distribution is the horizontal measurement from the mean to a point of inflection and equals the square root of these formulae (see diagram below).

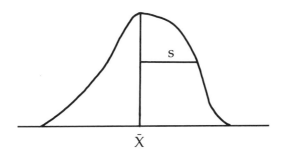

Transformations or non-parametric statistics
What if variation between individuals does not approximate the normal distribution? Often statistical transformations are used to smarten up data so that the variable becomes more acceptable in terms of being normally distributed. Square root, logarithmic, arcsin and probits are statistical transformations that are very useful because underneath them all is the original data which comes out in the statistical wash. If one is not prepared to spend the time transforming the data to simulate normality one is left in the field of what are generally called non-parametric statistics. Many statistical procedures based on the normal distribution have non-parametric counterparts.

Correlation and regression
Correlation means association between two or more variables. It can be positive, negative or non-existent. Positive correlation is where the variables tend to increase in size together. Where two variables are involved a scatter diagram may be used to represent the data. In positive correlation the dots tend to lie in the upper right-hand and lower left-hand quadrants, while in negative correlation the dots tend to lie in the other two quadrants. There is no preponderance of dots in any quadrant where correlation does not exist.

The two most frequently used correlation coefficients are Pearson's and Spearman's. Pearson's correlation coefficient is used when both variables are normally distributed. It is symbolised by 'r'. Spearman's correlation coefficient is used when either variable is not normally distributed, as well as when only ranks are available. It is not such an accurate measure as Pearson's and is symbolized by ρ (rho), which is calculated using the difference between rankings. Both r and ρ range from $+1$ to -1. They have sign and magnitude: $+1$ signifies maximum positive correlation; -1 signifies maximum negative correlation; and 0 means no correlation at all.

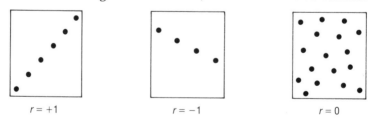

$r = +1$ $r = -1$ $r = 0$

The magnitude of correlation is indicated by how closely the dots approximate to a straight line (i.e how narrow the scatter is about an imaginary line) and not by their slope. If in fact the dots do approximate to a straight line which is sloped it is then meaningful to talk about the gradient of the slope, i.e. the *regression* coefficient. The regression coefficient is higher in the first diagram given above than in the second. This is the basic idea of regression by which, for example, we can predict the best value of one variable for a given value of the other.

Ideas about reliability

The population and samples
The 'population' is the entire group in which one is interested. A 'sample'

is a portion of that population. The population must be clearly and exhaustively defined before a sample is drawn from it. If you are not sure whether a certain type of patient is included in the population because the population is not fully defined, you cannot be sure that any conclusion based on the sample refers to that particular type of patient. Any conclusions based on information from the sample refer only to the particular population as defined, and this is particularly relevant in drug development.

Parameters and statistics
μ (mu) and σ (sigma) are parameters and refer to the mean and standard deviation in the population. $\bar{X}$ and s, which we have met already, are the equivalent statistics in the sample which can be used to estimate the parameters. The only accurate way of estimating parameters is a complete population enumeration. Sampling is cheaper and quicker and is occasionally the only method of estimation available. The inference about a parameter using statistics is always hazardous even with good samples.

Precision and bias in sampling
One of the characteristics of a good sampling is 'precision', where different samples would have their statistics lying close together. Precision is measured by

$$\frac{\sqrt{n}}{\sigma}$$

where n is the sample size and σ the standard deviation in the population.

$$\frac{\sigma}{\sqrt{n}}$$

is called the standard error of the mean and it estimates how precisely sample means will estimate the mean of the population, i.e. it is the standard deviation in the distribution of sample means.

σ can be estimated, if unknown, from a pilot survey. To increase precision the sample size must be increased. To double precision the sample size must be increased four-fold.

Precision and bias are entirely different entities. Precision describes how far *from each other* statistics from samples will be: they will approximate each other more if the samples from the same population are made bigger.

'Bias' produces unreliable results because the *statistics lie away from the parameter* which they are to estimate – they are off target. Statistics can be off target (biased) but precise or conversely on target and scattered but ideally they should be both precise and unbiased.

Randomization is the insurance against systematic bias arising at the sampling stage. Randomization does not eliminate bias but it does allow us to predict the size of the bias problem.

Precision does not affect bias that describes how far a statistic lies from the population parameter it is trying to estimate. If the sample or control group is wrongly selected so that the result is off target (i.e. systematic bias), increasing the sample size will not correct the bias – it will only make the study more expensive!

Sources of systematic bias

Retrospective (backward-looking) studies are generally more prone to systematic bias than prospective studies although they are usually smaller, cheaper and quicker to perform.

Subjective results (based on opinion rather than facts) are more prone to systematic bias than objective results. Randomized control groups (with a placebo in drug trials) and blind or double-blind experimental designs can be used to diminish the effect of systematic bias. The control group (yardstick) must be as like the group under investigation as possible save for the variable under consideration and one of the properties of randomization is to ensure matching of groups on both observed and unobserved characteristics.

Dissimilarities in age, sex, social class, etc. can be brought into line by a method called standardization. This is a rather spooky procedure whereby one estimates what would have been the picture had the groups been balanced, e.g. for age. It is spooky in the sense that instead of talking about real people we talk about ghosts!

Worst of all is the situation where no control groups are used at all. For example, a disease situation could be described in a particular group of people and we are left in the dark as to what is the normal picture in that place at that time for the general population of that age and sex. If there is no yardstick there can be no statistical conclusion.

Probability

Probability means likelihood, chances or odds. It has the symbol 'P' and ranges from 0 (impossibility) to 1 (inevitability). It is estimated from the formula:

$$\frac{\text{total number of occurrences of the particular target event}}{\text{total number of events}}$$

Laws of probability

The Addition Law of Probability applies to 'mutually exclusive' events, i.e. events such that the occurrence of one event excludes the possibility of any other taking place. The probability of one *or* more mutually exclusive event is the sum of the individual probabilities. If all possible mutually exclusive events are enumerated for a particular problem then their probabilities will sum up to one.

When the word *and* replaces *or* we use the Multiplication Law of Probability such that the probability of two or more events occurring together (e.g. Event A *and* Event B) is the product of their individual probabilities. This is only true if the probabilities are not associated in any way, i.e. if they are independent. When events can occur in more than one sequence the overall probability is the sum of the probabilities for the individual sequences.

Standard normal curve

Therefore, where the total area under a distribution curve is one unit, proportional area can be used to represent probability, *P*. All normal curves can be adjusted to the 'standard normal curve' so that the probability, P, of obtaining certain results or bigger can be calculated. The standard normal curve has mean equal to 0 and standard deviation equal to 1. In the standard normal curve, z equals the number of standard deviations a particular result lies from the mean.

Tables relating P to z are readily available. The P tabulated value is the probability of obtaining a result bigger than $+z$ or less than $-z$ added together. If you only want the probability at one end of the curve the tabulated P value is halved.

Confidence intervals and normal limits
A confidence interval can be used to predict a likely range of values for a parameter using statistics. The most commonly used confidence limits are used to predict the value of μ from $\bar{X}$. The 95 per cent limits in large random samples are between where $z = -1.96$ and $+1.96$.

By substituting results from a random sample in these formulae we have an interval within which we are 95 per cent confident μ falls on condition that the sample is fairly large (say bigger than 30).

Notice that it is usual that 5 per cent of results fall 'beyond the pale' or outside the confidence interval. Therefore an isolated pathological test result on a patient which is beyond the normal limits as quoted by the pathologist does not necessarily make the patient's result abnormal. On the contrary it is to be expected that a proportion of fit people will have sick results. Similarly, of course, normal results (i.e. within the expected normal limits) can arise in people whose diseases would cause one to anticipate results beyond the norm. Pathological results must be stressed in conjunction with the mathematical yardsticks proffered by the pathologists, but results fall both sides of these values in both sick and healthy individuals and so the rest of the clinical picture is important.

Significance tests

A short story, which is partly true.

A marketing manager and a drug company lawyer traditionally went to play golf on Thursday afternoons (time and weather permitting). At the nineteenth hole it was decided that they should each toss a coin. Should both toss 'heads' or both toss 'tails' they would re-toss their coins until the unfortunate threw a 'head' (and bought the drinks) and the other threw a very profitable 'tail'. On the first three occasions the marketing man tossed 'tails' and the lawyer 'heads'. The lawyer willingly bought the beverages but on the fourth successive occasion he emptied his pockets rather less willingly.

Returning home after the fifth successive Thursday's expenditure, the lawyer said to his wife: 'I am sure the sales manager is above board, but I do think there is something rather uncanny in his "tail tossing" ability'. However, the lawyer's wife was able to reassure her husband: 'It is obviously just bad luck on your part due entirely to chance – ignore it'.

The sixth week the lawyer tossed the unlucky 'head' yet again. Although feeling rather antisalespeople, he didn't comment. After the seventh game the lawyer's wife was faced with a very belligerent husband (even lawyers can be belligerent!). She agreed that enough was enough. Even though there was no proof that the sales manager was employing a trick (for these results could be entirely due to chance) it was very suspicious. 'The line must be drawn somewhere', she said. 'If it happens again, you must play golf with somebody else'.

Ideas like these are basic in analysing clinical trial data using significance tests, although the circumstances are different! The story has three statistical morals. First, any set of results involving data subject to random variation could be 'due entirely to chance' as the lawyer's wife pointed out. Statistics can never prove anything.

Second statisticians initially assume that chance is the only factor. Like the lawyer, they give the benefit of the doubt – they assume 'the possible guilty party is above board'. The lawyer's wife initially thought that the results were 'due entirely to chance' too.

Third, in statistical significance tests, as in the story, the time comes when 'the line must be drawn somewhere'. Otherwise, no conclusions can be drawn – no action taken. Chance could always be to blame, but the time comes when the evidence is such that it is more realistic to assume some other factor.

The science of statistics deals with material subject to inherent variability and helps by providing a measure of doubt about theories. These theories can never be proved. Significance tests enable research workers to draw conclusions based on preselected significance levels.

The stages in performing a significance test are: state the Null Hypothesis and its alternative; calculate P (the probability that the results are just due to chance); draw conclusions using significance levels.

The 'Null Hypothesis' states that the experimental results are not due to the theory, but only due to chance variation. It is not rejected until sufficient evidence is collected to do so.

Significance levels

The usual significance levels are 0.05 and 0.01. They are the yardsticks against which the evidence is measured. The 0.05 significance level means that 5 times out of 100 (a probability of 0.05) such an extreme value or more extreme value would occur by chance. The Null Hypothesis is rejected more often if the 0.05 level is used rather than the 0.01 level. At the 0.05 level more significant differences are found, but the Null Hypothesis is wrongly rejected in 5 tests out of 100. Statistically this is a type 1 error (risk of a false positive result). The failure to reject the Null Hypothesis when a difference is real is a type 2 error (risk of a false negative result). If we can be wrong all the time with significance tests you may doubt their value. Their value is only that they give us a measure for our doubts about the reality of observed differences.

Look back at the golfing story, where the lawyer was left puzzling about the sales manager's ability to toss 'tails' so consistently. After how many rounds should the surgeon's wife have persuaded her husband to call a halt?

Remember, if they both tossed heads or both tossed tails they threw again. Ignore the probability of this happening and just calculate, the Null

Hypothesis being assumed correct, the probability of one throwing heads and the other tails and vice versa for an increasing number of total times until the significance levels are passed.

The probability the first time was $\frac{1}{2}$ and the same was true for each successive throw. After five rounds P equalled $\frac{1}{32}$, which is $(\frac{1}{2})^5$, less than $\frac{1}{20}$, i.e. $P < 0.05$.

The P value for the experimental result is the probability of the actual experimental result or more extreme results arising by chance alone. Usually P includes the equally extreme results at both ends of the scale (a two-tailed test). In this case the significance levels also include both ends. If one end of the scale can be excluded on theoretical grounds the P value and significance levels only apply to the relevant end (a one-tailed test).

If $0.05 > P > 0.01$ the alternative is accepted at the 0.05 significance level, but not at the 0.01 level. An alternative to the Null Hypothesis accepted at 0.01 is more 'significant' than one at 0.05.

Occasionally results are significant at the 0.001 significance level, which is very significant. Even when this is so it does not prove that there is a real effect. It means that we should provisionally accept the idea of a real difference rather than suppose that a very improbable chance result has occurred.

Which significance test?
Simple tests involving 'z' and the standard normal curve are used when: the samples are random; the data is quantitative; the variable can be as-sumed to be normally distributed in the population. This test is only approxi-mate but is adequate when the samples involved are bigger in size than 30.

A more accurate method for significance testing was discovered by a man call Gosset in 1908. At the time he was employed by Guinness Brewery in Dublin. The firm's standard operating procedures required him to use a pen-name and he chose the name 'Student'; 't' was the symbol later introduced in connection with the distribution used, which is consequently known as Student's 't'.

Student's t-tests are not so straightforward as tests based on z as there are a series of 't' distributions which cannot all be standardized to one t distribution. If the results naturally fall into pairs the particular type of Student's t which must be applied is the Paired Student's t-test.

Examples where pairing may be appropriate include a drug trial with 'before' and 'after' results or animal experiments where two animals are taken from each litter. Some doctors match patients successfully for age/sex/severity of disease but if the matched people are not very alike this can be a mistake.

Most tests involving qualitative data depend on χ^2.

χ^2 (chi-squared) is the distribution used for testing data where: the samples are random; the data is qualitative; there is ideally no expected value less than 5.

$$\text{Calculated } \chi^2 = \sum \frac{(O - E)^2}{E}$$

where O is observed for each cell in the table of possible outcomes and E the result which would be expected under the Null Hypothesis.

As with the 't'-tests there are a series of χ^2 distributions which depend for χ^2 on the number of rows and columns in the table showing possible outcomes.

As always, the Null Hypothesis states that the differences between the observed and expected results are only due to chance variation. If the calculated value of χ^2 (or z or t) is greater than the significance value shown in the statistical tables, then P, the probability of a more extreme result arising by chance, is less than the equivalent significance level, the Null Hypothesis is rejected and the results are declared statistically significant and are thought of as representing a real difference.

Common statistical problems

Variability

In a clinical trial the ability to detect a difference between treatments is partly dependent on the variability of the results obtained. Three key areas where variability can be introduced into the treatment comparison are patient selection, trial procedures and measurement errors.

To get an accurate assessment of the difference between treatments it is natural to try and choose patients who clearly have the disease to be treated but do not have other problems that may interfere with the response to treatment. Although this will lead to less variable results, the outcome of the trial will not necessarily be applicable to a wide population of patients with the disease. A good example, here, is the treatment of asthma. It is possible to define the asthmatic patients required fairly closely in terms of lung function results and symptoms. However, the situation is complicated by the fact that asthmatic patients will typically be taking a number of anti-asthma medications before entry into the trial. In an ideal situation all these medications would be stopped pretrial so that the effect of trial treatment can be accurately observed. In practice, however, stopping all anti-asthma medication is likely to lead to a deterioration in the patient's condition that could be dangerous and would be ethically unacceptable. Two alternatives are possible. Trial entry could be restricted to those taking no other asthma medication. However, this would restrict recruitment to such an extent that trials would take many years to complete. In addition, such groups of patients would be completely different from the vast population of asthma sufferers. The other alternative is to allow certain types of asthma medication to be continued. This then potentially increases the variability of response to treatment and makes it much harder to detect differences. However, when detected the results will be applicable to a much wider population of patients. Every protocol has to select patients with these two alternatives in mind. Typically the trials in Phase II will concentrate on groups of patients with fewer problems apart from the disease in question. The consequence of this is that the variability of the results will tend to be lower, and treatment effects should be seen more clearly. In Phase III a wider selection of patients will normally be made, and the loss of sensitivity will be compensated for by performing larger trials.

The second major area where excess variability can be introduced into clinical trials is in trial procedures. It is important to standardize these as far as possible. In a later section on multicentre trials the importance is stressed of adopting established criteria to define the disease of interest, and of consistently applying assessment criteria in all centres. In addition it is important to consider what can go wrong and what can be done to prevent it. Timing is often a problem – patients do not always attend clinics on the day specified. In short-term healing trials, such as in duodenal ulcer disease, this timing is important and the protocol needs to be clear about what time window is acceptable around each visit. This will be less critical in longer term trials of antihypertensive agents where a 4-month visit after 19 weeks instead of 16 weeks may be of little consequence. Concomitant medication is often difficult to control, but it is important to specify what is acceptable in the protocol and to make sure investigators and patients are aware of this. If some additional medication for relief of pain or discomfort is likely to be needed then it can help to supply a standard preparation and to perform tablet counts to provide a degree of assurance that consumption was similar in different treatment groups. It is important that the trial procedures are not too complex and that only data that are really required are collected. Since clinic time is always limited the pressure to collect too much data is likely to lower the quality and increase the variability of the important items.

The final area where variability can be reduced is in measurement error. In many diseases the assessment of outcome has a high subjective component and it is vital that a common observer is used for successive assessments of one patient. Otherwise apparent improvements can be due to changes in observers rather than the treatment being taken. It is also preferable to have one, or a small number of trained observers assess every patient. Training is often neglected but it is a major issue since any difference between treatments can only be demonstrated if the observers can evaluate improvement consistently. If several observers are used then exercises to standardize their performance are also important. Even when the assessment is reasonably objective, such as the standard lung function tests, it is important to specify standard procedures in the protocol, e.g. the length of the resting period before the procedure is carried out. Finally, it is helpful to use internationally accepted standard methods whenever possible since these are likely to be known already to many investigators and probably represent the best and most consistent way in which a parameter can be measured.

Randomization

It is important that when treatments are allocated to patients in clinical trials there is no selection bias, i.e. that the physicians entering patients do not choose particular treatments for particular patients. If physicians are allowed to choose then consciously or subconsciously they may select one treatment for patients of a certain type (e.g. the more severe patients). This will mean that at the end of the trial the comparison of results will not be fair, i.e. there will be a bias in favour of one treatment. This can be avoided if a random procedure is used to allocate treatments.

It is important that the decision to enter the patient into the trial is made before the random treatment is selected. A random allocation of patients to treatments has two other important advantages. Following the randomization, on average the treatment groups formed will be balanced in terms of all observed and unobserved characteristics. So if there is a difference in outcome between two treatment groups, the randomization provides reassurance that this is unlikely to be due to differences in other characteristics. The randomization procedure is also a necessary requirement for the validity of statistical significance tests.

A randomization list consists simply of a series of patient numbers for each of which a treatment is selected at random. Usually this is accomplished by using a psuedo-random number generator on a computer or a table of random numbers. Trial supplies are then packaged using the patient number as the only identifier. If a completely random allocation is used the treatments may not be given to the correct proportions of patients, so a blocked randomization is usually used. A block size is determined, and within this block size patients are allocated in the correct proportions to each treatment. Shown below is a randomization list for two treatments using a block size of six patients and allocating equal numbers of patients to take A and B.

Block	Patient Number	Treatment Code
1	1	A
	2	B
	3	B
	4	A
	5	B
	6	A
2	7	A
	8	B
	9	A
	10	A
	11	B
	12	B
3	13 etc.	

The choice of block size attempts to balance two factors. If the block size is small, then before patients are entered it may be possible to guess which treatment will be allocated for the next patient. However, if the block size is large then there may be a long run of patients who by chance get allocated the same treatment. In practice, for two-treatment trials block sizes of 6, 8 and 10 are often used. It is also important to ensure that in multicentre trials each centre is allocated a complete number of blocks, so that the correct proportions of patients receive the trial treatments within each centre.

In some clinical trials it is known that one or more characteristics of the patients will have a profound effect on response to treatment. There may then be concern that randomization will allocate most of the patients of one type to one treatment making the trial results difficult to interpret. In trials involving hundreds of patients randomization will nearly always ensure an adequate balance between the treatment groups. In small trials, however, the concern may be real. Use of a stratified randomization will eliminate this possibility. The principle is to create a different randomization list for each patient subgroup. If, for example, sex and severity of disease (mild, moderate, severe) are known to be important determinants of outcome then six random lists will need to be prepared for the following six patient subgroups:

1. Male, mild disease
2. Male, moderate disease
3. Male, severe disease

4. Female, mild disease
5. Female, moderate disease
6. Female, severe disease

Patients are entered in the trial by selecting the next patient number in sequence from the list defined by their sex and disease severity. The disadvantage of the method is the extra complexity introduced by using many randomization lists and the need to supply more medication since the number of patients who will be entered with different characteristics cannot be known in advance.

Alternative techniques are available to ensure a balance of patient characteristics across treatment groups. These are generally called adaptive randomization procedures. As patients are entered a central organizer reviews the degree of balance achieved so far and randomizes further patients to maintain the best balance possible. Methods are described by Taves[1] and Pocock and Simon.[2] A wide overview of randomization and its properties is given in a series of papers by Lachin.[3]

Blinding

Knowledge of the treatment a patient is taking can be a major source of bias in the evaluation of response to treatment. This bias can be avoided by keeping patients, physicians and other medical staff involved in the trial unaware of the treatment being taken by any patient. A single-blind trial is one in which the patient is unaware of the treatment being taken although the physician does know. A double-blind trial keeps both physician and patient 'blind' to the treatment being taken by the patient. Another option is to use an observer-blind trial where the patient and a physician assessing response to treatment remain blind but a second physician prescribes treatment. When none of these options is possible an open trial can be performed, but this will usually be a last resort.

The double-blind trial is the design chosen whenever possible. To perform such a trial, the best method is to obtain supplies of the trial treatments that are indistinguishable. To do this it is necessary to match shape, size, marking, colour (external and internal), texture (external and internal), weight, taste and after taste and smell. This can be difficult and in many cases impossible. If it involves reprocessing of drug material to achieve the matching then it will be necessary to show that the reprocessed material has bioavailability equivalent to the original material.

When it is not possible to produce matching treatments a double-dummy method is used. For each of two treatments an active and placebo form is manufactured. Patients are given either:

Active form of A + Placebo form of B

or

Placebo form of A + Active form of B

With this technique it is possible to compare tablets with solutions, tablets with capsules and so on. Clearly, it will not be ideal when a drug has a clearly identifiable taste or smell that will not be present in its placebo form.

Blindness may be difficult to maintain for other reasons. If one drug produces a particular response or an identifiable side effect, then physicians may be able to conclude which treatment a patient is on. Usually this is not possible with complete assurance and an element of blindness remains. In addition, blindness will apply at the time of randomization, thus precluding any biased patient selection at that time.

Data processing

One of the important features in conducting a good clinical trial is the quality and speed of the data processing. Clinical trial data are complex and many of the data items are related to each other. The data have to be provided by busy physicians and nurses and there is a potential for data to be omitted or entered in error, and all data problems have the potential to distort the results of the trial. A high quality data base is an essential prerequisite for producing high quality reports and publications. In the pharmaceutical industry the data bases used are highly complex computer systems that can capture large amounts of data and can be programmed to identify errors and omissions requiring follow-up. They also provide a permanent record available in future years to generate new hypotheses and throw light on new questions.

It is important to realize that the aim in data processing is not a completely error-free data base. This is almost certainly impossible and the time invested in trying to achieve it will not be worthwhile. What is required is a level of accuracy high enough to know that any remaining errors will not affect the results reported for the trial. In small trials this may equate to no errors, but in large trials with hundreds of patients we must live with the knowledge that perfection is impossible.

Data management for these complex computer data bases is now a science itself and specialists in this work are now routinely involved in large clinical trials programmes. Their main functions are to:

1. Advise at the protocol and record form design stage so that data processing requirements are considered from the start of the process.

2. Set up the computer database so that it is ready to receive data from the trial.
3. Define in conjunction with clinical and statistical colleagues the computer checks that will be performed on the data. These generally fall into the area of checks for missing data, range checks to see whether a variable has values in an acceptable range and logical checks to see if different data items are consistent.
4. To load data into the data base, identify errors and ensure that these are resolved by reference to the investigator where necessary.
5. To perform quality control checks to ensure the quality of the data.
6. To feedback information on areas where quality is deficient as the trial progresses, so that steps may be taken to improve the data in these areas.
7. To work with statistical and clinical colleagues on the analysis and reporting of the trial from a perspective of day-to-day contact with the data base and knowledge of the problems involved in finalizing it.

The technical aspects of clinical data processing are covered now by many books most of which date from the 1980s.[4,5] The quantity of literature produced during the last decade, the existence of a common interest group within the pharmaceutical industry and the regular conferences and publications devoted to data management are all signals of the growing importance of data processing in clinical trial work.

Trial size
One of the key issues when designing a clinical trial is the number of patients to be recruited. It is vital to choose a trial size that is sufficient to enable useful conclusions to be drawn from the trial. This is achieved by using techniques based on the concept of 'power'.

When the trial protocol is being prepared, the statistician needs answers to seven key questions:

1. *What is the main aim of the trial?* Protocols should have one primary aim and the trial size should be chosen to give a high chance of achieving this aim.
2. *What is the primary measure of outcome?* Once the aim is clear it is important to be sure which outcome measure is the most important in terms of achieving the aim of the trial. In many trials there may be several ways of measuring a particular factor (e.g. lung function can be assessed using three or four lung function tests) and one of these must be designated as primary.
3. *How will the primary measure of outcome be analysed?* The statistician has to be aware of the method of analysis that will be used since this will affect the calculations required to determine sample size. In addition it is necessary to specify the level that will be used in the significance test – usually this will be 0.05 but sometimes other values such as 0.01 will be more appropriate.

4. *What results are expected for the standard treatment?* This may be obtainable from previous trials, from literature searches or from expert opinions. However, expert opinions are notoriously bad predictors of the results seen with standard treatments in clinical trials. In addition to information about the expected result for the standard, it is necessary to have an estimate of variance if the primary measure will be analysed using procedures such as the 't' test. Previous trials are invariably the best source for estimates of variance.

5. *What results are expected for the new treatment?* It is necessary to know the size of the treatment difference the trial should detect. If treatment differences are very large then only a small trial will be needed. Conversely, very small differences can be detected only if the trial is very large. To enable the trial size to be chosen sensibly it is important to define what size of difference one would be unhappy to miss. This is a clinical decision. In some minor diseases a difference of a few per cent in healing rates would not be clinically useful whereas a reduction in mortality of a few per cent could be very important.

6. *What degree of certainty is required that the above treatment difference will be detected?* Even in very large clinical trials there is a chance that an inaccurate answer will be obtained. However, the bigger a trial is, the more likely it is that the result will be reliable. This idea is encapsulated in the concept of power. This is the probability of detecting the difference specified in point 5 above, i.e. the probability that a significant difference will be obtained at the end of the trial. Typically we want the power to be high and values of 0.80 or 0.90 are frequently used.

7. *What proportion of patients may not provide suitable data for analysis?* Often some patients will be recruited but will not provide data that can be analysed. These may be included in any case in an intention-to-treat analysis (see pp. 133–4), but the effect of this can then be to reduce observed treatment differences. If an analysis excluding those with unsuitable data is carried out then power will be reduced as the number of patients used will be less. To account for these problems it is wise to increase the trial size based on an estimate of the expected number of patients with unsuitable data. Typically between 10 and 30 per cent of patients may fall into this category. If 10 per cent is the estimate then the calculated number of patients required should be increased by 100/90 and if 30 per cent is the estimate an increase of 100/70 is needed.

Once this information is obtained standard formulae can be used to calculate the trial size. To describe these a certain amount of mathematical notation is required. Let:

θ_1 = expected proportion of successes on the standard treatment (where outcome is success or failure)

θ_2 = expected proportion of successes on the new treatment (where outcome is success or failure)

μ_1 = expected mean value for the standard treatment (where the outcome is quantitative)

μ_2 = expected mean value for the new treatment (where the outcome is quantitative)

σ^2 = estimate of variance (where the outcome is quantitative)

α = level of the significance test used for detecting a treatment difference (often this is called the type 1 error and it represents the risk of a false positive result)

$1-\beta$= power to detect a difference (β is often called the type 2 error and it represents the risk of a false negative result)

It is also necessary to refer to the normal cumulative distribution curve with mean 0 and standard deviation 1 to obtain two probabilities.[6] $z_{\alpha/2}$ is found so that the probability of obtaining a value greater than $z_{\alpha/2}$ is $\alpha/2$. If α is 0.05 then $z_{\alpha/2}$ is 1.96, and if α is 0.01 then $z_{\alpha/2}$ is 2.58 (Table 5.1). z_β is found so that the probability of obtaining a value greater than z_β is β. If β is 0.20 then z_β is 0.84, and if β is 0.10 then z_β is 1.28 (Table 5.1). In many calculations a standard multiplier SM (α, β) is required which is a combination of these two values – $(z_{\alpha/2} + z_\beta)^2$ and for convenience these standard multipliers are also shown in Table 5.1.

Trial size for a success/failure outcome in a parallel group trial
The number of patients required for each treatment can be calculated as:

$$n = \frac{\theta_1 \times (100 - \theta_1) + \theta_2 \times (100 - \theta_2)}{(\theta_2 - \theta_1)^2} \times SM\,(\alpha, \beta)$$

Example
A trial was designed to compare the ability of two anti-emetic drugs to control nausea and vomiting caused by radiotherapy.[7] The primary outcome measure was defined in the protocol to be the proportion of patients vomiting less than twice in the first 24 hours. For the standard therapy the success rate was predicted to be 0.60, and it was expected that the new therapy would lead to a success rate of 0.80. A power $(1-\beta)$ of 0.80 was selected with a significance level α of 0.05. Thus the number of patients needed in each group was calculated to be:

Table 5.1   Values of standard multipliers (α, β)

	Significance level 'α'	
	0.05 ($z_{\alpha/2} = 1.96$)	0.01 ($z_{\alpha/2} = 2.58$)
Power $1-\beta$		
0.50 ($z_\beta = 0.00$)	3.84	6.63
0.80 ($z_\beta = 0.84$)	7.85	11.68
0.90 ($z_\beta = 1.28$)	10.51	14.88
0.95 ($z_\beta = 1.64$)	13.00	17.81

$$n = \frac{0.60 \times 0.40 + 0.80 \times 0.20}{(0.80 - 0.60)^2} \times 7.85$$

$$= 79$$

To allow for a possible 10 per cent of cases providing unsuitable data a randomization for 176 patients was performed.

Trial size for a success/failure outcome in a crossover trial
Although the calculations for a crossover are still relatively simple some preparatory work is necessary.[8] In a crossover trial of this kind the analysis concentrates only on patients who succeed on one treatment but fail on the other. If there is no difference in the efficacy of the treatments then in those showing a preference the probability of the new treatment being the one preferred should be equal to 0.5.

Suppose that θ_1 and θ_2 are the proportions of successes expected on the two treatments. Then in the crossover trial (assuming there are no effects due to the period in which treatments are taken) the probabilities of success on one treatment and not the other are

$$\theta_1 (1 - \theta_2) \text{ and } \theta_2 (1 - \theta_1)$$

So, given that attention is confined only to patients who succeed on one treatment and not the other, the probability of preferring the new treatment (which will be called θ) is

$$\theta = \frac{\theta_2 (1 - \theta_1)}{\theta_1 (1 - \theta_2) + \theta_2 (1 - \theta_1)}$$

Also if n patients enter the crossover trial then

$n \times [\theta_1 (1 - \theta_2) + \theta_2 (1 - \theta_1)]$ will show a preference and

$n \times [\theta_1 \theta_2 + (1 - \theta_1) (1 - \theta_2)]$ will not show a preference.

The significance test that will be performed assesses whether the proportion of patients preferring the new treatment is 0.5. If the proportion is θ, then a high power is required to detect the difference between θ and 0.5.

To achieve a power of $1-\beta$ will require

$$\left[\frac{0.50 \, z_{\alpha/2} + z_\beta \sqrt{\theta (1 - \theta)}}{\theta - 0.50} \right]^2$$

patients who succeed on one treatment and not the other.
To achieve this will require

$$n = \left[\frac{0.50 \, z_{\alpha/2} + z_{\beta} \sqrt{\theta (1 - \theta)}}{\theta - 0.50} \right]^2 \div [\theta_1 (1 - \theta_2) + \theta_2 (1 - \theta_1)]$$

patients to be entered in the crossover trial.

Example
Two anti-emetic drugs were compared for the control of nausea and vomiting caused by cancer chemotherapy in a two-period crossover design.[9] The proportions of successes expected were $\theta_2 = 0.70$ on the new treatment and $\theta_1 = 0.50$ on the comparator. A power $(1 - \beta)$ of 80 per cent and a significance level of 0.05 were chosen.
   Based on the expected proportions of successes, the probability of prefering the new treatment in patients where one treatment succeeds and the other fails is

$$\theta = \frac{0.70 \, (1 - 0.50)}{0.50 \, (1 - 0.70) + 0.70 \, (1 - 0.50)} = 0.70$$

So

$$\left[\frac{0.50 \times 1.96 + 0.84 \sqrt{0.70 \times 0.30}}{0.70 - 0.50} \right]^2 = 46.6$$

patients who succeed on one treatment and not the other are required. Hence:

$$46.6 \div (0.50 \times 0.30 + 0.70 \times 0.50) = 93$$

patients were required in the crossover trial. A total of 120 patients were randomized to allow for unassessable cases.

Trial size for a quantitative outcome in a parallel group trial
The number of patients required for each treatment can be calculated as

$$n = \frac{2 \sigma^2}{(\mu_2 - \mu_1)^2} \times SM(\alpha, \beta)$$

Example
A trial was designed to compare a new bronchodilator with a standard bronchodilator in the treatment of asthmatic patients. The primary outcome measure was mean daily morning peak flow recorded by patients

at home. The trial was designed to detect a difference of 15 l/min between the mean morning peak flow on new and standard therapy. Previous trials had shown that the standard deviation to be expected was 50 l/min. A power $(1 - \beta)$ of 0.95 was required with a significance level α of 0.05. The number of patients in each group was calculated to be:

$$n = \frac{2 \times 50^2 \times 13.00}{15^2} = 289$$

Data were therefore needed on nearly 600 patients and to allow for the relatively high expected rate of 25 per cent for patients not providing complete data, 800 patients were recruited.

Trial size for a quantitative outcome in a crossover trial
The formula for trial size in a crossover trial is similar to that for a parallel group trial, except that some preparatory work is required.

The analysis of a crossover trial is based on the treatment difference observed for each patient. This means that the estimate of the standard deviation must relate to the treatment difference calculated for each patient. This will usually be obtainable from previous crossover trials where differences for individual patients can be calculated.

With this proviso about the standard deviation the number of patients required for the crossover trial will be

$$n = \frac{\sigma^2}{(\mu_2 - \mu_1)^2} \times SM (\alpha, \beta)$$

This number of patients will be split into $n/2$ patients taking the two different treatment sequences.

Example
A trial was designed to compare a new inhaled bronchodilator with an oral bronchodilator. The primary outcome measure was mean daily morning peak flow.

A power of 0.95 was required to detect a difference of 20 l/min between treatments. The standard deviation of the treatment difference calculated for each patient was estimated to be 64 l/min. A significance level α of 0.05 was assumed. The number of patients required for the trial was

$$n = \frac{64^2}{20^2} \times 13.00 = 133$$

To allow for a relatively high expected rate of 25 per cent for those patients not providing complete data, 180 patients were recruited into the trial.

Trial size for survival studies

In some trials the key parameter of interest is the time until a particular event occurs. In cancer trials this may be time to relapse or death; in maintenance trials with duodenal ulcer it may be time to recurrence of the ulcer. Trials of this kind are analysed using special methods that allow data to be used for patients whose follow-up period is censored, i.e. they are known to be well at a particular follow-up time but no information about their subsequent condition is available. This can often occur because the trial is terminated before they have a relevant event. Methods for analysing data of this kind are described by Pocock.[10]

A simple approach to this situation is to use survival at a particular time point as the key parameter. If 2-year survival is chosen and estimates of 2 years of survival for two treatments can be obtained then the methods appropriate to a success/failure outcome can be used. This will tend to overestimate the number of patients required, since the analysis will not take account of the extra information concerning the actual time of each event. However, for practical purposes this method will give a reasonable estimate of trial size. More precise methods are available (see for example Machin and Campbell[6]).

Trial size when seeking to show equivalence

Most trials are designed to try and demonstrate that one treatment is superior to another. However, in some instances the opposite is true. A treatment may be developed which has no benefit in terms of efficacy but has a better side effect profile. In this case it is necessary to demonstrate that the new treatment is equivalent in terms of efficacy to existing treatments. Clearly a small study will almost certainly lead to the conclusion that the treatments are not significantly different. However, this does not prove equivalence since calculation of a confidence interval will show that the data are consistent with a very large difference – the trial is just too small to detect it.

One way out of this dilemma is to proceed as before. Define a treatment difference which, if it existed, would lead a clinician to conclude that the treatments were not equivalent. Then design the study to have high power to detect this difference. A no difference result to such a trial is more convincing since the trial would be expected to detect a clinically important difference if it existed.

Makuch and Simon[11] describe a method which is more directly aimed at the equivalence problem. This centres on the confidence interval that will be derived from the trial. For a success/failure response an estimate of the overall proportion of successes, θ, that will occur in the trial is required. A value d is then defined and a trial size is to be chosen so that with probability $1-\beta$ the $100 (1-\alpha)$ per cent confidence interval for the difference between the proportion of successes will lie within the interval $-d$ to $+d$ if there is no treatment difference. The required number of patients on each treatment is then

$$n = \frac{2\theta \times (1 - \theta) \times SM(\alpha, \beta)}{d^2}$$

A similar formula will apply for trials with quantitative outcome. The interest here will be in the 100 $(1-\alpha)$ per cent confidence interval for the difference between the two treatment means. The trial size is to be chosen so that with probability $(1-\beta)$ this lies within the interval $-d$ to $+d$ if there is no difference between the treatments. The appropriate formula requires an estimate of the variance σ^2 of the observations:

$$n = \frac{2 \times \sigma^2 \times SM\,(\alpha,\ \beta)}{d^2}$$

In practice this method gives very similar results to the standard approach when the same value for d is used in both.

Example
A trial was designed to compare the 4-week duodenal ulcer healing rate for a standard twice daily regime of an ulcer healing drug with the rate when the total dose was given once at night. The overall proportion of patients healed was expected to be 0.75. The trial was designed so that the 95 per cent confidence interval for the difference in proportions healed should not exceed ± 0.10. A probability $(1-\beta)$ of 0.80 was required that this would occur if there was no real treatment difference. The trial size required for each treatment is

$$n = \frac{2 \times 0.75 \times 0.25}{0.10^2} \times 7.85 = 296$$

Suppose we design the trial in the conventional way to detect a difference of 0.10 between the proportions of patients healed and assume that for the standard therapy the healing rate will be 0.75. Then to obtain power $(1-\beta)$ of 0.80 with a significance level α of 0.05 the number of patients needed is

$$n = \frac{(0.75 \times 0.25 + 0.85 + 0.15)}{0.10^2} \times 7.85$$

$$= 249$$

Clearly the formulas are very similar and the trial sizes that result will also be approximately the same.

Unequal randomization in the treatment groups
Most trials allocate equal numbers of patients to the different treatment groups. For any trial size this gives the maximum power to detect differences. Other considerations may arise which lead to the suggestion that more patients be allocated to one treatment than the other. It may be necessary to collect more safety data on a new treatment and to do this a 2:1 randomization or a 3:2 randomization may be appropriate.

Moderate imbalances of this kind have a very small effect on power. For success/failure outcomes, Cohen[12] notes that if n_1 and n_2 are the number of patients in two treatment groups then the power of the trial is

equal to that for two groups each with $\dfrac{2n_1 n_2}{n_1 + n_2}$ patients.

So, the power of a trial with 200 on one treatment and 100 on the other is equivalent to that of a trial with 133 patients in each group. Clearly this loss of power is not appreciable and can be a small price to pay if other reasons suggest that an unequal randomization is preferable.

Trial design when equivalence is expected

The previous section discusses the calculation of trial size when the trial is designed to demonstrate equivalence rather than superiority. The general point is that it is just as difficult to establish the former as the latter, and often large trials are needed. There are additional difficulties, however, with trials directed at equivalence. The first of these relates to the performance of the standard comparator in this situation. It is often the case that, even when a treatment is known to be effective in a disease, any one particular trial against placebo may show no treatment difference. Of course, if many trials are done then many will demonstrate a difference, but there will still be some inconclusive ones. If a new treatment is being compared to a standard then a no difference result may be obtained. However, this might mean that both treatments worked equally well or that both were completely ineffective. Without a placebo arm in the trial there is no way of knowing which of the explanations is correct.

The second problem with equivalence trials is that poor study methodology may increase variability and make a difference undetectable. So, contrary to the normal type of trial designed to show a difference, for an equivalence trial poor methodology appears to be an advantage. Although in some situations the increase in variability may be observable, this will often not be the case for success/failure variables, and it is hard for a reviewer to evaluate the quality of the methodology in a trial. The investigator's attitude to evaluating response will also be indifferent in trials directed at equivalence. The presumption will be that most patients will improve and so there is less need for care in evaluating the response to treatment. These issues are discussed in more detail by Temple.[13]

Group sequential designs

When trials are in progress there is often a desire to know how the trial is progressing. It is important to monitor the safety of the patients on a regular basis, particularly when a treatment being used is new and has not been widely tested. There is no problem with such safety moni-toring and it is usually an ethical requirement. Whenever possible this safety monitoring should be carried out by a group who are not in day-to-day contact with investigators so that the trial remains blind.

There is sometimes also a desire to examine the efficacy results as they accumulate. This can be due to simple curiosity, or because there is a desire to stop the trial if one treatment is clearly superior, or because some information is required so that further clinical trials can be started. However, examination of efficacy data in this way leads to a number of problems. Some of these are at a practical level. It must be remembered that results from interim analyses are unreliable. Since a trial is designed so that with all patients recruited the power to detect a difference is high, it is clear that at an interim stage there is unlikely to be sufficient power to detect some differences of clinical interest. In addition, patients available for an interim analysis may not be representative of all patients who will eventually be recruited. They may tend to come from a few centres who are recruiting fast; they may be patients easily available for recruitment because their disease severity ensures they are attending clinics regularly; there may not be equal allocation within centres to the different treat-ments since whole randomized blocks may not yet have been entered. Additional problems relate to the maintenance of blindness. If interim efficacy results are known to clinical trial monitors it may be possible for them to influence recruitment in such a way that the sample selected is distorted (e.g. by recruiting more patients of a certain type). Although this is a possibility that can be discounted if reputable scientists are involved in the clinical trial, it is a concern of regulatory authorities that cannot be discounted. The existence of positive or negative interim results may also have profound effects on the enthusiasm with which the trial progresses. These reasons imply that interim analyses always reduce the credibility of the trial results.

The other major problem with interim analyses of efficacy depends on the reason for the interim analyses. To start with, curiosity is never a sufficient reason to perform an interim analysis. Scientists are always curious, but this should not be accepted as a reason to weaken the credibility of the trial results by performing an interim analysis. The second possible reason for an interim analysis is to stop the trial if one treatment is clearly superior. The problem then relates to the nature of the significance tests used to compare results for the treatments. If a significance test is carried out at the 5 per cent level of significance, then five times out of a hundred a significant result will be declared when there is actually no real difference between the treatments. If a number of interim analyses are performed, then on each occasion there is a chance of declaring a difference when the treatments are truly the same. So performing a number of interim analyses and stopping as soon as we observe a significant difference will lead us to identify many more spurious treatment differences. Armitage *et al.*[14] looked at this problem, and showed for example that if five interim analyses are carried out with significance tests at the 5 per cent level, then there is a 14 per cent chance of claiming a difference between the treatments when there is no real difference at all. As the number of interim analyses increases, so does the chance of finding spurious differences between treatments.

The implication of this discussion is that if interim analyses are required, it is necessary to be conservative at each interim analysis and only stop the trial if the preference for one treatment is very marked. It will also be necessary to use a more stringent significance level at the final analysis, if the trial is not terminated early, so that in only five trials out of a hundred will the whole procedure lead to a claim of a treatment difference when the treatments are truly the same. Designs that formalize this idea are called Group Sequential Designs. In the trial protocol the number of interim analyses is defined and for each of these the level of statistical significance required before the trial is stopped is also defined. Typically, a level of significance far below the conventional 5 per cent level will be chosen. The problem then reduces to deciding how many interim analyses are needed and what significance levels to use. Unless a trial is very large or will take a very long time, it is usually sufficient to have just one interim analysis and one final. Occasionally it may be reasonable to perform two or three interim analyses but rarely is it sensible to perform more. There are a number of procedures for selecting significance levels to be used at the interim stages. It is preferable to use a procedure that only permits stopping at an interim analysis if differences are very marked. O'Brien and Fleming[15] suggest a procedure with this property and with the additional advantage that, if the trial proceeds to the end, the final significance test can be carried out at a level which is virtually unchanged from the conventional 5 per cent. Discussion of other procedures for selecting significance levels can be found in Pocock.[10]

A third reason for performing an interim analysis is to plan future trials rather than to stop the current trial. If the current trial is showing promising results, further trials may be started to gain more clinical experience with the treatments. This is a difficult issue to resolve. All interim analyses weaken the credibility of the results whether or not the intention is to stop the trial. If an interim analysis of this kind is proposed, then it is important to refer to it in the protocol, stating that the trial will continue to the end whatever the result of the interim analysis. However, this may not be sufficient to prevent regulatory authorities taking the view that the trial might have been stopped if the results had been sufficiently clear and requiring a smaller significance level to be achieved at the final analysis.

There are some additional practical issues to bear in mind when carrying out interim analyses. It is important that at the time of the interim analysis all available results are collected and processed. It is advisable to confine attention to one or two key efficacy variables, partly to clarify decision making but also to reduce the extra workload caused by the interim analysis. Finally, it is important to have a plan of action defined before the interim analysis is carried out that takes account of the clinical importance of the differences observed as well as the statistical significance.

Multicentre trials

A very high proportion of clinical trials are carried out on a multicentre basis, where a number of different medical centres cooperate to conduct one clinical trial. The reason for this is simple. It can often be impossible to recruit enough patients in one centre to show differences between treatments; in statistical terms many centres are needed to provide adequate statistical power. If this is the case it is pointless to carry out a trial in one centre since it will inevitably be inconclusive. The solution is to include a number of different centres since this will provide additional statistical power. It will confer the added advantage that the results from the trial will be likely to apply more broadly and will not be specific to one centre only.

Unfortunately, the use of several centres in one clinical trial leads to a number of practical problems. The first key issue is to design a protocol that all participating centres will be able to follow. Typically, it can be difficult to specify inclusion and exclusion criteria to which all centres will be able to agree and which will also lead to a reasonable recruitment rate in all centres. It is often useful to arrange investigator meetings to finalize the protocol. Another important issue is to use established criteria for the disease of interest. There are internationally accepted definitions for many diseases[16,17] and use of these will ensure conformity in trials conducted in several countries as well as many centres. There are also internationally accepted guidelines for the conduct of clinical trials in particular diseases.[18,19] The design of the record form is also important since if anything in the form can be misunderstood then it is likely to be by at least some of the centres.

The second key issue is the need to ensure consistency in the application of assessment criteria in the different centres. A detailed review of the assessment criteria is essential for all the staff participating. In some trials it may be possible to provide training in the use of assessment scales. This can be useful, for example, in anxiety and depression where videos of patients can be assessed using standard rating scales and consistency can be reviewed. Feedback on data quality is also essential to ensure that centres are working to the same standards.

The third key issue in multicentre trials concerns part of the analysis when the trial is complete. It is important to examine the consistency of any treatment difference across the centres. The concern is that an apparent difference in favour of one treatment might arise because of a large effect in a few centres with little difference in the remainder. This would suggest that the difference might not be observed in many centres outside of the clinical trial situation. Of course, it is likely that not every centre will show the treatments to be different, but it is important that there is a reasonable degree of consistency. Statisticians call a lack of consistency a 'treatment-by-centre interaction' and statistical analyses can be performed to examine this.[20] It can also be useful to tabulate treatment differences in the centres and assess them informally. If there is evidence of a treatment-by-centre interaction, then an explanation should be sought. It might relate to the characteristics of patients in different centres and further analyses may reveal this. However, usually the interaction cannot be explained and its existence will reduce the impact of the trial results. The concern about a treatment-by-centre interaction also has implications for sample size in each centre. It is preferable to have a moderate number of centres with more patients than a large number of centres with few patients. In the latter case, statistical methods for examining treatment-by-centre interaction are not reliable. From this point of view, it is preferable to have at least 20 patients per treatment in each centre. Where this is not achieved it may not be possible to test for treatment-by-centre interaction. However, some impression of consistency may be achieved by combining centres appropriately. In particular, country in international trials, or region or city in single country trials, may be appropriate groupings.

Subgroup analyses

Clinical trials are designed to investigate a few simple questions, and the primary analysis must be directed at answering these questions. However, there is always a temptation to ask additional questions about particular subgroups such as: 'Is there a treatment difference for males and not for females?' Analysis of subgroups of this type is dangerous when the subgroups are not defined beforehand. The reason is simple. Data on many patient characteristics are collected, and using these data it is possible to define hundreds if not thousands of patient subgroups. It is very likely by chance alone that some of these subgroups will show apparently interesting treatment differences. Differences found as part of this type of 'data dredging' exercise, where the subgroups are not defined in the protocol, should be treated with extreme scepticism.

Although great care is needed in looking at patient subgroups, the exercise can have a place. If a difference between treatments is found in a trial it is useful to demonstrate that the result is broadly consistent in major patient subgroups defined, for example, by factors such as sex, age, centre and disease characteristics. The intention here is to provide assurance that the result is likely to apply to a broad cross-section of patients. Examination of subgroups can also suggest new hypotheses. If there appears to be evidence that the size of the treatment difference is dependent on a particular patient characteristic, then new trials to look at this hypothesis can be designed. Without confirmation from new trials, however, the finding can have no scientific validity.

It is important that the correct statistical method is used to look at treatment differences in patient subgroups. It is not appropriate to perform a separate significance test for each subgroup. The data in Table 5.2 are results from a comparison of ranitidine and placebo in the prevention of gastric damage caused by non-steroidal anti-inflammatory drugs.[21] Although the difference between ranitidine and placebo is similar for males and females, only the significance test for females approaches

Table 5.2   Patients with gastric or duodenal damage graded as two or more on a four point scale.

	Ranitidine	Placebo
Females	14/79 (18%)	24/79 (30%)
Males	19/58 (33%)	20/47 (43%)

Test for interaction $P = 0.617$

significance ($P = 0.064$); that for males ($P = 0.304$) does not. This is primarily because there is a larger subgroup of females. The correct procedure is to perform a test for consistency of the treatment difference across the males and females – in statistical terms to perform a test for treatment by sex interaction. In this case the test is clearly non-significant, showing that the treatment difference is consistent for males and females. Methods for performing such tests can be found in the paper by Koch and Edwards.[22]

If there are factors that are of interest in terms of their interaction with trial treatment, it is helpful to specify them in advance when writing the protocol. Knowledge of the disease and previous trials carried out is important if relevant factors are to be selected. Usually, analyses directed at interactions will be specified as secondary in the protocol. If this approach is adopted then findings of interest are at least not subject to the criticism that they were found only after review of hundreds of possible subgroups.

Intent-to-treat

It is an unavoidable fact that in clinical trials with human patients it is impossible to perform a flawless trial: some patients may not take the trial drug to which they were randomized; patients may fail to return to the clinic and if they do return they may report that they have taken other drugs as well as the trial drug; investigators may fail to make key observations at certain visits; and worst of all it may come to light that the patient did not have the disease of interest at all. One of the most difficult issues in clinical trial methodology is what to do about these deficiencies in the conduct of the trial.

The first thing to do is to avoid as many of the problems as possible. The protocol must define eligible patients clearly and the trial procedures must try and ensure that only those patients are randomized. Follow-up procedures can be arranged so that data is obtained on patients who fail to return. Clear guidance can be given about concomitant medication and if it is an important issue additional unscheduled clinic visits can be allowed to give patients advice if they feel they need more therapy. Careful thought at the time of writing the protocol and the use of expert and committed investigators will minimize the problems occurring with a trial.

Despite the best effort of all involved, there will still remain a number of patients who have not followed the trial protocol satisfactorily. There is much controversy about what should be done with these patients when analysing the trial. The problem revolves around the randomization procedure, which guards against bias in the allocation of treatments to patients, leads to treatment groups that are on average balanced for all observed and unobserved characteristics and is a prerequisite for the validity of significance tests used in analysing the data. If patients are omitted from analyses following randomization then these properties of the randomization procedure are compromised. The intent-to-treat view is that all patients randomized should be analysed so that the benefits of the randomization still apply.

The alternative view is that including patients in the analysis who did not take the drug or did not satisfy all the inclusion criteria or failed to return because of a road traffic accident makes little biological sense. It is not reasonable to expect a drug to show a benefit for the disease in question in these circumstances and so such cases should be excluded. Analysis is then confined to a 'per protocol' analysis, i.e. only patients who fulfill all the major protocol requirements.

The intent-to-treat principle can also be seen to coincide with pragmatic trials.[23] In pragmatic trials the purpose is to determine which is the better treatment to be used in general medical practice. A treatment seen to be better on an intent-to-treat analysis represents the best option for a physician to initiate with the intention of continuing with the regime if possible. An explanatory trial is more concerned with mechanisms of action and as such a per protocol analysis may be more relevant.

The issue of intent-to-treat versus per protocol analysis is still very controversial. An excellent discussion and many additional references are given by Fisher *et al.*[24] There is fairly general support for the intent-to-treat analysis being considered as the primary one and the per protocol analysis as secondary. This approach is now being recommended in many regulatory guidelines. Food and Drug Administration (FDA) guidelines[25] specifically state that an intent-to-treat analysis must be submitted.

Even when an intent-to-treat analysis is the target, there is still room for dicussion about the detail. In general patients will be included whether or not they fulfill all the inclusion/exclusion criteria. Where patients fail to meet the criteria only due to a matter of degree (e.g. they have moderate but not severe symptoms) they would normally be included in the intent-to-treat analysis. However, if the trial is looking at the healing of duodenal ulcer then the intent-to-treat principle would probably be modified to exclude a patient entered with a gastric ulcer for whom no assessment of duodenal ulcer healing is possible. In short-term efficacy trials, such as in the treatment of depression, some assumption has to be made about the response if patients withdraw early. Approaches such as carrying forward the last available response will allow randomized patients who never return to be included in the analysis. Finally, the issue of patients with incomplete data has to be tackled. The only data for these are prerandomization. They can be included in the analysis and classed as failures. Alternatively, if it can be assumed that failure to return is not related to treatment response (a difficult assumption to justify) then a modified intent-to-treat analysis may be appropriate, omitting patients with no follow-up data. Analyses making assumptions about the response in these cases can then be accommodated in the spirit of sensitivity analyses to see the degree to which the modified intent-to-treat analysis will be affected if these cases are put back into the analysis. The Division of Neuropharmacological Drug Products of FDA adopt this approach by defining intent-to-treat as an 'analysis with all patients randomised to treatment who received at least one dose of the assigned treatment and had a subsequent rating on the treatment.'[26]

Meta-analysis

Meta-analysis is a broad term to describe statistical procedures that interpret data arising from several similar clinical trials. It can be a useful way of illuminating controversial areas, particularly where treatment effects are moderate and trials are directed at important but relatively rare events such as death. There are many examples of meta-analyses in the literature and the paper by Boissel *et al.*[27] provides both a detailed review of methodology and examples.

There are three major problems in performing a meta-analysis. The first is the difficulty experienced in finding all trials carried out relevant to the particular issue. In particular, authors may not submit results for negative trials for publication and if they do editors may not accept them. Thus, it can be difficult to be sure that all trials have been included and there may well be a tendency towards positive bias in the trials available. In some areas this problem is being approached by maintaining registers of all trials in progress so that none are lost to sight.

The second problem is that protocols may vary even though the Null Hypothesis is the same. Inclusion/exclusion criteria may be different, the definition of end-points may be different and so on. Even basic criteria such as randomization may not be carried out in all trials. Even if all trials are tracked down there will be decisions to be made in terms of whether to use only randomized trials or only trials with a common end-point definition. The outcome of the meta-analysis is likely to be highly dependent on the trials selected for inclusion.

A third problem relates to the quality of the trials available. This will not be the same for all trials and the logic of mixing high quality trials likely to detect differences with others using poorer methodology is questionable. However, it can be difficult to assess trial quality and so selection of trials on this basis can again be rather subjective. The quality of published information will also be variable and a considerable effort is likely to be required to get original data from investigators.

There seems to be little place for formal meta-analysis in drug development. In most therapeutic areas it is possible to perform a number of distinct multicentre clinical trials all with high power to detect treatment differences. If the results of these are equivocal, it is unlikely that a formal meta-analysis will rescue the situation. It is possible that in some rare situations differences in patient populations and medical practice may obviate a multicentre trial with centres following a common protocol. It would only then be possible to conduct single centre trials with low power trying to ensure sufficient common features to allow a meta-analysis.

Finally, it is of course true that data presented in a submission to a regulatory authority are subjected to an informal meta-analysis. Efficacy and safety overviews are produced because there is a perceived need to bring together all the evidence from all trials. However it is rare for this to require any of the formal analysis techniques used in meta-analysis.

Repeated measures

In clinical trials it is frequently the case that the patient response is measured at a number of time-points. In asthma, for example, patients may record their peak flow daily on diary cards for the duration of the trial. In trials of antidepressants, rating scales will be completed at weekly intervals. Data of this kind are referred to as repeated measures and pose a number of statistical problems. It is not usually correct or useful to perform a significance test at every time-point separately. To do so increases the number of significance tests and consequently the chance of a false positive result. In addition, if a significant result is obtained at a few time-points but not at others it is difficult to know how to react.

The basic principle in handling this situation is to develop a summary to measure the aspect of the response of interest. A number of different summaries are available. It may be appropriate to analyse the last time-point if interest is concentrated on the final condition of the patient. Alternatively, if the general level on treatment is of interest then measures like the average over all the time-points or the 'area under the response curve' may be appropriate. Other possibilities are the maximum or minimum value and the time for which the response is above a critical threshold. Once a summary measure is defined then the analysis is based on significance tests and confidence intervals for the summary. To accompany this plots of the response against time for individual patients are valuable and a plot of the mean response against time may also be useful provided individuals have broadly similar response curves.

The final important point here is that the approach to be adopted to handle the multiple time-points must be specified in the protocol. If attention is concentrated on one time point then this must be designated as the primary end-point in the protocol. If a summary measure is to be used it must be clearly defined in the protocol.

Particular statistical problems in monitoring drug safety

Most would agree that we are better, statistically, at determining whether a medicine is effective than we are at measuring its safety. The problems in measuring efficacy are fewer; a clear hypothesis, agreed scientific models, statistical consensus, volunteers or patients who are disciplined by protocols, well behaved investigators, etc. In trying to decide whether

a medicine is safe we are uncertain about the hypothesis, debate definitions of terms such as serious, probable, etc., require statistical input that
is not readily forthcoming, observe patients who take advice and therapy
from their helpful neighbours and rely on a medical profession whose time
is already heavily committed.

The problems will not go away if we ignore them, nor will they be solved
by writing about them here! But in the hope that statisticians will help
us agree better models, methods and yardsticks for measuring safety we
conclude this chapter by bringing some of the problems out into the open.
Everybody within the industry needs to be clear about the shortcomings
of our current procedures.

The problems are presented in the following order: overall aim, methods,
results and conclusion.

Overall aim in assessing drug safety

Our concept of an adverse reaction is wrong because we focus on
individual patients with case histories possibly warranting a formal report
to some regulatory authority. The more important elements – the drug and
its totality of users – seem of secondary importance. An adverse reaction
is better thought of as a clinical situation suspected to be due to a drug
at a sufficient frequency and level of severity for the medical profession
to wish to be cautioned in order to provide better medical treatment of
patients. Our main focus in assessing drug safety should be the medical
profession and patients rather than regulatory authorities. Therefore, one
problem area is whether we have our emphasis correct.

Methods

Many of our methods for measuring safety are inappropriate. In the past
everybody panicked whenever the media turned to a problem of drug
safety. Our current methods result more from panic than realism – the
data bases are filled with much bureaucratic nonsense and white noise,
the result of political and ethical needs for something to be seen to be done
rather than of decisions about the best scientific methods.

We do not clearly distinguish between our methods for trying to identify
the type A (pharmacologically related, dose-dependent i.e. directly drug-
related reactions) from the more serious type B which occur in a few
susceptible patients.

Type A adverse reactions (the 'augmented')

Type A reactions are better studied along with efficacy in Phase II and
Phase III trials. We need to develop our clinical trial methodology to get
better insight into whether there are any patients at particular risk, such as
the elderly: after all, efficacy studies are used to see if there are subgroups
of people particularly likely to benefit.

We do not need more than a few hundred patients to determine whether
β-blockers can be used to treat hypertension (an efficacy parameter) and
we do not need more than that to determine whether they tend to cause

bradycardia (a safety parameter). To have more than two studies measuring efficacy is scientifically inappropriate (if the study is statistically sound and the trialists trusted), and the same is largely true for typical type A reactions.

To some extent we are assessing type A side effects in clinical trials already, but are we doing it with sufficient determination? Can we not collectively better agree which we should monitor and in how many patients?

Do we underestimate the potential usefulness of withdrawals from clinical trials? Although a good way to identify type A reactions is during clinical trials, even a statistically significant type A effect need not be medically important. A drug may cause bradycardia, but does it matter?

If the end-point of safety is to decide whether we should warn the profession, there seems a lot to be said for using withdrawals for medical reasons as a basis for pooling medically significant as opposed to statistically significant safety information across all clinical trials.

Not only does a medical withdrawal represent a significant degree of incapacity, but, if the clinical trialist decides on drug withdrawal, then this implies a degree of suspicion that the drug could be causing this medically significant event. Clinical trial withdrawals for medical reasons are therefore much more important in estimating safety than some realize. This is especially so if the information is collected internationally on an ongoing basis. Many fairly large Phase IIIb and IV studies are set up prospectively all over the world and many have a control group. Industry could accumulate medical withdrawals from all its controlled drug studies internationally so that one could improve our evaluation of type A adverse reactions.

As we have control data the clinical trial exercise largely involves counting, with the number of patient years' exposure as the denominator. We could largely do away with our perceived need to collect a lot of clinical detail for each clinical withdrawal within each study. Only when we have targeted a particular adverse reaction need we follow up relevant patients in more detail to decide the type of patient, reversibility, time to onset, etc.

Some would say that we are not following up important trial withdrawals adequately (to determine for example the outcome after the drug is discontinued, i.e. whether there is a positive or negative de-challenge, etc.). If this follow-up could be targeted on a limited number of relevant patients with an accepted medical need, trialists might be more motivated to follow up significant patients after a study was 'complete'.

Type B adverse reactions (the 'bizarre')

Where our methods are particularly inappropriate is when we try to use clinical trials to search for type B adverse reactions. Here, clinical trials are inappropriate. Part of the belief that we need data on more than 3000 patients before a marketing licence is approved, with all the extra work involved, is that our gut feeling tells us that we ought to use them to try to seek type B reactions. It is clear statistically that clinical studies are the wrong way to seek type B reactions because the events are too rare for clinical trial methodology. Remember, these are the type of adverse reactions that occur once in, for example, a thousand times. (The patients rather than the drug are unsafe!)

It is also largely misspent effort looking for them in PMS studies as currently designed. Many publications describe how little is achieved, or can be expected to be achieved, when we monitor even 10 000 subjects so far as these type B adverse reactions are concerned. As the Duke of York found in his campaigns, even 10 000 men can be too few!

It is obviously inappropriate that we ignore these rare but very important type B adverse reactions. Where is the most appropriate place to find them? An appropriate place is for consultants nationally, and within each speciality, to keep registers of drugs taken by people presenting with each well recognized type B reaction. This is increasingly being appreciated and registers are being developed in Europe. If the haematologists all over the country could each be persuaded to keep six to eight registers on specific blood dyscrasias (e.g. an agranulocytosis register), each could forward centrally some means of patient identification and the drugs each had taken over a predetermined but relevant time interval. There could be other registers kept by other specialities, e.g. a Stevens Johnson register.

If this information were pooled centrally (possibly by the relevant Royal College) we could all very soon get an idea about whether any new or old drug was overrepresented in any register in relation to its sales. Everybody else's well intentioned methods, which are statistically weak, could be phased out.

There are five main advantages to registers for identifying typical type B reactions: one would not need to wait for an expensive cohort study in a large number of patients to have had continuous exposure over a period of time; although there is no formal control group the pattern of drugs listed on the other registers would serve as a yardstick; not much information would need to be collected at patient registration and the hospital clerk could possibly complete a short slip, including concomitant drugs taken over a predetermined time span; as the hospital clerk would in any case need to inform the patient's general practitioner that their patient had been registered, the general practitioners could possibly be relieved of the task of forwarding a report to the regulatory authority for their patients known to have been incorporated into the registers. Finally, the standards of diagnosis should improve because consultants are better trained in their speciality and have more time for each patient.

Methods for other adverse reactions

If type A adverse reactions were monitored in trials by trialists and by industry pooling clinical trial withdrawals internationally, and well recognized important type B adverse reactions were identified by consultants using registers, what else? The only area where there remains a need for a further method of detection is for very uncommon and novel serious adverse reactions that do not have a register (e.g. practolol's sclerosing peritonitis).

This could be the major role for the general practitioners and the regulators. The appropriate place to detect these formally, apart from publications, is by such as the Yellow Card Scheme, which would have an improved potential for identifying rare unusual reactions immediately postmarketing if the type A and registered type B were excluded. Such government-run schemes are inexpensive and could continue to be used to monitor drugs indefinitely and be applied to all drugs. An optimist could also hope that if reporting were more focused the medical profession could respond by reporting more responsibly.

Record linkage
There has recently been a lot of discussion about the feasibility of record linkage in general practice as a means of simultaneously pooling events of safety import for different drugs. The hope is that we can all use this information to monitor drug safety and some believe that it is simple and feasible because the 'nuts and bolts' exist in computers and the means of linking them are known. You must ask yourself whether you believe that general practitioners have the motivation and resources to feed information of PMS import into some black hole, where subsequent handling seems insufficiently planned in some cases. From the point of view of doctors and patients, goodwill could be lost if such systems were introduced and then did not work. The good conscientious doctor may also stop supporting existing spontaneous schemes which, despite having faults, are currently the best available contribution to the PMS scene made by people in the UK.

Analysing results

The safety hypothesis
Those handling efficacy start from the hypothesis: 'this drug is effective'. One of the problems in drug safety is that we sometimes forget that we do have a vague safety hypothesis which we are testing. It is the same general hypothesis whether evaluating a single case or a group of similar events.
    A clinical situation subsequent to patient(s) receiving a particular drug is due to one of six causes: (i) an adverse reaction to the subject drug; (ii) another coprescribed drug; (iii) an interaction between drugs; (iv) the disease which is being treated by the subject drug; (v) another illness; or (vi) chance or coincidence, i.e. it is a new independent condition. The Null Hypothesis, as for efficacy, should be that the drug does not cause the effect, i.e. that the first of the above options is not true.

Statistical versus medical analysis
Another problem is to determine who is responsible for analysing safety results where a potentially serious issue is thought to exist. Take, for example, a situation where there is a safety committee in a large international double-blind controlled clinical trial. If there is a safety problem, there may well be a conflict of interest between medical members of the safety committee and the statisticians, and this will particularly be the case if the safety committee is doing its monitoring work properly before

the problem becomes statistically significant.

On the one hand we have the medical members of the safety committee wanting appropriate patients to be investigated quickly in considerable clinical detail. The statisticians quite rightly get increasingly bothered by the repeated code breaks, interim data reviews and general interference with Good Clinical Practice (GCP) statistical niceties. Even the hypothesis becomes a subject of debate because the statisticians are there to ensure that the original hypothesis remains the subject of statistical analysis. The safety committee meanwhile suddenly switches its attention to the exact cause of death and identification of particular people at risk. Indeed a *'P'* value with a known pharmacological mechanism seems to me to be medically different from a *'P'* value where the mechanism is not clearly understood.

In analysing safety we need to take into account the specific medical description of particular serious events, the consistency of time to onset between patients, the effect of discontinuing treatment (de-challenge), etc. Statistically the best mathematical models to perform these analyses do not seem to be being discussed, let alone agreed upon.

This is not a criticism of the statisticians, who have been tremendously effective in benefiting the pharmaceutical industry in relation to comparing the efficacy of drugs. Their idea of analysis by intent-to-treat seems appropriate in measuring efficacy – but less so perhaps in monitoring safety. How should a rash be counted against a drug because the person was intended to be treated with a drug but wasn't? How should a death, x months after a drug has been discontinued, be scored in contrast to one occuring at the appropriate time after starting treatment? Statisticians have achieved a tremendous amount for efficacy and I hope soon they will come and help us monitor safety.

The conclusions

We are all fully aware of the difficulties in drawing conclusions in drug safety. For example, the yellow cards are no more than 'floating numerators'. Case control studies only generate 'relative risks', i.e. the rates among those with the effect divided by the rates of those who are controls. They give us the 'odds ratio' – the so-called causal 'force'.

Cohort studies are used to measure 'absolute risks' – they are expensive but do give us the size of the risk. So far so good (if we can get there!).

Ideally we ought to move on, even from measures of absolute risk to consideration of the size of the population potentially at risk. A large risk in few patients, particularly if there is no other treatment available, may be well worth taking. However, even a small risk in a very large potentially exposed population may be too high a price for society to pay. We ought really to be extrapolating medical significance to costs to the total community. We should think in terms of community health rather than results of a study.

Finally, we seem to operate without any notion of epidemiologically agreed yardsticks which can be used to make a decision one way or the other in relation to drug safety. Although a safety conclusion may occasionally be pretty obvious, unless we can come to a consensus as to what we mean by 'significant risk', political and media pressures are going to remain such that an occasional drug is withdrawn from circulation unnecessarily.

Overall summary

People in regulatory authorities, academia and the industry all basically care about the patient and work hard and mean well. The sooner we all can agree to collect more focused safety information, pool it sensibly, follow up appropriate case reports, fulfill our own role well, and look at the data openly and collectively against predetermined yardsticks, the sooner we will be in the position to control the situation. We will then be better able to advise the medical profession and through them protect the patients, our drugs, ourselves and our industry from pressure from lawyers and the media.

References

1. Taves DR (1974). Minimisation: a new method of assigning patients to treatment and control groups. *Clinical Pharmacology and Therapeutics* **15**: 443–53.
2. Pocock SJ, Simon R (1975). Sequential treatment assignment with balancing for prognostic factors in the controlled clinical trial. *Biometrics* **31**: 103–15.
3. Lachin JM (1988). Properties of randomisation in clinical trials: foreword. *Controlled Clinical Trials* **9**: 287–8.
4. Date CJ (1985). An introduction to database systems. Boston, MA: Addison-Wesley.
5. Stern K, Lienthal J, Sauermann W *et al*. (1989). Requirements on an integrated DBMS for data for clinical trials. *Drug Information Journal* **23**: 23–5.
6. Machin D, Campbell MJ (1987) *Statistical Tables for the Design of Clinical Trials*. Oxford: Blackwell.
7. Priestman TJ *et al*. (1990). Results of a randomised, double blind comparative study of ondansetron and metoclopramide in the prevention of nausea and vomiting following high-dose upper abdominal radiation. *Clinical Oncology* **2**: 71–5.
8. Hills M, Armitage P (1979). The two period crossover clinical trial. *British Journal of Clinical Pharmacology* **8**: 7–20.
9. Marty M, Pouillart P, Scholl S *et al*. (1990). Comparison of the 5-hydroxytryptamine (serotonin) antagonist ondansetron (GR38032F) with high-dose metaclopramide in the control of cisplatin-induced emesis. *New England Journal of Medicine* **322**: 816–21.
10. Pocock SJ (1987). *Clinical Trials – A Practical Approach*. Chichester: John Wiley.
11. Makuch R, Simon R (1978). Sample size requirements for evaluating a conservative therapy. *Cancer Treatment Reports* **62**: 1037–40.
12. Cohen J (1977). *Statistical Power Analysis for the Behavioural Sciences*. New York: Academic Press.
13. Temple R (1983). *Difficulties in Evaluating Positive Control Trials*. Proceeding of the Bio-pharmaceutical Section, American Statistical Association (ASA), 143rd Annual Meeting, Toronto, Canada: 1–7.
14. Armitage P, McPherson K, Rowe BC (1969). Repeated significance tests on accumulating data. *Journal of the Royal Statistical Society, A* **132**: 235–44.

15. O'Brien PC, Fleming TR (1979). A multiple testing procedure for clinical trials. *Biometrics* **35**: 549–56.
16. American Psychiatric Association (1987). *Diagnostic and Statistical Manual of Mental Disorders*, 3rd edn, revised: APA.
17. IMS (1988). Definition of migraine. *Cephalalgia* **8 (suppl 7)**.
18. FDA (1977). *Guidelines for the Clinical Evaluation of Anti-infective Drugs*. HEW (FDA) 77–3046. Rockville, ML: FDA.
19. WHO Drug Guideline Series (1983). *Guidelines for the Clinical Investigation of Anxiolytic Drugs*. Copenhagen: WHO.
20. Fleiss JL (1986). Analysis of data from multiclinic trials. *Controlled Clinical Trials* **7**: 267–75.
21. Ehsanullah RSB *et al.* (1988). Prevention of gastroduodenal damage induced by non-steroidal anti-inflamatory drugs. Controlled trial of ranitidine. *British Medical Journal* **297**: 1017–21.
22. Koch GG, Edwards S (1988). *Clinical Trials with Categorical Data. Biopharmaceutical Statistics for Drug Development*. New York: Marcel Dekker.
23. Schwartz D, Lellouch J (1967). Explanatory and pragmatic attitudes in therapeutic trials. *Journal of Chronic Diseases* **20**: 637–48.
24. Fisher LD, Dixon DO, Herson J *et al.* (1990). *Intention to Treat in Clinical Trials. Statistical Issues in Drug Research and Development*. New York: Marcel Dekker.
25. FDA (1988). *Guideline for the Format and Content of the Clinical and Statistical Sections of New Drug Applications*. Rockville, ML: FDA.
26. Leber P (1985). *Form and Content of NDA Reviews: Strategies for the Efficacy Analysis*. Rockville, ML: FDA.
27. Boissel JP, Blanchard J, Panak E (1989). Considerations for the meta-analysis of randomised clinical trials: summary of a panel discussion. *Controlled Clinical Trials* **10**: 254–81.

6

Adverse reactions, postmarketing surveillance and pharmacoepidemiology
Judith K. Jones and Juhana E. Idänpään-Heikkilä

By 1990 it was appreciated that some type of postmarketing monitoring is needed for essentially all prescription pharmaceuticals released onto the market, an awareness bolstered in part by our growing understanding of when and how we learn about the safety and use of pharmaceuticals. We gain a major proportion of the safety information after a drug enters the market and is prescribed in variable ways to a much more diverse population who, in turn, take the drug for durations and on schedules clearly not described or tested before approval. Inevitably, new adverse effects are discovered in this setting and the occurrence of new, unexpected and severe adverse drug reactions (ADRs) leading to widespread publicity has become part of our daily life, affecting patients and their doctors, the pharmaceutical company concerned, regulatory agencies, and even the legal system. Furthermore, in the last two decades such events have invariably become international issues, and it is this latter factor that has both helped increase options for understanding and preventing ADRs, but has also enlarged and complicated the practical solutions.

The past two decades have provided instructive examples, summarized in Table 6.1, which, while creating difficult problems for patients, regulators and manufacturers, clearly have provided the stimulus for expanding research and the beginnings for better benefit/risk decisions.

Why are these events only discovered in the postmarketing phase despite modern methods of drug development, sophisticated medicine

Table 6.1 Some examples of important adverse drug effects

Drug	Effect
Practolol	Oculomucocutaneous syndrome[1–3]
Clioquinol	SMON (subacute myelo-optic neuritis)[4]
Stilboestrol	Vaginal cancer in the second generation[5,6]
Clozapine	Agranulocytosis[7,8]
Phenformin	Lactic acidosis[9,10]
Benoxaprofen	Hepatic and renal disease[11,12]
Zomepirac	Severe allergy and anaphylaxis[13,14]
Osmosin	Bowel perforation[15]
Zimeldine	Guillian–Barré Syndrome[16]

and high technology? After its discovery and synthesis, a new chemical entity (a new drug, therapeutic substance) has to pass relevant toxicological studies in animals and then clinical trials. A product license, registration or new drug approval issued by a health authority is required in most countries before the marketing and prescribing of a new medicine. Although the preclinical and premarketing investigations are carefully performed and assessed, these tests of new and novel medical products do not always discover all possible effects in all patients who will ultimately use the products.

Limitations of premarketing studies

Animal testing

Before exposing humans to new products, animal testing is carried out on healthy, non-diseased animals which are carefully selected, controlled and fed. The overall value of these tests in the development of a drug has long been debated, due to the variable ability to extrapolate findings in animals to humans. The experimental toxicity studies in animals sometimes eliminate otherwise promising therapeutic substances before clinical trials in humans. In other cases, extensive testing has failed to show or predict toxicity that unfortunately occurs when the medicine is used in patients. Many known toxic reactions in humans are not reproducible in animals.[17] Thus, laboratory tests on animals do not provide a wholly reliable method of predicting human toxicity.

Premarketing clinical trials

Phase I–III clinical trials are performed in well controlled conditions in which all effects – both therapeutic and adverse – are carefully recorded (Table 6.2). There are a number of reasons why this extensive clinical research often fails to discover drug safety problems which appear after marketing, as illustrated in Fig. 6.1. In general, the conditions in clinical trials are often artificial, restricted and thus fail to mimic the actual situation when patients are taking their medicine at home. Typically only highly selected relatively healthy patients with clear-cut syndromes are admitted to many trials which are designed primarily to establish efficacy. When drugs are ultimately marketed and prescribed routinely to patients there are many differences from the clinical trial situation that will affect both the actual occurrence and detection of associated adverse events (Table 6.2). The condition of the patients and their drug intake are no longer so well controlled, except in the recent limited experiments with monitored release (such as clozapine in the USA in 1989). Selection of patients is less strict and a wide spectrum of associated diseases and medications are present and may cause interactions or otherwise alter expected effects.

There are several discrete limitations.

- The number of patients exposed to a drug *and* the duration of exposure is limited. Only a few hundred patients may be exposed and ADRs

Table 6.2 Challenges to detecting and quantitating the spectrum of a drug's associated adverse effects: differences between conditions in clinical trials and routine prescribing

Type of data collection	Clinical trials	Routine clinical setting
Setting of observation	Well controlled conditions Limited number of patients Short-term observation	Less or not controlled Wide spectrum of subjects Long-term therapies
Patient factors	Highly selected cases, diseases	Multiple underlying diseases
	Subgroups excluded (e.g. elderly, pregnant) Other unusual concomitant drugs excluded	Variations in diet, race, environment Other concomitant drugs; new indications
Data analysis	Interpretation of observations, focus on efficacy Sparse adverse effect data not easily analysable	Efficacy assumed; events may be over- or underdetected, attributed, reported Interpretation of effects requires epidemiological data often not available yet

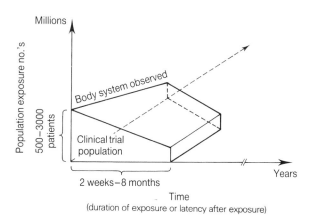

Fig. 6.1 Diagram illustrating the relatively small numbers of patients and the limited data collected in clinical trials prior to marketing a pharmaceutical. In the frontal plan, the progressively smaller numbers of patients observed on chronic use of a drug are shown; thus, seldom are there more than 500 patients observed on a drug for more than 6–12 months, despite the fact that most drugs are tested on over 2000 patients. The third dimension of the diagram illustrates the fact that most trial designs capture data on only a limited number of body systems, so that events occurring may not be observed.

occurring less frequently than 1:100 are therefore not often discovered.

- Clinical trials seldom explore the effects of long-term treatment and reactions that are long delayed remain undetected.
- Elderly subjects, pregnant women, children and infants, and severely ill patients and other subgroups (e.g. hypertensives with type I diabetes, who would clinically be a candidate for an antihypertensive) may be excluded.
- The trial design may limit observation to certain measurements, such as blood count and blood pressure, and miss events not in the protocol (such as muscle pain, menorrhagia or visual changes).
- In some circumstances during premarketing trials the investigator as well as the manufacturer (sponsor) may be biased – good effects are anticipated and adverse effects tend to be neglected, or discounted, except in double-blind studies.

Furthermore, no group of trials, even on thousands of patients, can expect to capture all of the individual differences and idiosyncratic responses which may occur due to such things as variations of diet, use of other drugs or herbs, genetic background and living environment and which are unavoidable.

Thus, when pharmaceuticals are used in larger populations, many new effects may be observed which may be attributed to the drug, and a portion of these events are truly undiscovered drug effects (and a portion are ultimately shown to be manifestations of the underlying disease, especially in complex patients). Furthermore, it is expected that latent and rare or slowly developing reactions may possibly be discovered only after large numbers of patients (up to thousands or millions) are exposed to the drug. These are the conditions that have made the arena of postmarketing drug surveillance (PMS), or 'pharmacoepidemiology' a major challenge in the coming decade. The term 'pharmacoepidemiology' was coined in the early 1980s to more explicitly describe the study (usually postmarketing) of adverse reactions and/or use of drugs in populations. Although to some extent the term has supplanted 'postmarketing surveillance (PMS)', both terms will be used in this discussion. In contrast, the term 'Phase IV', refers to *all* activities involving a drug after marketing, including clinical trials, market open label studies and surveys, as well as pharmacoepidemiology studies.

Need for expeditious approval of promising new drugs

The considerable time necessary for pharmaceutical development, testing and regulatory review for market approval, at present carried out under patents of limited duration, has long been a commercial stimulus for more expedited drug approval. The stimulus has been strengthened by a growing public demand for a more expeditious access to drugs. Both demands have raised the question of a possible 'trade-off' between more rapid approval, and the availability of a truly effective PMS 'system' has long been conceptualized as a potential 'safety net' which could ensure that any undiscovered effects could be routinely discovered after marketing.* However, despite an interest dating back to the late 1970s,[18] and the belief that a 'turn-key' method would serve this purpose, it has since been discovered that discovery, characterization, verification and quantitation of the majority of adverse effects require a 'system' of surveillance with coverage of most diseases and populations. Such a system has been in the process of developing, and will be described briefly in this chapter; however, it is recognized that the ability to predictably capture all new effects of a drug after marketing is still imperfect. Nonetheless, prospects are improving, and recognition of this monitoring capability is likely to ultimately affect the process of drug approval.

Appreciation of the need for population data

With the gradual emergence of epidemiology and data on larger populations than are captured in clinical trials has come appreciation of the growing ability to find and describe much less common events in the natural setting. This has been particularly manifest with use of the large population (e.g. 300 000 to millions) and automated data bases that enable study of a drug in 10–50 000 patients under a variety of conditions. Although the use of data crossnationally for decision making in the approval process has not occurred to any great extent, it is possible it will gain value, as described below.

Recent recognition of the value of postmarketing data for premarket planning

For a number of years, the majority of pharmaceutical manufacturers' marketing departments have used data collected by marketing data firms, notably IMS (International Medical Statistics Plymouth PA; London, and elsewhere) which collects population samples of drug prescribing and dispensing in the majority of developed countries. Use of these and related data concerning drugs similar to a drug positioned for approval and prescribers likely to use the drug has often been part of market planning. With the emergence of epidemiology, it has increasingly been recognized that population-based data describing diseases, their treatment and the behaviour of prescribers and patients with an indicated disease can be of great value both for more effective marketing[19] and for predicting potential problems after marketing (e.g. identifying the morbidity profile of a disease indication, which will be reflected in

---

*It could be argued that the emergence of the formal regulatory definition of the Treatment Investigation New Drug as well as the Phase IIIb trial of drugs involving monitoring large numbers of diverse patients before market approval are variants of answers to this demand, but these topics are beyond the scope of this chapter.

spontaneous reports). This method has had limited exploration using traditional epidemiology data, but its usage promises to increase in the future.

An overview: basic methods and a brief history

Components of PMS

Once a drug is approved for marketing and has an approved data sheet, or label, some type of PMS is operating in almost all developed countries (and many others as well, in the form of various public health surveillance programs, some supported by the World Health Organization (WHO)). The typical modes of surveillance describe the stepwise progression from suspicion of a problem to the actual verification of its causal association with a drug, and finally, quantitation, as follows:

- *Signal generation and collection*, almost always by spontaneous reports of suspected drug reactions
- *Signal verification, hypothesis strengthening and evaluation of potential public health significance*, carried out by evaluation of supporting information in reports on the same or related drugs, careful evaluation of the pharmacology and biological plausibility and, sometimes, actual scrutiny of the cases or records at the medical site, and finally, in some cases, an initial epidemiological study, such as use of an automated population data base, or examination of trends in the suspected disorder relative to expected trends; all of which may contribute to this evaluation of the verity and significance of the signal
- *Hypothesis testing and quantitation*, by one or more structured studies, either epidemiological and/or experimental depending upon the questions

In almost all cases, the initial 'signal' of an ADR continues to be the anecdotal and spontaneous description of unknown and unexpected drug reactions reported to regulatory agencies, pharmaceutical manufacturers or to medical journals. Primary observations can initiate a cluster effect – cumulative reporting of similar cases. These may or may not be based on true associations of the event with a drug. It has now become well accepted that such reports constitute only a 'signal' which:

1. cannot have quantitative meaning, and
2. as outlined, requires complementary data from other sources to allow interpretation, and where needed, quantitation.[18]

Although regulatory decisions are of necessity sometimes made on this preliminary data, it is the appreciation of the pitfalls of single and aggregate ADR reports that has stimulated the growth of structured studies, usually epidemiological, and the emergence of the discipline of 'pharmacoepidemiology' devoted to this area.[20,21]

The pharmacoepidemiological view of this process can best be summarized by a 2 × 2 table categorizing the types of information needed to understand the risk of a drug, as illustrated in Fig. 6.2. As shown in Fig. 6.2a, spontaneous reports of suspected problems primarily represent cases where the disease occurs in persons exposed to the drug; however, there is a potential for misclassification in two ways: (1) the patient may actually *not* be exposed to the suspect drug (or not for an adequate time, or dose); and (2) the patient may not have the designated disease (e.g., the rash is a viral exanthem rather than a drug rash). Furthermore, almost never is there information in a spontaneous reporting system about the precise numbers exposed (A + B) and with (A + C) or without (B + D) the disease. Nor do studies of only the numbers of events in a

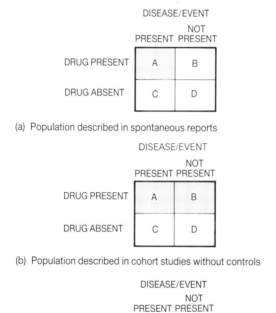

(a) Population described in spontaneous reports

(b) Population described in cohort studies without controls

(c) Population described in case control and controlled cohort studies

Fig. 6.2 Description of a pharmacoepidemiological data using a 2 × 2 table of data on patients exposed to a drug with the event (A); exposed and without the event (B); not exposed and with the event (C); and not exposed and without the event (D). (a) Population described in spontaneous reports; without knowledge of B, C and D no estimate of incidence can be made. (b) Population described in cohort studies without controls; incidence of an event is A/A + B but event cannot be attributed to exposure. (c) Population described in case control studies is roughly equal to the odds ratio [OR = (A × D)/(C × B)].

drug-exposed population (A/A + B; Fig. 6.2b), such as those carried out in the early postmarketing study of cimetidine,[22] provide any information that determines whether the cases found were associated with the drug, or the underlying disease.

The basic methods of pharmacoepidemiology are described by using data from the entire table, (Fig. 6.2c). Thus, *case control* studies start from the *Event* of interest and determine drug exposure in those *with*, and *without*, the defined event. Since case control studies do not estimate the frequency of exposure or frequency of disease in a whole population, they only allow an estimation of *Relative Risk* of a disease or event in the exposed versus that in a non-exposed person. This is estimated roughly by the odds ratio [OR = (A × D)/(B × C)]. This does *not* provide an estimate of incidence. These studies are particularly useful for the study of rare disorders, if there is sufficient drug exposure.

The estimation of incidence of the drug-associated event is possible through *Cohort studies*, which follow forward in time those exposed and (matched patients) not exposed to identify the occurrence of defined events (e.g. liver disease). Since many drug-related events are relatively uncommon (e.g. <1/5000), it is often difficult to carry out sufficiently large cohort studies to appropriately estimate incidence of these rare events, although the availability of large population data bases has helped to increase the limits.

Both types of studies are challenging, often expensive and time consuming, and difficult to conduct, but over the last 10–15 years, more and more such efforts have been launched, gradually creating a growing body of information and useful data on the characteristics, risk factors and frequencies of drug-associated effects. Recent publications have summarized varied explorations of these types of studies[23] as well as standard approaches and calculations for carrying out such studies,[21] and these should be consulted for more thorough discussions and detailed examples of the methods.

After a brief overview of the history of how these approaches to monitoring drug safety evolved, this chapter will first describe the international spontaneous report monitoring as it currently exists, and then provide an overview of the various pharmacoepidemiological approaches and data sources which have developed, concluding with a view of future developments in the postmarketing assessment of drugs.

A brief history

Initial approaches to capturing information on postmarketing experience with drugs were restricted to various efforts to collect reports of suspected problems from clinicians through medical societies (as in the American Medical Association[18] and its counterpart, the Arzneimittelkommission in former West Germany) and through national regulatory bodies such as those of the US Food and Drug Administration (FDA),[18,24] and the UK Yellow Card System,[25] which is one of the earlier well organized national systems which continues to the present).

In 1963 the World Health Assembly urged member states to notify WHO of any steps taken to stop or restrict the use of a drug on account of its supposed dangers and agreed that WHO should inform all members when any such notice was received. This passive attitude later developed into more active monitoring of ADRs in 1968 when a feasibility study was undertaken for a proposed collaborative international scheme.[26] Thereafter member states operating spontaneous reporting systems started to submit ADR records to the WHO Coordinating centre where they were collated and tabulated. WHO now receives 2000 ADR reports every month from over 35 member states and WHO ADR records involve over 1 million reported cases.[27]

Thus, spontaneous notification, or voluntary reporting of ADRs, has, for almost 30 years, been the most widely used national and international method for drug safety monitoring (Table 6.3).

Table 6.3 Some systems used for postmarketing surveillance (PMS) of drug-associated events

Approaches to PMS	Countries
Voluntary reporting	Most European, North American, Japan, Australia, New Zealand, some other Asian, Middle East, S. Africa
Intensified adverse drug reaction reporting	New Zealand
Special registries of drug-associated disorders	USA, Switzerland, Germany, Japan, The Netherlands
Intensive hospital monitoring	USA, Germany, Italy, Switzerland
Multiple case control surveillance	USA, participants in single studies in multiple countries, e.g. Sweden, Spain, etc.
Disease-based case control surveillance	UK, France, other Europe: birth defects. Germany: Stevens Johnson/Lyell Syndrome
Medical record linkage	USA, Canada, UK, The Netherlands (beginning)
Prescription event monitoring	UK; other countries considering
Computers in physician's offices	UK, The Netherlands, Germany

Complementing the early beginnings in spontaneous reporting, a second early approach initiated in the mid 1960s was intensive hospital-based surveillance of ADRs.[28–31] This approach, initiated in Boston and extended internationally, developed a useful data base which provided one of the first sources of quantitative information on ADRs in a postmarketing setting, and the book summarizing the experience[32] continues to serve as a useful resource for understanding general ADR rates for older drugs commonly used in the hospital setting (e.g. penicillins, narcotics). Unfortunately, this Boston-based effort did not continue beyond the 1970s except in selected studies[33] although the Boston Children's Hospital Drug Surveillance program,[21] modelled in a similar manner, continues. A similar, smaller scale effort in Switzerland, the Comprehensive Hospital

Drug Monitoring Berne, has continued to collect useful information to the present.[34] In the 1980s there was a paucity of detailed information in the USA on experience with hospital use of drugs, but this has been addressed more recently.[34-37]

The Boston effort was later extended to survey drug exposure in *ambulatory* populations admitted to hospital for specific disorders which might be drug associated (multiple case-control surveillance).[38] At this time, and thereafter, a number of specific case-control studies of drug-associated conditions such as birth defects were launched, and some are ongoing, especially in the birth defect field.

Also complementing the Boston effort were those of FDA to encourage the development of methodologies to survey drugs. A notable example, later to become a major methodological approach, may have emerged before its value was fully appreciated. One of the earliest *record-linkage* efforts was the FDA funded project at Kaiser Oakland, which collected medical and prescription information on over 140 000 patients from 1969 to 1973.[39] Although not appreciated at the time and discontinued, the data have subsequently been a valuable resource, and retrospectively the approach also, although the need for very large size populations for significant power to detect many drug effects was less well appreciated at the time. In the mid 1970s this same concept of using previously collected diagnosis and prescription data and linking them to discover associations was explored further in the UK and re-emerged in the USA.[8,18,40-42]

Several other types of schemes developed for prospective event-monitoring in general practice such as Registered Release. In 1977 the New Zealand drug regulatory agency launched an Intensified Adverse Drug Reaction Reporting Scheme in which selected drugs are monitored and their ADRs intensively reported using the normal voluntary ADR reporting system.[43] In the UK the concept of 'event recording' was introduced and a Prescription-event Monitoring Programme was started in 1980.[44]

The 1980s saw a literal flurry of activity in the area, with spontaneous reporting increasing several-fold,[45,46] stimulated by the 'epidemic' of drug withdrawals,[47] the development of guidelines for reporting and increased public attention. With increasing activity, the emergence of regular international meetings of the WHO Collaborating Centre for Drug Monitoring, and scientific meetings and publications by what became the 'International Society of Pharmacoepidemiology' (ISPE) in 1989,[20] the proliferation of new approaches has continued, as outlined below.

Voluntary reporting, or spontaneous notification of suspected adverse effects

Overall status worldwide

Beginning in 1969 national systems for spontaneous notification of ADRs were established in Australia, the UK (Yellow Card System), Germany, the USA, Canada, The Netherlands, New Zealand and Sweden, followed by Czechoslovakia, Ireland, Finland, Norway, Japan and many other countries. At present, there are more than 27 countries with organized spontaneous reporting systems, and a number of other countries are beginning to develop systems.[46]

The reporting or spontaneous notification is generally based on the voluntary cooperation of physicians and in the USA some other health care personnel who observe or are told of an event. The word 'spontaneous', or 'voluntary', indicates that not all reactions are reported, for a variety of reasons.

The reporting of ADRs is compulsory for physicians in Sweden,[48] and is an expected professional responsibility of physicians in Germany, who report to either their medical organization (Arzneimittelkommission) or to the government (Bundesgesundheitsamt; BGA). In the USA FDA drug regulations require reporting of all events brought to a manufacturer's attention about their drug. Accordingly, the majority of US ADR reports (85 per cent) are sent to FDA via the pharmaceutical industry[49] while in the UK most of the ADR reports (also 85 per cent) are received directly from doctors.[25] In France there are 33 regional Pharmacovigilance reporting centres staffed by clinical pharmacologists who interact with the reporters to exchange information. Reports collected in the French system are entered directly into the national computer system on a daily basis to allow ongoing current assessment.[50]

Thus, one could describe at least three types of models for spontaneous reporting.

1. *Reports directly to the Health Authority Centre.* This is most often the traditional system in many countries; however, some centres are not in the direct mainstream of drug regulatory activity and drug approval.
2. *The 'Collegial' Model.* In this case, exemplified in France and being tested elsewhere, reporting is to a regional centre, often academically based, as are the French Pharmacovigilance centres, which carry out a dialogue with the reporter as the information is gathered and may provide additional information at that time. Other variants of this exist, e.g. in The Netherlands or in the German Arzneimittlekommission, where the centre may often be able to obtain detailed clinical information on cases of interest.
3. *The Intermediary Model.* This is the predominant model in the USA, where reports are obtained via detail persons or letters and calls to the manufacturer. Since all events are to be reported, this results in a large number of notifications, e.g. 85 per cent of the 60 000+ reports to the US FDA.

It can be argued that each type of system may result in qualitatively and quantitatively different reports. Since the FDA requirement is for reporting of *all events*, whether related of not, this results in a large number of reports which must be evaluated at the agency. This is likely to increase the sensitivity of the surveillance, but makes the data less specific. In contrast, the smaller direct and collegial systems potentially have the capability of capturing higher quality and more complete data. These may be more specific for likely cases, but may also be relatively sensitive, if reporters are alerted. Both types of systems can be biased by many things, ranging from activities of pharmaceutical detail persons to special interests at other centres.

Handling and evaluation of spontaneous reports

Reporting and managing incoming reports
Almost universally a relatively simple form is used to report the suspected ADR to the ADR centre. In most countries the data in ADR report forms and the name of the reporting physician are kept confidential. The majority of national forms request similar information but often differ somewhat. However, two processes have helped develop a consensus on the minimum desired information.

1. The WHO Collaborating Centre for Drug Monitoring, located in Uppsala, has long required a standardized set of information for its international computer data base, and this form was updated in the early 1980s. All data reported to the Centre is provided using this format and standardized WHO terminology.
2. Subsequently, in an effort to simplify the reporting process for multinational companies required to report to multiple countries, a multidisciplinary committee of the Council of International Organizations of Medical Science (CIOMS), composed of both regulators and representatives of the pharmaceutical industry in Europe and the USA, developed a standardized form that is accepted by the regulatory bodies of many countries.[51] An example of this form is shown in Fig. 6.3.

The first report of a suspected drug reaction may only contain some of the data needed, and it is often the task of the collector/evaluator to encourage the busy physician to collaborate with the centre. In a busy regulatory or manufacturer ADR data centre, the decisions about which reports to pursue, and how (letters, calls, faxes, visits), become a continually challenging task. It is generally known, especially in the USA, that follow-up data may be difficult to obtain from busy physicians with many patients whose records may be in one of several sites.

Is there a cause–effect relation?
Regarding those reports describing significant, serious, and especially new or unexpected reactions,* many feel that determination of the likelihood of drug causation is important. Clinical pharmacologists and physicians working in the drug industry, drug regulatory agencies or in clinical

---

*The US FDA regulations require that a report of an association of an event which is unexpected (not in the label) and serious (death, hospitalization, prolonged disability) must be reported within 15 days. [US Codes of Federal Regulations 21:314.80; Federal Register 50(30): 7500, 1985.]

IN CONFIDENCE — REPORT ON SUSPECTED ADVERSE REACTIONS

1. Please report all suspected reactions to recently introduced drugs (identified by a black triangle in the British National Formulary), vaccines, dental or surgical materials, IUCD's, absorbable sutures, contact lenses and associated fluids, and serious or unusual reactions to all agents.

2. Record all other drugs etc, including self-medication, taken in the previous 3 months. With congenital abnormalities, record all drugs taken during pregnancy, and date of last menstrual period.

3. Do not be deterred from reporting because some details are not known.

4. Please report suspected drug interactions.

NAME OF PATIENT (To allow for linkage with other reports for same patient. Please give record number for hospital patients.)	Family name					SEX	AGE or DATE OF BIRTH	WEIGHT (Kg.)
	Forenames							

DRUGS, VACCINES (Inc. Batch No.), DEVICES, MATERIALS etc. (Please give Brand Name if known)	ROUTE	DAILY DOSE	DATE STARTED	DATE ENDED	INDICATION
Suspected drug, etc.					
Other drugs, etc. (Please state if no other drug given.)					

SUSPECTED REACTIONS	STARTED	ENDED	OUTCOME (eg. fatal, recovered)

ADDITIONAL NOTES	REPORTING DOCTOR (Block letters please)
	Name:
	Address:
	Tel. No: Specialty:
	Signature: Date:

If you would like information about other reports associated with the suspected drug, please tick box —

AR/20   250,000 2/83 / 52/4286   C.BROS(N/C) Ltd.

Fig. 6.3 An adverse drug reaction (ADR) report form used in the UK.

research or practice are increasingly confronted by this dilemma. On many occasions this evaluation is further complicated because of wide publicity of the problem and lack of time for in-depth investigations before preliminary decision making. The necessity and importance of a valid and reliable method for identification of an ADR and its cause–effect relation to drug treatment has been strongly emphasized, and a recent review of the various approaches to causality has been carried out.[52,53]

The following basic instructions and guidelines have been useful in assessing the possible cause–effect relation between the suspected drug and the reported adverse reaction. Given that one of the major values of spontaneous notification has been to capture *new* information on new drugs released to market in a very heterogeneous population, the general stance taken by many centres has been to consider a reaction possibly 'drug-related' and then to seek evidence against this theory, in order to avoid missing new, unusual and potentially serious problems such as the practolol syndrome, which initially presented as 'dry eyes'.[3]

Most causality assessments are based on a few simple questions.

1. Did the subject or patient take the drug before the event occurred?
2. Is there a temporal relation between the drug's actual prescription and the suspected reaction? (For example, agranulocytosis, alopecia or jaundice on the second treatment day is not appropriate, but rash or anaphylaxis may well be.)
3. Did the subject or patient improve with withdrawal of the drug (de-challenge)?
4. Was the suspected drug restarted and, if so, did the reaction recur or exacerbate (re-challenge)?
5. Are there concomitant diseases or other drugs (including non-prescription (over-the-counter) drugs, herbs, cosmetics, special diets, etc.) that could also produce this effect or function as a confounding factor?
6. Has this reaction or some of its symptoms occurred in the patient before/after taking this drug or a related drug?
7. Is the event a well known and accepted reaction to this or related drugs (reports in literature, mentioned in labelling or data sheet)?
8. Were drug levels in body fluids or in tissues measured?

Furthermore, data on the following questions is often included.

9. Do the experimental animal studies or the pharmacological actions of the drug support a relation to ADR (biological plausibility)?
10. Did the Phase III clinical trials uncover any similar or related reactions?
11. Has the reaction ever been reported in another country either to the manufacturer or to national ADR registries?
12. Does the reporting doctor agree with my final judgement?
13. Do two or three qualified independent evaluators agree with my judgement?

No consistently reliable method for assigning responsibility of a clinical event to a drug has been devised. The new ADRs are seldom specific and it is known that evaluators differ both in their assessments of them and in their own knowledge and experience and attitudes to drugs. Despite several unsolved problems there have been promising attempts to develop special criteria for ADR evaluation.[54] Some of the more recent approaches have a higher degree of inter-rater agreement, but Pere *et al*,[55] in a very comprehensive analysis of these methods and sources of disagreement, found a considerable complexity in causes of disagreement between methods. The most comprehensive approach to causality is reflected in the Bayesian method for assessing the probability of causation.[56,57] This method assesses the probability of a discrete clinical event, given drug causation, versus the probability of the event, given non-drug causation. This probability is a product of: (1) the Prior Probability, which is based on known data (ideally incidence of drug-caused and non-drug caused); and (2) the Likelihood Ratios of each component of the event (its timing, characteristics, behaviour on de-challenge, and re-challenge). Although controversial because of its difficulty, it has now been automated in varying ways, and is in practical use in premarketing drug evaluation.

Coding of spontaneous reports

The age of computers and the entry of the many reports of suspected reactions into computers, beginning the late 1960s, has necessitated the use of various coding systems to assure the data can be retrieved in some standardized way. One example illustrating this is the following hypothetical report:

> A 40-year-old woman has presented with complaints of nausea, diarrhoea, itching of the skin, fever, malaise, headache and sore tongue 3 days after starting an antibiotic. Over the next 5 days, she subsequently developed jaundice, anorexia and abdominal pain, and became comatose.

Such a report contains many signs (fever, jaundice, coma), and symptoms (nausea, diarrhoea, itching, malaise, headache, sore tongue, anorexia, abdominal pain); however, the practical limitations for many centres with large numbers of reports* requires that a limited number of terms describing the reaction must be used for computer recording (and future retrieval) of the report, even if the entire report is maintained in a file. Thus, the adverse reaction specialty field has required, for both pharmaceutical manufacturers and ADR centres, that some type of standardized coding system be used. Accordingly, with the presence of FDA's adverse reaction staff and WHO's initial data collection system existing in close proximity in Northern Virginia in the late 1960s, the first of an evolving series of adverse reaction thesauri were developed. The initial efforts by FDA resulted in versions of DART (Drug Adverse

*According to FDA, approximately 75 000 reports were received in 1990 (FDA Division of Epidemiology, Office of Epidemiology and Biometrics, personal communication, 1991).

Reaction Terminology) and soon thereafter, COSTART (Coding Symbols for Thesaurus of Adverse Reaction Terms), which were mirrored by WHO's similar but different thesaurus; both have evolved over the years with new versions[58] and, most recently, dictionaries bridging the two have been developed.[59]

Typically, these systems require a limitation on numbers of terms, and most develop conventions for choice of terms (e.g. most serious, no assumptions about syndromes unless designated by original reporter, etc.). Thus, a report such as the above would likely be coded:

FEVER, JAUNDICE, COMA, with possibly other terms added (e.g. NAUSEA, DIARRHOEA, etc.)

As can be seen, retrieval of data in these systems with multiple descriptors, or COSTART terms, can result in a misleading account of events, and this provides the potential for variable interpretations of the *profiles* of drug effects. For example, a computer printout of reports by body system, which includes the above case, might show the following:

'Partial Tabulation of Events'

BODY SYSTEM:	GENERAL	GI	CNS	... etc.
Fever	Jaundice	Coma		

suggesting three discrete events. The appropriate analysis of data in the growing computer banks at the WHO and national centres constitute an interesting challenge to arrive at descriptions of the *actual* types of events associated with a drug.

Uses of spontaneous reports: identification of new hazards, risk evaluation and in-depth studies: using ADR data, drug exposure data to characterize and strengthen a hypothesis

Several events have demonstrated that spontaneous reporting of ADRs can provide a rapid identification of previously unsuspected drug reactions. There are usually three situations that are most likely to produce a hypothesis of a new significant ADR. First, in some cases the reports may describe serious events or findings. Second, the ADR findings or events themselves may be of an unusual nature. Third, the reports may appear more numerous than would be expected in the patient population under treatment. In the following examples (see also Table 6.4), two or all three of these apply at the same time.

- In 1976 The Netherlands Bureau of Adverse Reaction Monitoring had received, in about 4 years, 32 reports of anaphylactic reactions attributed to the use of glafenine – an anti-inflammatory derivative of anthranilic acid.[60] Based on these findings a warning was issued to physicians and the data sheet was accordingly revised. Since then over 100 similar cases have been reported to the same monitoring centre.

- Six patients who developed agranulocytosis while taking aprindine – an anti-arrhythmic drug – were reported to the ADR register in The Netherlands.[60] Two patients died. Since aprindine had been available only for a relatively short time it seemed likely that the drug induced an unacceptably high incidence of this serious complication. A warning was issued. Later more cases were reported and other equally or more efficacious and safer alternative drugs were recommended.
- Tienilic acid, or selacryn, a new uricosuric diuretic was introduced in the USA in 1979. In 1980 it was withdrawn because more than 50 cases of liver damage, including at least four fatalities, had been reported in patients taking the drug.[62] The causal link appeared very probable since liver changes reappeared in cases re-exposed to the drug.
- Zomepirac, a non-steroidal anti-inflammatory drug, was introduced in the USA in 1980 and since then it was prescribed for more than 15 million patients to relieve moderate to severe pain. By February 1983 many hundreds of allergic reactions had been reported to FDA.[13,63] Among them were five deaths due to anaphylaxis. In March 1983 the company withdrew zomepirac temporarily from the market.[14] Subsequent epidemiological study of the phenomenon

Table 6.4 Examples of spontaneous reports as early warning of new adverse drug reactions (ADRs)

Centre and drug	ADR	Outcome/conclusion
The Netherlands (NARD) Glafenine (Glafenan)[60]	Anaphylactic shock	Warning issued to physicians; data sheet revised
Aprindine (Fiboran)[61]	Agranulocytosis	Warning issued
The USA (FDA)		
Tienilic acid (Ticrynafen)[62]	Hepatic injuries	Withdrawal
Zomepirac (Zomax)[63]	Accumulation of serious allergic and anaphylactic reactions	Suspension from the market by the manufacturer
The Finnish ADR Centre		
Clozapine (Leponex)[65]	Agranulocytosis, leukopenia	Withdrawal
Bromocriptine (Parlodel)[67]	Pulmonary infiltrations, pleural effusions and thickening	Warning issued
The UK		
Benoxaprofen (Oraflex,[66] Opren)	Serious liver, gastro-intestinal tract, bone marrow and nail reactions	Suspension of product license (later also elsewhere)
Oestrogen content of oral contraceptives[68–70]	Thromboembolic complications	Move from high-dose to low-dose preparations

suggested that the risk was primarily associated with specific indications, and probably intermittent use of the product.[64]

- Clozapine, a promising antipsychotic drug was approved in Finland in January 1975. Five months later the first case of fatal agranulocytosis in connection with the drug was reported.[65] Within about 7 weeks seven cases of neutropenia and ten cases of agranulocytosis (eight fatal) were reported in Finland. The risk of agranulocytosis was estimated to be 0.5–0.7 per cent on the basis of drug utilization data. The risk was considered unacceptable and clozapine was withdrawn from the Finnish market.[65] Thereafter the drug was withdrawn from several other countries where it had been marketed. However, this product symbolizes a new trend in addressing the known risks of drugs, since it has now been approved for marketing in the USA with a mandated monitoring programme – a new effort to 'manage' risk. The results of this experiment are not yet known, except that the effort to manage this in the USA by required blood tests has been controversial because of cost.

- In an open study of long-term efficacy and safety of high dose (from 20 to 90 mg daily) bromocriptine alone or with levodopa in Parkinson's disease carried out among 123 patients, seven developed pleurisy accompanied by effusion, pleural thickening and pulmonary infiltrations.[67] A warning was issued and these discoveries have initiated further studies to assess the relation of the reports to therapy.

- On the advice of the British Committee on Safety of Medicines (CSM), the Licensing Authority suspended the product license of benoxaprofen in August 1982. The suspension was issued on the basis of over 3500 total ADR reports.[66] Serious ADRs to benoxaprofen (61 deaths) affected various organ systems, particularly the gastrointestinal tract, the liver and bone marrow, skin, eyes and nails.[12]

Between-drug comparisons of the profiles or patterns of ADRs may reveal significant differences among alternative therapeutic agents. Because of under-reporting the absolute incidence of ADRs cannot be measured by a voluntary reporting system. In some instances crude information on comparative safety can be derived by estimating reports per population exposed, although this does not give an estimate of true incidence. If several similar drugs have been introduced to the market at about the same time and, if there are no biases that account for selective reporting of ADRs of one or other of the drugs, comparisons between drugs can be useful to generate or refine hypotheses.

- Inman[44] used the 'Yellow Card' System in the UK (Fig. 6.3; Table 6.4) to study the correlation of morbidity and mortality trends with the various oestrogen containing oral contraceptives.[68,69] Using ADR and sales data from the UK and the Nordic Countries he concluded that there was a clear trend towards a greater risk of thromboembolism with the high-dose oestrogen preparations.[70] These findings early in 1970 contributed in an important way to the safety of oral contraceptive drugs. The low-dose new preparations containing oestrogen 30

1970 contributed in an important way to the safety of oral contraceptive drugs. The low-dose new preparations containing oestrogen 30 μg or less have been introduced. This ADR study also illustrated the value of international cooperation between ADR centres in order to gather sufficient material to permit corroboration of findings.[64]

- The reported lactic acidosis cases and other ADRs to various biguanides between 1965 and 1975 were analysed in Sweden in relation to sales figures and prescriptions (Table 6.5).[9] No differences in age and sex between patients receiving phenformin and metformin were discovered. Between 1975 and 1977 both drugs were used in similar quantities in Sweden. Significantly more cases of lactic acidosis and deaths were reported with phenformin.[9] Phenformin was withdrawn but metformin was left on the Swedish market. Follow-up studies have shown that the risk of lactic acidosis has significantly decreased in the same patient population.
- The Australian Registry of Adverse Drug Reactions received a number of reports between 1972 and 1973 of a neurological syndrome possibly associated with the ingestion of bismuth subgallate powder.[71] Medical practitioners were invited to report details of any similar cases of which they were aware. The additional reports collected defined bismuth encephalopathy, a previously unrecognized or misdiagnosed

Table 6.5 Spontaneous adverse drug reaction (ADR) reports which have led to in-depth drug safety studies and clinically significant conclusions

Centre and drug	ADR	Outcome/conclusion
The Swedish Register		
Biguanides-phenformin[9]	Lactic acidosis deaths	Phenformin withdrawn and replaced with metformin
Phenylpropanolamine[76,77]	Psychic reactions, psychoses in children	Description of reaction; warning; change in product information
The Australian Registry		
Bismuth subgallate[71]	Encephalopathy	Description of bismuth encephalopathy; change in product information
The Finnish and UK Centre		
Emepronium bromide[72,73]	Oesophageal ulcers	Detection of oesophageal erosions and ulcers; change in dosing instructions and product formulation
The Swedish and Finnish Registry		
Nitrofurantoin[78–80]	Eosinophilic lung reaction	Description of the clinical reactions, picture of disease and other ADRs; change in product information

syndrome. Interestingly, a similar syndrome appeared in certain regions in France in the late 1970s, but essentially in no other places, despite use of the compound in other areas.

- Phenylpropanolamine (norephedrine) has been mainly used in mixtures with antihistamines to produce nasal decongestion. In the USA phenylpropanolamine is available in about 60 different over-the-counter preparations (non-prescription drugs) for colds and appetite suppression and is widely used. It is claimed to have relatively little central nervous system stimulating effect, although it is structurally similar to amphetamine. Phenylpropanolamine preparations for paediatric use were increasingly reported in Sweden to cause psychiatric irritation, restlessness, aggression, sleep disturbances and even psychoses in children.[76] These reactions may have been masked by the same kind of symptoms common in paediatric infections.[77]
- The willingness of doctors to report nitrofurantoin-induced eosinophilic lung reactions has offered valuable material for in-depth studies of this syndrome both in Sweden[48] and Finland[78,79] as well as in the UK and Holland.[80]

ADR profile of a drug can differ from country to country. In the past history of ADR surveillance there have been a number of examples suggesting that the ADR profile for a given drug can differ from area to area and from country to country. The occurrence of subacute myelo-optic neuropathy as a reaction to clioquinol primarily in Japan,[4,81] blood dyscrasias to clozapine seen more frequently in Finland[65] and the different incidences of aplastic anaemia due to chloramphenicol[82] are classic, inadequately explained, examples. In addition, the incidence rates of hepatic and thromboembolic complications with oral contraceptives,[83,84] granulocytopenic responses caused by pyrazolone derivatives[85] as well as the tienilic acid (selacryn)-associated hepatic disorders and methyldopa-induced haemolytic anaemia have been claimed to vary from one geographic area to another.[86,87] During the past 10 years the pulmonary hypersensitivity reactions with nitrofurantoin have been reported increasingly in Finland[88] and Sweden[79] whereas this reaction has rarely been reported in former West Germany, the UK or Holland.[80]

There are many possible reasons for these differences.

1. In some cases, there appears to be reasonable suggestion that true genetic differences may exist, as for clioquinol.
2. Geographic differences in the incidence rates of some ADRs may be real and the consequence of other drugs, or dietary or other environmental influences.
3. Reporting is probably never reliably related to the actual occurrence, or incidence, of the events. Studies in Sweden have revealed that only 5–10 per cent of all significant ADRs and about 30–40 per cent of serious ADRs are reported.[89] This may be due to the inability to recognize the ADR, especially if the disease is serious or similar to the ADR. This was clearly seen in the practolol oculomucocutaneous syndrome.
4. On some occasions variations in estimated reports per million

prescriptions may be due to misleading estimates resulting from lack of reliable, precise and comparative drug consumption data. It is well known that prescribing habits and drug utilization figures differ from one country to another.

5. Some doctors are unwilling to cooperate with a government or national agency. Fear of involvement in litigation may decrease the motivation to report ADRs. Many physicians are anxious to publish their discoveries and they may then forget to report them to the centre. The mistaken belief that only safe drugs are allowed on the market and lack of interest or time are other reasons for failure to report suspected drug-induced reactions.

6. They may also be caused by various methodological approaches in ADR monitoring or ADR studies or by more careful attention at one centre or in one country than in others. In smaller countries the members of the medical community generally have more frequent contacts and new observations can be more effectively and easily transmitted, which increases alertness and reporting frequency. Thus, drug monitoring may function more effectively than in countries having a high number of physicians from a variety of educational backgrounds.

It is therefore important to be aware that any novel, new or unexpected adverse reaction or drug event as well as many known reactions may differ widely in the reported rate from one country to another. Clearly there is a need to exercise caution in trying to extrapolate data on ADRs from one area to another.

Spontaneous reporting: advantages and disadvantages

Many events have proved that spontaneous reporting can operate as an effective rapid early warning system, covering the entire population exposed, for previously unknown ADRs; this has not always been the case, however, as contended in Venning's review of spontaneous reports.[74,75,90] This has been especially important where new, recently marketed medicines have caused unexpected, serious side effects. The process of spontaneous reporting is relatively easy and inexpensive, and if the notification card is well designed and understood, it minimizes the physician's time. Phone and computer alternatives to reporting have also been under evaluation. For centres collecting physicians' reports directly, as in most European countries, the process is straightforward. However, centres such as FDA and the German BGA, which must handle a much wider range of 'events', both national and international, have progressively more work as the large number of reports requiring handling increases.

Many published investigations show that ADR data serve as useful starting material for in-depth studies. Accumulation of a large number of case reports sometimes provides valuable additional and complementary data on rare reactions to drugs (Table 6.6), which is one reason that registries have been valuable mechanisms for gathering a better understanding of drug-induced disease.

Table 6.6   Advantages and difficulties with spontaneous reporting

Advantages	Disadvantages

Early warning system
    Most cost effective way to survey
        entire exposed population
    Simple and rapid
    Cheap
	Reporting low
	    Fear of involvement in litigation,
	        'big brother'
	    Guilt feelings toward the patient
	    Anxious to publish first
	    Lack of information on reporting process
	    Time constraints, or lethargy

Qualitatively comprehensive
    Captures data on all body systems
 	
    Provides 'snapshot' of exposed with
        specific problems
    Can provide descriptions of unique
        biological potential risk factors for
        hypothesis testing
	Seldom if ever, quantitative
	    Only 0.01+% of serious adverse
	        drug reactions reported
	    Many factors determine reporting:
	        detection, attribution, actual reporting
	    Industry reporting requirements may
	        skew data

Useful for qualitative overview
    Enables rough qualitative
        comparisons: between drugs,
        patient, countries
    Starting material for in-depth studies
    Complementary data of possible rare
        drug disorders
	Data quality
	    Often incomplete reports
	    Poor understanding by reporter of
	        critical information
	    Reporters may be unwilling to cooperate
	        on detailed follow-up

What reports are optimally desired?

The primary goals of a Spontaneous Reporting System are to:

- Identify unexpected or unknown serious ADRs as soon as possible; when a drug is new it is important to know all possible reactions connected with the new substance.
- Collect sufficient reports, and data on *each report* to evaluate reports in context, in order to make decisions about further study and public health.

It is important to remember that several weak suspicions strengthen each other and when taken together may identify a previously unknown adverse reaction. In many instances spontaneous reporting systems, in particular, have produced the first suspicions of a possible adverse reaction. The isolated suspected reaction has been diagnosed independently by several doctors and in each instance can be associated with prescription of the same drug. If the ADR centre is able to recognize this from the reports, a new ADR may be easily found. Sometimes this is not easy, as we remember in the case of practolol. However, especially in a very new chemical entity, and/or when a drug is being used in a very different population (e.g. neonates) or at a higher dose, all suspected drug-associated reactions or events should be reported.[91] This of course increases the number of signals or 'early warnings' which are often very difficult to evaluate and differentiate from the 'background noise' at the ADR centre.

An important factor in attaining the goals of a spontaneous reporting system relates to the understanding of the potential reporter about how to report, what to report, and when. This was particularly illustrated in the USA, where it was found that many physicians did not know of the FDA reporting process.[92] Furthermore, very few medical schools in most countries teach about ADR reporting, although Australia has made a useful educational film for students and physicians which explains the importance of reporting.

There is a general consensus that certain types of reports should be reported. Listed below are those medical conditions which it may be important to report to the ADR centre.

- When an ADR or drug-induced event is suspected
- Fatal ADRs
- ADR associated with prolonged hospitalization or disability
- Rare, new or unusual ADRs not described in data sheet
- All clinically significant events in newer (<3 years) drugs, especially new chemical entities.

Epidemiological methods to strengthen and test hypotheses

In selected cases where suspicion of a drug effect clearly indicates the need for further investigation, efforts are then made to further investigate and quantify the effect. As described above, almost all efforts have involved application of either cohort or case-control methodology to a particular problem, in a particular population or clinical setting. The choice of method, setting and population has been dependent upon many factors. First, it was limited to sites where the ability to monitor drug intake and clinical events was being carried out, and later, these specific efforts were made in ad hoc studies. With recognition of the importance of linking clinical data with drug use, a search, continuing today, began for those sources where prescriptions were linked by patient identifier to clinical events and outcome, so-called 'record linkage'. Each of these efforts have contributed to the development of a vast array of data resources that can be used in pharmacoepidemiology. Recently a compilation of these resources has been made for several developed countries.[93] This section will consider a few of the major milestones in the development of usable methods and data resources. For a more complete coverage of examples, the reader is referred to some of the excellent compilations appearing in the late 1980s.[18,20,21]

Intensive hospital monitoring

The research programme which in 1971 was named the Boston Collaborative Drug Surveillance Program (BCDSP) has been collecting and analysing information on clinical drug effects since 1966. In the 1970s, over 40 hospitals in seven countries participated in the acute hospital monitoring programme, in which data were collected by nurses who attended ward rounds.[30] This methodology has been described in detail elsewhere.[31]

From the large number of published findings of this programme the following may be mentioned as examples; reactions to large volumes of parenteral fluid,[94] to potassium chloride,[95,96] and to spironolactone, as well as studies on bleeding from heparin in women,[57] reserpine and breast cancer[8,97,126] and oversedation caused by flurazepam in the elderly.[98]

A limitation of acute hospital monitoring is the rather short duration of drug exposure; since a vast majority of drugs are used by outpatients it was concluded in the mid 1970s that hospital monitoring alone may be insufficient for a wide spectrum of ADR surveillance.[99,100] This led to a number of innovative efforts in epidemiological, population monitoring.

Population monitoring

A variety of types of population monitoring have developed over the past two decades. Approaches have been either *ad hoc* or ongoing, usually using the case-control methodology to capture cases of interest. Some examples illustrate this:

- In 1975 the Drug Epidemiology Unit (DEU), now the Slone Epidemiology Unit, of Boston University, began to develop and implement the method of multiple case control surveillance.[38] The strategy involves the interviewing of hospitalized patients with diseases which may be drug-induced and with control diseases to determine prior *outpatient* exposure to drugs. Since multiple suspect diseases served as cases, this approach was developed to provide for the discovery of serious drug-induced illness and the testing of hypotheses, whether generated from within the surveillance system itself or from other sources such as animal experiments, clinical observations, anecdotal reports or ADR registries. The Slone Epidemiology Unit has published a number of studies on birth defects, [101–103] association of myocardial infarction with oral contraceptives,[104] acetylsalicylic acid,[105] oestrogens,[106] coffee drinking[107] and cigarette smoking[108,109] as well as risk factors of various types of cancer.[110,111]
- The Center for Disease Control, charged with monitoring a wide variety of diseases in the US population, has conducted two types of population monitoring of birth defects; one in the local Atlanta Georgia area,[112] the other nationally, in a sample of hospitals, to look for trends in types of birth defects.[113] In the Atlanta survey, ongoing case control surveillance with interview of mothers of deformed infants has been carried out for a number of years, and has been one of the many types of studies that have contributed to a growing understanding of birth defects and the role, or the lack thereof (in the case of Bendectin, or Debendox), of ADRs.[114]

These case control studies are especially useful for study of rare adverse drug reactions, untoward effects occurring after a long duration of use (such as endometrial cancer associated with chronic oestrogen use) and ADRs occurring after a long interval between drug use and adverse event (such as vaginal carcinoma as a next generation malignancy).

Medical record linkage

Modern society with computers and advanced health care has generated a large number of records of vital events (such as birth, marriage and death) and medical events (such as prescriptions for drugs, vaccinations, admissions to hospital, hospital discharges, birth defects, diagnosed cancers, records on morbidity and mortality).[8,115] In some countries these records are nationwide; in other countries they may represent a relevant sample of the population. The greatest advances have been in the USA and Canada, due to development of methods to protect privacy while still using the data for epidemiological research, but in recent years systems have been developing in the UK and The Netherlands, and the potential exists for a number of other efforts. Examples of record linkage in use of the past decade include:

- The Medicaid system in the USA, which provides for payment of medical care for approximately 26 million indigent and/or disabled people of all ages. This is managed through collection of diagnosis and procedure claims from practitioners and health care institutions and prescription claims from pharmacies, which are maintained in computer files by each state.[41] A number of studies by different investigators have been carried out using this data source from different states.[116–119]
- After it was recognized that the inpatient hospital data was not enough, the BCDSP identified a population with records linking outpatient drug use and hospitalizations. This population, the 300 000+ member Health Maintenance Organization of Puget Sound, in Seattle, Washington, has now been a prime source of pharmacopidemiology data for over a decade.[120] A number of studies, by multiple investigators, have described the relation of oestrogens to endometrial cancer,[121] and many other drug disease associations.
- More recent additions to the array of record linkage resources have included the Harvard Health Plan,[122] United Health Care of Minneapolis in the USA, the Saskatchewan Health Care Data source[123] in Canada, and the MEMO, VAMP and AAH Meditel (now IMS International) data sources in the UK[124].

Another type of record linkage is possible in countries that have relatively small populations; a well organized and regulated national health care system coupled with a health insurance system covering the whole country offer selected opportunities for pharmacoepidemiological research. In these countries, the main goal of health care surveillance and morbidity statistics has been to provide data for the further planning and development of the health care system. However, during the past 10 years some use of these registries has been extended to the study of drug safety. The linkage is possible if every person has a single individual identification code in all records and data sources. The most commonly applied personal code has been the social security number.[8] The linkage of existing records does not require special facilities for data collection. In fact in many of the existing systems the 'raw data' are notified to the data bank as a routine part of the daily work on patient medical records.

A typical application of medical record linkage was the testing of the hypothesis suggested by previous studies,[124,125] namely that treatment with reserpine (rauwolfia) may increase the risk of breast cancer. Linkage between two nationwide health surveillance registries in Finland (Cancer Registry and the Drug Embursement Register of Health Insurance System) identified patients with and without breast cancer who had received drugs for hypertension.[126] The relative risks from the use of reserpine, methyldopa and any other synthetic antihypertensive or diuretic as main antihypertensive ranged between 0.19 and 1.11. Thus there was no consistent association found based on this nationwide surveillance.

Record linkage has advantages and disadvantages. The advantages include:

1. Access to *unbiased* data, collected for other reasons, that describe drugs and events.
2. Access, in the large automated sources, to very large cohorts and to rare diseases, thus expanding the horizon of studies of drug effects.
3. Some speed in determining certain factors important when making judgments about studying a problem, since the data is automated and simple questions can be searched rapidly (though actual studies are much more time consuming).

The major disadvantages of record linkage methods in drug safety surveillance are:

1. The strict confidentiality of the data.
2. The fact that the primary data collection is not to capture drug use and ADR but rather for billing purposes, and so has limited accuracy.
3. Because of this latter fact, for any epidemiological study that is testing hypotheses, it is almost always essential to obtain access to medical records to verify diagnosis data, which is often imprecise. In many cases this is difficult.

Prescription event monitoring

A new type of large scale event monitoring was set up in 1980 within the Faculty of Medicine at the University of Southampton.[44] This Drug Safety Research Unit (DSRU) is an independent, non-governmental and non-regulatory unit totally dedicated to the study of the safety of drugs in a large population of patients after the drugs have been released for marketing.

Inman has proposed an event reporting system.[44] According to Inman the term 'event' includes 'any new diagnosis, unexpected deterioration in pre-existing condition, accident or complaint of symptoms which were not present before the treatment was started and which are of sufficient severity to be recorded in the patient's notes, or which lead to referral for a consultation or to hospital admission'.

Prescription event monitoring is dependent on identifying doctors and their patients as the prescriptions pass through about 2000 pricing clerks at the national Prescription Pricing Authority. Relevant prescriptions (i.e. those of study drug and control drug) are photocopied for transmission to DSRU. In the second phase a simple questionnaire is sent to the prescribing doctors asking for a note of any 'events' that may have occurred during the treatments. These events may have been accidental, a change for the better or worse in the patient's condition, a new diagnosis or a suspected ADR reported to the doctor that may have led to referral to hospital. In an ideal situation approximately 10 000 patients both in the study group and control group would be recorded to detect a risk of 0.1 per cent in this system. In the third phase the pattern of events experienced by patients taking the test and control drug are compared in the light of ADR experience from other sources such as from spontaneous ADR registries and morbidity and mortality statistics. If at this stage one or more classes of events appear to be unexpectedly frequent, the preliminary patient data are used for more detailed investigation. The first experiment of DSRU involved about 9000 general practitioners and a preliminary analysis of about 15 800 patients treated with two newly marketed, non-steroidal, anti-inflammatory agents.

One of the major benefits of this method is that the doctors are not aware when the prescription is written that the drug is being monitored and therefore the system is free from selection bias. Therefore prescription event monitoring may both generate and test hypotheses. This system is so far limited to England, which has a suitable national prescription coding procedure. However, the number of drugs that could be monitored at any one time may be limited to four or six per year. Furthermore, prescription event monitoring will probably not be used as a method for surveillance of parenteral drugs, topical preparations or drugs used only intermittently.

Drug surveillance within the pharmaceutical industry[127–131]

Pharmaceutical companies have established a variety of systems to monitor drug safety. The manufacturers receive spontaneous reports of their products directly from patients, hospitals, doctors and pharmacists, and in many countries, reporting of these to the regulatory agency is required, as for the USA.

The great increase in activity in drug monitoring and pharmaco-epidemiology has resulted in the major growth of this discipline within the industry in North America, the UK, Europe and more recently, Japan. A large proportion of research on postmarketing drug safety is funded by the pharmaceutical industry safety departments and, most recently, a consortium started by one company, the RADAR (Risk Assessment of Drugs – Analysis and Response) has now evolved into a foundation funded by many multinational companies with the objective of expanding the knowledge and understanding of drug risk and benefit.[132-134] One major legacy of this has been the formation of national working groups of industry pharmacoepidemiologists, as well as an organization, EPI (Epidemiologists in the Pharmaceutical Industry).[135]

Furthermore, in some countries the drug control legislation may make some form of PMS a condition for an approval of a new drug. This was considered in the late 1970s, and just recently, in early 1991, has been re-introduced as a possible concept for expediting drug approval.[136] In the 1970s Dantrolone sodium, cimetidine, cyclobenzaprine and prazosin were subject to these studies,[137] but the surveillance was claimed to be rather expensive, often promotional and to have seldom been controlled because a competitor is unlikely to agree to the use of his product for what may turn out to be an adverse comparison. Following a period when these studies were viewed negatively, the growth of pharmacoepidemiology and available data and the realization of the crude nature of these studies appears to have resulted in a possible second look at this notion.

Communication of information

It is the duty of the ADR centre to disseminate relevant information on reported cases to the collaborating doctors. In most ADR centres the evaluation of the single report is carried out by a group of reviewers (pharmacologists, clinicians, etc.) using WHO causality grading and terminology.[138] The reporting doctor may receive this evaluation with a letter from the ADR centre. This is important to encourage the practitioner to collaborate with the centre and report his findings in the future.

The Finnish National Centre has tested over 3 years an information program in which the individual reported ADR is released to the manufacturer of the drug but without the name of the reporting doctor and without the name of the patient.[91] This is based on the fact that the manufacturer should know everything about his product including suspected adverse reactions reported to the national ADR centre. Each manufacturer receives annually a computer printout of those ADRs that involve their products. If the company requests additional information the national ADR centre transfers the inquiry to the reporting physician. On some occasions the physician may agree to discuss the topic directly with the manufacturer. However, frequent supplementary requests to the same physician seem to decrease the reporting activity and particularly if disagreements and conflicts between the reporting physician and the manufacturer occur repeatedly.

The ADR centres in the Nordic Countries have regular contact during the year. The Northern European regulatory agencies meet annually and the WHO has, since 1979, arranged every second year an international meeting for drug regulatory agencies. Furthermore, the current ADR findings are discussed in annual WHO meetings for national representatives of those member countries which have ADR monitoring programmes or which are actively interested in ADR surveillance.

Many national centres report back the main ADR discoveries to the doctors and health personnel annually through articles or statements in medical journals.[139] Several clinics and university institutes have research projects in common with ADR centres to investigate in depth some actual and important ADR problems.

The future of postmarketing drug monitoring

There is good reason for optimism about pharmacoepidemiology. A major driving force is the *need* for the type of information that can be provided by fully developed pharmacoepidemiology research. The recognition that fair and unbiased decisions about the benefit and risk of pharmaceuticals, their value and cost in diverse populations, can *only* be made on the basis of adequate studies of these populations, is growing to a consensus. Seldom can spontaneous reports suffice as a basis for judgment, except when the condition is so rare and the use so infrequent that there are not epidemiological alternatives.

This need is supported by growing *means* for carrying out such studies, attributed to the rapid growth of computers and data on populations in many sectors. It is further supported by *more researchers*, who are developing an understanding of epidemiological methods, although this will require much further development.

Countering these *needs, means, and researchers* are important barriers to progress that must be addressed. These include:

1. The typical *need for more than one study* in a separate population to provide answers for difficult problems and to overcome the presence of bias in even the most elegant research designs. Although this applies to most experimental studies, including clinical trials, the cost and time consuming nature of pharmacoepidemiological studies makes this more difficult. Early recognition of this factor may address the delay in providing answers, and further methods to diminish bias are likely to evolve. Meanwhile, general education of decision makers as to the values and limitations of the data will help in understanding this need.
2. The lack of access to important medical data. This problem occurs nationally in certain countries where privacy protection laws prevent access to medical data even under the strictest precautions. It also occurs due to destruction or loss of medical records after 5–10 years. These are both problems which are potentially solvable in the next decade.

In the next decade the field of pharmacoepidemiology is likely to grow, and it is likely that bridges from this field will extend to diverse areas reflecting this hybrid specialty's origins. Thus, some research may bridge to economics, to studies of computers in the medical environment and other social research, to communications research, and certainly to environmental epidemiology and to pharmacological, pharmacokinetic, pharmacodynamic, genetic, and molecular biology research, as the need for biological plausibility lurks behind each epidemiological finding.

In this age, where worldwide communication and advanced computerization creates a propitious environment not present in earlier years, pharmacoepidemiology, the *study of pharmaceuticals* (complex in themselves even in simple organisms) *in populations* (whose complexity is not yet appreciated), provides an exciting challenge, not only for the decade, but likely for many years thereafter.

References

1. Felix R, Ives FA (1974). Skin reactions to practolol. *British Medical Journal* **2**: 333.
2. Wright P (1974). Skin reactions to practolol. *British Medical Journal* **2**: 560.
3. Brown P, Baddley H, Read AE *et al.* (1974). Sclerosing peritonitis. An unusual reaction to a β-adrenergic blocking drug (practolol). *Lancet* **2**: 1477–81.
4. Tsubaki T, Homna Y, Hoski M (1971). Neurological syndrome associated with clioquinol. *Lancet* **1**: 696.
5. Herbst AL, Ulfelder H, Poskanzer DC (1971). Adenocarcinoma of the vagina. Association of maternal stilbestrol therapy with tumor appearance in young women. *New England Journal of Medicine* **284**: 878–81.
6. Herbst AL *et al.* (1975). Prenatal exposure to stilbestrol. *New England Journal of Medicine* **292**: 334.
7. Idänpään-Heikkilä J, Alhava E, Olkinuora M *et al.* (1977). Agranulocytosis during treatment with clozapine. *European Journal of Clinical Pharmacology* **11**: 193–8.
8. Idänpään-Heikkilä J (1977). Population monitoring: medical record linkage for drug safety surveillance. In Gross FH, Inman WHW (eds.) *Drug Monitoring*. London: Academic Press: 17–26.
9. Bergman U, Boman G, Wilholm BE (1978). Epidemiology of adverse drug reactions to phenformin and metformin. *British Medical Journal* **2**: 464–6.
10. Korhonen T, Idänpään-Heikkilä J, Aro A (1978). Biguanide induced lactic acidosis in Finland. *European Journal of Clinical Pharmacology* **15**: 407.
11. Anon (1982). Lilly suspends benoxaprofen worldwide. *Scrip* **717**: 1.
12. del Favero A (1983). Anti-inflammatory analgesics and drugs used in rheumatoid arthritis and gout. In Dukes MNG (ed.) *Side Effects of Drugs, annual 7/1983.* Amsterdam: Exerpta Medica: 109–12.
13. Anon (1983). FDA's Zomax ADR reports. *Scrip* **776**: 13.
14. Anon (1983). Zomax withdrawn from market after fatal reactions. *The Pharmaceutical Journal* **230**: 299.
15. Anon (1983). *Scrip* **82**: 1.
16. Anon (1983). Bulletin from Swedish Adverse Drug Reactions Advisory Committee 39/40.
17. Gross FH (1982). The scientific basis of drug safety regulations. In Auriche M *et al.* (eds.) *Drug Safety, Progress and Controversies.* London: Pergamon Press: 9–18.
18. Jones JK, Faich GA, Anello C. (1985). Post-marketing surveillance in the general population – the U.S.A. In Inman WHW (ed.) *Monitoring for Drug Safety,* 2nd edn. Lancaster: MTP Press Limited: 153–63.
19. Guess H (1989). Personal communication.
20. Edlavich S (1990). Pharmacoepidemiology: a Banner Year. *Journal of Clinical Research and Pharmacoepidemiology* **4**: 107–11.

21. Strom BL (ed.) (1989). *Pharmacoepidemiology*. New York: Churchill Livingstone.
22. Humphries TJ, Myerson RM, Gifford LM *et al*. (1984). A unique postmarket outpatient surveillance program of cimetidine: report on phase II and final summary. *American Journal of Gastroenterology* **79**: 593.
23. Edlavich SA (1989). *Pharmacoepidemiology*, Vol 1. Chelsea, MI: Lewis Publishers.
24. Faich GA (1986). Adverse drug reaction monitoring. *New England Journal of Medicine* **314**: 1589.
25. Inman WHW (1980). The United Kingdom. In Inman WHW (ed.) *Monitoring for Drug Safety*. Philadelphia: JB Lippincott Company: 9–48.
26. Royall BW (1971). International aspects of drug monitoring: role of the World Health Organization. *WHO Chronicle* **25**: 445.
27. ten Harn M (1992). WHO's role in international ADR monitoring. *Post Marketing Surveillance* **5**: 223–30.
28. Slone D, Jick H, Horda I *et al*. (1966): Drug surveillance utilizing nurse monitors. *Lancet* **2**: 901.
29. Lawson DH, Shapiro S, Slone D *et al*. (1979). Drug surveillance: problems and challenges. *Pediatric Clinics of North America* **19**: 117.
30. Jick H (1977). In-patient hospital surveillance for acute effects. In Colombo F *et al*. (eds.) *Epidemiological Evaluation of Drugs*. Amsterdam: Elsevier: 47–53.
31. Lawson DH, Beard K (1989). Intensive hospital-based cohort studies. In Strom B (ed.) *Pharmacoepidemiology*. New York: Churchill Livingstone: 135–48.
32. Miller RR, Greenblatt D (1976). *Drug Effects in Hospitalized Patients*. New York: John Wiley & Sons.
33. Jick H, Andrews B, Tilson H *et al*. (1989). Atricurium – a post marketing surveillance study: methods and U.S. experience. *British Journal of Anaesthesiology* **62**: 590–95.
34. Torok M, Zoppi M, Winzenried P *et al*. (1982). Drug-related death among 17,285 inpatients in the divisions of internal medicine of two teaching hospitals in Berne, 1974–1980. In Manell P, Johansson SG, (eds.) *The Impact of Computer Technology on Drug Information*. Amsterdam: North Holland Press: 79.
35. Jones JK (1989). Inpatient data bases. In Strom BL (ed.) *Pharmacoepidemiology*. New York: Churchill Livingstone: 213–28.
36. Grasela TH, Schentag JJ (1987). A clinical pharmacy-oriented drug surveillance network: I. Program description. *Drug Intelligence and Clinical Pharmacology* **21**: 902–08.
37. Evans RS, Larsen RA, Burke JP (1986). Computer surveillance of hospital acquired infections and antibiotic use. *Journal of the American Medical Association* **256**: 1007–11.
38. Slone D, Shapiro S, Miettinen OS (1977). Case-control surveillance of serious illness attributable to ambulatory drug use. In Colombo F *et al*. (eds.) *Epidemiological Evaluation of Drugs*. Amsterdam: Elsevier: 59–70.
39. Friedman G (1989). Kaiser Permanente Medical Care Program: Northern California and other regions. In Strom BL (ed.) *Pharmacoepidemiology*. New York: Churchill Livingstone: 161–72.
40. Skegg DCG (1980). Medical record linkage. In Inman WHW (ed.) *Monitoring for Drug Safety*. Philadelphia: JB Lippincott Company: 337–48.
41. Westerholm B, Wiholm BE (1982). Experiences of Registries in drug safety assessment in Sweden. In Auriche M *et al*. (eds.) *Drug Safety, Progress and*

Controversies. Oxford: Pergamon Press: 93–103.

42. Jones JK, van de Carr SW, Rosa F *et al.* (1984). Medicaid drug-event data: an emerging tool for evaluation of drug risk. *Acta Medica Scandinavica* **683**: 127–34.

43. Phillips JS (1982). Post-marketing safety assessment, New Zealand experience. In Auriche M *et al.* (eds.) *Drug Safety, Progress and Controversies*. Oxford: Pergamon Press: 143–50.

44. Inman WHW (1981). Postmarketing surveillance of adverse reactions in general practice. I: Search for new methods. *British Medical Journal* **282**: 1131. II: Prescription-event monitoring at the University of Southampton. *British Medical Journal* **282**: 1216.

45. Baum C, Anello C (1989). The spontaneous reporting system in the United States. In Strom BL (ed.) *Pharmacoepidemiology*. New York: Churchill Livingstone: 107–18.

46. Wiholm B, Olsson S (1989). Spontaneous reporting systems outside the United States. In Strom BL (ed.) *Pharmacoepidemiology*. New York: Churchill Livingstone: 119–34.

47. Panel Discussion (1990). The impact of drug withdrawals. In Naranjo C, Jones J (eds.) *Idiosyncratic Adverse Drug Reactions: Impact on Drug Development and Clinical Use After Marketing*. Amsterdam: Excerpta Medica: 78.

48. Boman G (1980). The Nordic Countries. In Inman WHW (ed.) *Monitoring for Drug Safety*. Philadelphia: JB Lippincott Company: 109–13.

49. Jones JK (1981). Suspected drug-induced hepatic reactions reported to the FDA's adverse reaction system. *Seminars in Liver Disease* **1**: 157.

50. Moore N, Paux G, Begaud B *et al.* (1985). Adverse drug reaction monitoring: doing it the French way. *Lancet*: **ii**: 1056–8.

51. CIOMS (1990). *International Reporting of Adverse Drug Reactions. Final Report of the CIOMS Working Group*. Geneva: Council of International Organizations of Medical Science.

52. Jones JK (1989). Determining causation from case reports. In Strom BL (ed.) *Pharmacoepidemiology*. New York: Churchill Livingstone.

53. Jones JK (1991). Approaches to evaluating causation of suspected drug reactions. In Strom BL, Velo G (eds.) *Drug Epidemiology and Post-Marketing Surveillance*. NATO ASI Series. New York: Plenum.

54. Jones JK, Herman RL (eds.) (1986). The Future of Adverse Drug Reaction Diagnosis: Computers, Clinical Judgement and the Logic of Uncertainty. Proceedings of the Drug Information Association Workshop, Arlington, VA February 1986. *Drug Information Journal* **20**: 383–566.

55. Pere JC, Begaud B, Harumbaru F *et al.* (1986). Computerized comparison of six adverse drug reaction assessment procedures. *Clinical and Pharmacological Therapy* **40**: 451.

56. Naranjo CA, Lanctôt KL, Lane DA (1990). The Bayesian differential diagnosis of neutropenia associated with antiarrhythmic agents. *Journal of Clinical Pharmacology*, **30**: 120–27.

57. Lane DA, Kramer MS, Hutchinson TA *et al.* (1987). The causality assessment of adverse drug reactions using a Bayesian approach. *Pharmaceutical Medicine* **2**: 265.

58. FDA (1990). *COSTART (Coding Symbols for Thesaurus of Adverse Reaction Terms*. Rockville, MD: FDA.

59. Nissman EF, Iezzoni DG (1989). Report on a WHO ART-COSTART Translation Project. *Drug Information Journal* **23**: 75.

60. Meyboom RHB (1976). Anafylaxie na het bebruik van glafenine. *Nederlands Tijdschrift voor Geneeskunde (Amsterdam)* **120**: 296.

61. van Leeuwen R, Meyboom, RHB (1976). Agranulocytosis and aprindine. *Lancet* **2**: 1137.
62. Anon (1980). Ticrynafen recalled. *FDA Drug Bulletin* **10**: 3.
63. Anon (1983). McNeil asking for return of Zomax from patients to pharmacies until relabelling on anaphylactic reaction is complete: less than 0.01% incidence. F–D–C Reports. *The Pink Sheet* **45**: 19.
64. Strom BL, Carson JL, Morse ML *et al.* (1987). The effect of indication on hypersensitivity reactions associated with nonsteroidal anti-inflammatory drugs. *Arthritis and Rheumatism* **30**: 1142.
65. Idänpään-Heikkilä J (1990). Clozapine-induced blood disorders in 1975–1989 in Finland: a review of a drug from withdrawal to re-approval with restrictions. In Naranjo C, Jones J (eds.). *Idiosyncratic Adverse Drug Reactions: Impact on Drug Development and Clinical Use after Marketing.* International Congress Series 878. Amsterdam: Excerpta Medica: 45–56.
66. Anon (1982). Lilly suspends benoxaprofen worldwide. *Scrip* **717**: 1.
67. Rinne UK (1981). Pleuropulmonary changes during long-term bromocriptine treatment for Parkinson's disease. *Lancet* **1**: 44.
68. Inman WHW (1970). Role of drug-reaction monitoring in the investigation of thromboembolism and 'The Pill'. *British Medical Bulletin* **26**: 248.
69. Inman WHW, Vessey MP (1968). Investigation of deaths from pulmonary, coronary and cerebral thrombosis and embolism in women of childbearing age. *British Medical Journal* **2**: 193.
70. Inman, WHW, Vessey MP, Westerholm B *et al.* (1970). Thromboembolic disease and the steroidal content of oral contraceptives. *British Medical Journal* **2**: 203.
71. Lowe DJ (1974). Adverse effects of bismuth subgallate. A further report from the Australian Drug Evaluation Committee. *Medical Journal of Australia* **2**: 664.
72. Puhakka HJ (1978). Drug-induced corrosive injury. *British Medical Journal of Laryngology and Otolaryngology* **92**: 927.
73. Collins FJ, Matthews HR, Baker SE *et al.* (1979). Drug-induced oesophageal injury. *British Medical Journal* **1**: 1673–6.
74. Venning GR (1983). Identification of adverse reactions to new drugs. I. What have been the important adverse reactions since thalidomide? *British Medical Journal* **286**: 199–202.
75. Venning GR (1983). Identification of adverse reactions to new drugs. II. How were 18 important adverse reactions discovered and with what delays? *British Medical Journal* **286**: 289–92.
76. Norvenius G, Widerlow E, Lonnerholm G (1979). Phenylpropanolamine and mental disturbances. *Lancet* **2**: 1367.
77. Lopatin AS (1981). CNS stimulants and anorectic agents. In Dukes MNG (ed.) *Side Effects of Drugs*, Annual 5. Amsterdam: Excerpta Medica: 9–11.
78. Sovijarvi ARA, Lemola M, Stenius B *et al.* (1977). Nitrofurantoin-induced acute, subacute and chronic pulmonary reactions. *Scandinavian Journal of Respiratory Diseases* **58**: 41.
79. Holmberg L, Boman G, Bottiger LE *et al.* (1980). Adverse reactions to nitrofurantoin. Analysis of 921 reports. *American Journal of Medicine* **69**: 733–8
80. Penn RG, Griffin JP (1982). Adverse reactions to nitrofurantoin in the United Kingdom, Sweden and Holland. *British Medical Journal* **284**: 1440.
81. Dukes MNG (1981). The paradox of clioquinol and SMON. In d'Arcy PF, Griffin JP (eds.). *Iatrogenic Diseases*, Update 1981. Oxford: Oxford University Press: 105–13.
82. Gross FH (1980). The clinical pharmacologist. In Inman WHW (ed.) *Monitoring for Drug Safety*. Philadelphia: JB Lippincott Company: 627–35.

83. Jick H *et al*. (1969). Venous thromboembolic disease and ABO blood type. *Lancet*, i: 539.
84. Sherlock S (1972). Liver disease due to drugs. In Meyler L, Peck HM (eds.) *Drug Induced Diseases*, Vol 4, Amsterdam: Elsevier: 256
85. del Favero A (1981). Anti-inflammatory analgesics and drugs used in rheumatism and gout. In Dukes MNG (ed.). *Side Effects of Drugs*, Annual 6. Amsterdam: Excerpta Medica: 88–117.
86. Burke EJ (1981). Diuretic drugs. In Dukes MNG (ed.) *Side Effects of Drugs*, Annual 5. Amsterdam: Excerpta Medica: 228–31.
87. Sedat YK, Vawda EI (1986). The Coombs' test and methyldopa. *Lancet* i: 427.
88. Idänpään-Heikkilä J, Tuomisto J (1983). Miscellaneous antibacterial and antiviral drugs. In Dukes MNG (ed.) *Side Effects of Drugs*, Annual 7. Amsterdam: Excerpta Medica: 301–7.
89. Böttiger LE, Westerholm B (1979). Drug induced blood dyscrasias in Sweden. *British Medical Journal* 3: 339.
90. Venning GR (1983). Identification of adverse reactions to new drugs. III. Alerting processes and early warning systems. *British Medical Journal* **286**: 458–60.
91. Idänpään-Heikkilä J (1982). Spontaneous notification. In Auriche M *et al*. (eds.) *Drug Safety, Progress and Controversies*. London: Pergamon Press: 73–82.
92. Scott HD, Thacher-Renshaw A, Rosenbaum SE *et al*. (1990). Physician reporting of ADR's – Rhode Island. *Journal of the American Medical Association* **263**: 1785–8.
93. Jones JK (ed.) (1989). *International Drug Benefit/Risk Resource Handbook*, vol I: U.S. & Canada; vol II: UK; vol III: Europe. Washington DC: Pharma International & The Degge Group, Ltd.
94. Lawson DH (1977). Intravenous fluids in medical inpatients. *British Journal of Clinical Pharmacology* 4: 299.
95. Jick H, Slone D, Borda IT *et al*. (1968). Efficacy and toxicity of heparin in relation to age and sex. *New England Journal of Medicine* **279**: 284.
96. Greenblatt DJ, Koch-Weser J (1973). Adverse reactions to spironolactone. *Journal of the American Medical Association* **225**: 40.
97. Boston Collaborative Drug Surveillance Program (1974). Reserpine and breast cancer. *Lancet* 2: 669.
98. Greenblatt DJ, Allan MD, Shader RI (1977). Toxicity of high dose flurazepam in the elderly. *Clinical Pharmacology and Therapeutics* 21: 355.
99. Dollery CT, Rawlins MD (1977). Monitoring adverse reactions to new drugs. *British Medical Journal* 1: 96
100. Lawson DH, Henry DA (1977). Monitoring adverse reactions to new drugs: restricted release or monitored release? *British Medical Journal* 1: 691.
101. Hartz SC, Heinonen OP, Shapiro S *et al*. (1975). Antenatal exposure to meprobamate and chlordiazexopide in relation to malformations, mental development and childhood mortality. *New England Journal of Medicine* **292**: 726.
102. Shapiro S, Slone D, Hartz SC *et al*. (1976). Anticonvulsants and parental epilepsy in the development of birth defects. *Lancet* 1: 272.
103. Heinonen OP, Slone D, Monson RR *et al*. (1977). Cardiovascular birth defects and antenatal exposure to female sex hormones. *New England Journal of Medicine* **296**: 67.
104. Shapiro S, Slone D, Rosenberg L *et al*. (1979). Oral contraceptive use in relation to myocardial infarction. *Lancet* 1: 743.
105. Rosenberg L, Slone D, Shapiro S *et al*. (1982). Aspirin and myocardial

infarction in young women. *American Journal of Public Health* **72**: 389–91.

106. Rosenberg L, Slone D, Shapiro S *et al.* (1980). Noncontraceptive estrogens and myocardial infarction in young women. *Journal of the American Medical Association* **244**: 339.

107. Rosenberg L, Slone D, Shapiro S *et al.* (1980). Coffee drinking and myocardial infarction in young women. *American Journal of Epidemiology* **111**: 675.

108. Slone S, Shapiro S, Rosenberg L *et al.* (1978). Relation of cigarette smoking to myocardial infaction in young women. *New England Journal of Medicine* **298**: 1273.

109. Rosenberg L, Kaufman DW, Shapiro S *et al.* (1980). Cigarette smoking and risk of premature myocardial infarction. *Primary Cardiology* **6**: 11.

110. Shapiro S, Kaufman DW, Slone D (1980). Recent and past use of conjugated estrogens in relation to adenocarcinoma of the endometrium. *New England Journal of Medicine* **303**: 485.

111. Helmrich SP, Slone D, Shapiro S *et al.* (1983). Risk factors for breast cancer. *American Journal of Epidemiology* **1**: 35.

112. Cordero JF, Oakley GP, Greenberg F *et al.* (1981). Is Bendectin a teratogen? *Journal of the American Medical Association* **245**: 2307–10.

113. Centers for Disease Control (1988). *Congenital Malformations – Surveillance (Atlanta, GA).* Washington DC: US Department of Health and Human Services, Public Health Service.

114. McCredie J, Kricker A, Elliot J *et al.* (1984). The innocent bystander: doxylamine-dicyclomine/pyridoxine and congenital limb defects. *Medical Journal of Australia* **140**: 525–7.

115. Skegg DCG (1978). Use of record linkage for drug surveillance: a progress report. In Ducrot H *et al.* (eds.) *Computer Aid to Drug Therapy and to Drug Monitoring.* Amsterdam: Elsevier: 77–83.

116. Ray WA, Griffin MR, Shaffner W *et al.* (1987). Psychotropic drug use and the risk of hip fracture. *New England Journal of Medicine* **316**: 363.

117. Carson JL, Strom BL, Soper KA *et al.* (1987). The association of nonsteroidal antiinflamatory drugs with upper gastrointestinal tract bleeding. *Archives of Internal Medicine* **147**: 85.

118. Strom BL, Ravikiran MT, Morse ML *et al.* (1986) Oral contraceptives and other risk factors for gall bladder disease. *Clinical and Pharmacological Therapy* **39**: 335.

119. Avorn J, Everitt DE, Weiss S (1986). Increased antidepressant use in patients prescribed beta-blockers. *Journal of the American Medical Association* **255**: 357.

120. Jick H, Madsen SK, Nudelman PM *et al.* (1984). Postmarketing follow-up at Group Health Cooperative of Puget Sound. *Pharmacotherapy* **4**: 99.

121. Jick H, Watkins RN, Hunter JR *et al.* (1979). Replacement estrogens and endometrial cancer. *New England Journal of Medicine* **300**: 218.

122. Platt R, Stryker WS, Komaroff AL (1988). Pharmacoepidemiology in hospitals using automated data systems. In Tilson H (ed.) Progress in Pharmacoepidemiology. *American Journal of Preventitive Medicine* **4 (suppl. 2)**: 39

123. Strand L, West R (1989). Health data bases in Saskatchewan. In Strom BL (ed.) *Pharmacoepidemiology.* New York: Churchill Livingstone: 189–200.

124. Heinonen OP, Shapiro S, Tuominen L *et al.* (1974). Reserpine use in relation to breast cancer. *Lancet* **2**: 675.

125. Armstrong B, Stevens N, Doll R (1974). Retrospective study of association between use of rauwolfia and breast cancer in English women. *Lancet* **2**: 674.

126. Aromaa A, Hakama M, Hakulinen T *et al.* (1976). Breast cancer and use of rauwolfia and other antihypertensive agents in hypertensive patients:

a nationwide case-control study in Finland. *International Journal of Cancer* **18**: 727.

127. Crawford M, Berneker G-C, Pinto O de S (1980). The pharmaceutical industry. In Inman WHW (ed.) *Monitoring for Drug Safety*. Philadelphia: JB Lippincott Company: 165–88.

128. Venulet J (1977). Methods of monitoring adverse reactions to drugs. *Progress in Drug Research* **21**: 231.

129. Frisch JM (1972). Monitoring of adverse reactions by a pharmaceutical company after marketing. In Richards DJ, Rondel RK (eds.) *Adverse Drug Reactions: Their Prediction, Detection and Assessment*. Edinburgh: Churchill Livingstone: 33–9.

130. Jouhar AJ (1977). *An Example of Post-marketing Drug Surveillance by a Pharmaceutical Company*. Presented at the Oxford Drug Monitoring Conference (Symposium on Drug Monitoring in General Practice), June 23rd–24th, 1977. Oxford.

131. Steichenwein SM, Blomer R (1982). Computer documentation of adverse drug reactions within a multinational pharmaceutical company. *Drug Information Journal* **16**: 109.

132. Horisberger B, Dinkel R (eds.) (1989). *The Perception and Management of Drug Safety Risks*. Berlin: Springer-Verlag.

133. Shimizu YU, Tanaka Y, Jones JK et al. (1990). *Improving Drug Safety: The Assessment, Management and Communication of the Therapeutic Benefits and Risks of Pharmaceutical Products*. Tokyo: Pharma International.

134. Dinkel R, Horisberger B, Tolo K (eds.) (1991). *Improving Drug Safety – A Joint Responsibility*. Berlin: Springer-Verlag.

135. Bruppacher R, Tilson H (1991). Personal communication.

136. *The Pink Sheet*, Jan 21, 1991.

137. Ruskin A, Anello C (1980). The United States of America. In Inman WHW (ed.) *Monitoring for Drug Safety*. Philadelphia: JB Lippincott Company: 115–27

138. Dunne JF (1980). World Health Organization. In Inman WHW (ed.) *Monitoring for Drug Safety*. Philadelphia: JB Lippincott Company: 133–9.

139. Kimbel KH (1980). The Federal Republic of Germany. In Inman WHW (ed.) *Monitoring for Drug Safety*. Philadelphia: JB Lippincott Company: 67–72.

7

The regulation of medicines in the UK
David B. Jefferys and Gerald Jones

Introduction: definitions

Although various statutes have governed the manufacture and distribution of drugs for centuries, it is largely true that until recent times no limitation was placed on the freedom of individual manufacturers to put new medicinal products on the market. Most established manufacturers did carry out various tests and trials before marketing but they were not obliged to do so by law. The thalidomide tragedy in the early 1960s led to a re-appraisal of the existing controls in the UK and this culminated in the passage of the *Medicines Act* in 1968.[1] At the same time the first of the EC Pharmaceutical Directives (65/65) was being introduced. The initial major provisions of this Act came into force in 1971. From 1964 to 1971 interim voluntary arrangements for the control of drug development existed in the UK; pharmaceutical companies agreed not to market any new drug without the prior approval of the Committee on Safety of Drugs. These voluntary arrangements were superseded in 1971 by the statutory provisions associated with the Act.

The Act provides for a comprehensive system of licensing under which it is unlawful for the products concerned to be manufactured, sold or supplied in or imported into the UK except in accordance with the appropriate licences, clinical trial certificates or exemptions. The Act controls all medicinal products (see below) and various other substances and articles brought within the licensing system by statutory orders under the Act. A *product licence* is needed for relevant dealings in any medicinal product to which the Act applies, including import. This licence must be held by the person 'responsible for the composition' of the product. An individual engaged in manufacturing or assembling medicinal products must hold a *manufacturer's licence*. Wholesale dealing requires a *wholesale dealer's licence*. Retail dealers are not required to hold licences unless they engage in any of the activities referred to above.

Licences are issued by the *licensing authority* which consists of the Health and Agriculture ministers (Secretary of State for Health, Secretary of State for Scotland, Minister of Agriculture Fisheries and Food, Department of Health and Social Services (DHSS) N. Ireland, Department of Agriculture N. Ireland). In practice the licensing of human medicines is handled by the Medicines Control Agency (MCA; an Executive 'Next Steps' Agency) of the Department of Health (DoH) and veterinary medicines by the Veterinary Medicines Directorate of the Ministry of Agriculture Fisheries and Food.

In determining whether licences should be issued and the conditions under which they should be issued the licensing authority obtains advice on the quality, safety and efficacy of medicinal products from various *advisory committees*. These committees consist of independent experts, not the staff of Department of Health, and are appointed by Ministers on the advice of the Medicines Commission (see below). Currently these statutory (Section 4) advisory committees are:

1. *Committee on Safety of Medicines (CSM)*. This committee advises the licensing authority on questions of the safety, quality and efficacy of new medicines for human use. It is also responsible for collecting and investigating reports on adverse reactions to medicines already on the market. A number of subcommittees have been established to assist the main committee in its work.
2. *Committee on Dental and Surgical Materials (CDSM)*. This committee, as its name implies, provides advice on a range of products which fall outside the expertise of the CSM. It will lose some of its current work with the introduction of the Devices Directive in 1993.
3. *Veterinary Products Committee (VPC)*. This committee provides advice on veterinary products.
4. *Committee on the Review of Medicines (CRM)*. This committee advised the licensing authority on the review of the safety, quality and efficacy of products already on the market with so-called Product Licences of Right (PLRs). It completed its work in March 1991 and has been disbanded.
5. *British Pharmacopoeia Commission (BPC)*. The BPC is responsible for preparing future editions of the British Pharmacopoeia and for selecting non-proprietary names for medicinal substances.

The *Medicines Commission* is a separate advisory body that has a more broadly based membership than the advisory committees described above. The Commission provides advice to the licensing authority on all matters relating to the implementation of the Medicines Act and to medicines in general. Its specific duties are:

(a) To make recommendations on the constitution and functions of committees to be set up under the Act.
(b) To recommend persons well qualified to serve on such committees.
(c) To review the number or functions of such committees.
(d) To receive representations, in certain circumstances, from applicants for product licences or clinical trial certificates, or from existing licence or certificate holders.
(e) To act as an advisory committee on particular products or problems if an appropriate committee does not already exist.
(f) To direct the preparation of certain publications, e.g. the British Pharmacopoeia.

The relation of these bodies to the licensing authority and its activities are illustrated in Fig. 7.1.

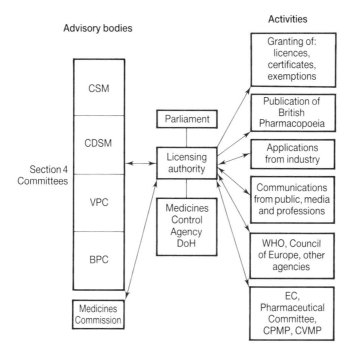

Fig. 7.1 The regulatory agency, the advisory bodies and their main activities. (For names of Section 4 committees see text).

Scope of control

The Act defines a *medicinal product* as a substance or article intended for use mainly or wholly for a medicinal purpose for administration to humans or animals. A medicinal purpose is defined as any of the following:

(a) Treating or preventing disease.
(b) Diagnosing disease or ascertaining the existence, degree or extent of a physiological condition.
(c) Contraception.
(d) Inducing anaesthesia.
(e) Otherwise preventing or interfering with the normal operation of a physiological function.

The above definition includes all those chemicals commonly regarded as drugs by the medical profession. It is worth noting that the ability of a chemical to produce toxic or adverse effects when administered to animals or humans is not a necessary or sufficient criterion for inclusion. Also, with certain exceptions mentioned below, the term 'medicinal product' does not include instruments, appliances or devices.

Other substances or articles may be brought within the scope of licensing by statutory orders. The following classes of product have been covered by the appropriate orders:

1. Certain biological substances for use as ingredients in the manufacture of medicinal products (required to ensure the quality and safety of biological products where control of the starting material is essential).
2. Absorbable surgical materials, and surgical ligatures and sutures of animal origin.
3. Dental filling substances.
4. Contact lenses, blanks from which they are made, contact lens fluids and intrauterine devices.

Licensing controls are not applied to chemicals or other substances used in the manufacture of ingredients of a medicinal product nor to bulk ingredients supplied to manufacturers with the exception of substances mentioned in point 1 above. Generally a substance or article becomes subject to licensing at the point at which it is manufactured or assembled for sale or supply or exportation as a medicinal product.

Although most human medicines are clearly medicinal products and subject to licensing there are *borderline cases*. In doubtful cases advice should be obtained from the staff of the MCA but the following notes may be helpful:

1. A substance that is for use solely as a toilet preparation, food, beverage or disinfectant is not within the scope of the Act.
2. Foods or cosmetics that are sold or supplied for a medicinal purpose may be exempt from licensing.
3. Bandages and other surgical dressing are not included except where the dressings are medicated and the medication has a curative function.

In many cases, e.g. hair restorers, antismoking preparations, alcoholic beverages, etc. the nature of the claims made or indications given on the labels or promotional material may be crucial in deciding whether the purpose of administration is wholly or mainly medicinal.

European licensing

The first pharmaceutical directive was issued in 1965 before the UK Medicines Act. This framework Directive 65/65 set out the general conditions for the licensing of medicines in the EC. An EC directive takes precedence over national laws. The next chapter will describe in detail the European legislation; however, it is important to recognize the extent to which EC law already impinges upon the regulation of pharmaceuticals in the UK. This will significantly increase over the next few years when the future system proposals (which at the time of writing are still under discussion) are enacted as part of the Internal Market programme.

The existing directives have been brought into UK law by the use of secondary legislation under the Medicines Act. This has been possible because the directives have either been complementary to the UK Medicines Act or have introduced new elements not covered under the Act. The major directives are listed below.

65/65, the general framework directive
75/318, which was concerned with approximating the technical standards for the testing of proprietary medicinal products
75/319, which established the Committee on Proprietary Medicinal Products (CPMP), the original Multi-State procedure, the expert report procedure and the framework for patient information leaflets.
83/570: this amended the Multi-State procedure and, in particular, introduced the SPC (summary of product characteristics)
87/19 established the regulatory committee procedure
87/21 established the procedure for abridged applications and the protection of innovation in the Community.
87/22 established the high technology and biotechnology concertation procedures
89/341, 89/342, 89/343 and 89/381 have brought immunological products, blood products, radiopharmaceuticals and vaccines into the scope of Directive 65/65 and introduced the requirement for the review of these products by January 1993.

The future system proposals envisage the creation of a centralized licensing procedure based on a European Medicines Evaluation Agency (EMEA) and a reinforced CPMP. The proposals suggest that all biotechnology products as currently defined in Annex A of Directive 87/22 will be considered through this procedure and in addition it will be open to all new active substances and other products of significance as defined within the current Annex B of Directive 87/22. The licence for these products would be issued by the Commission on the advice of the CPMP and after a regulatory committee consultation. The European licence would be valid throughout the Community and the legal and political responsibilities would lie with the EMEA. This will introduce into the UK a new type of licence to exist alongside national licences.

The so-called decentralized procedure will have at its heart the concept of binding arbitration by the reinforced CPMP. This means that if there is a difference of view between member states as to whether a licence should be granted, then this will be resolved through a process of binding arbitration and then the licences will be issued nationally. These proposals are still under discussion at the time of writing this chapter, but will need to be transposed into UK law and will have significant impact upon drug regulation in the second half of this decade.

Scope and types of licences

The main types of licences granted by the licensing authority are product licences, manufacturers' licences, wholesale dealers' licences and clinical trial certificates (or animal test certificates).

Product licences

A product licence authorizes the holder, in relation to the product in question, to:

(a)   sell, supply or export the product,

or (b)   procure the sale, supply or export of the product,

or (c)   procure the manufacture or assembly of the product for sale, supply or export,

or (d)   import the product.

The most common case will be as in (a) above. The other cases apply where the licence holder has made arrangements for a supply that is manufactured elsewhere. The product licence thus covers all the main activities associated with the marketing of a pharmaceutical preparation. A product licence may be granted to a person who is 'responsible for the composition' of the product, or imports it or first sells or supplies it after it has become a medicinal product. The person 'responsible for the composition' of the product is either the person to whose order the product is manufactured or, in any other case, the manufacturer.

Applications for product licences are made to the licensing authority. They must be accompanied by the relevant supporting data relating to pharmaceutical quality, and safety and efficacy in the proposed indications. Detailed guidelines on quality, preclinical testing and clinical trial requirements used to be issued by the DHSS. Since 1987 no new national guidelines have been issued. The requirements for licensing are now contained in Volume 2 of the CPMP Notice to the Applicants[2] and the technical requirements for quality, preclinical testing and efficacy are to be found in the CPMP guidelines. These are issued in Volume 3 of the Notice to the Applicants and an addendum of new or updated guidelines is issued each year. In 1989 an edition of MAL-2-Revised[3] was issued which contains purely national requirements and lists those national guidelines which have not yet been superseded or replaced by CPMP guidelines. Even these national requirements are diminishing, particularly since the CPMP has now agreed a common EC application form. The licensing authority must satisfy itself regarding the quality, safety and efficacy of the product before issuing a licence. The 'need' for the product, its price and its efficacy compared with existing products are not relevant issues for consideration. If the licensing authority wishes to refuse an application it must consult the appropriate advisory committee – for most medicinal products this will be the CSM. The applicant has the right to make representations, in writing or orally, to the Committee if the licensing authority intends to refuse the application. The applicant also has the right to make further representations to the Medicines Commission if the licensing authority still intends to refuse the application after considering the representations made before the Committee. Rarely the applicant may also make representations before a person appointed by the licensing authority. In all cases the various advisory bodies can only provide advice – the licensing authority is the only body with the power to grant or withhold licences, although the advice of the advisory committee is nearly always accepted.

In practice applications are assessed initially by the professional staff in the MCA and, in appropriate cases, referred to the advisory committee. Apart from those cases where referral to an advisory committee is mandatory all product licence applications involving new chemical entities are in fact routinely referred to an advisory committee. Consideration by advisory committees is usually preceded by detailed consideration by subcommittees.

Manufacturers' licences
Manufacture includes any process carried out in the course of making a medicinal product. Dilution of the product or mixing it with another substance are manufacture unless they are performed for the purpose of administering it to a patient. A manufacturer's licence is also needed to cover assembly, i.e. filling or labelling the final container for the product.

A manufacturer's licence covers the manufacture of broad classes of product rather than individual products. The licence holder must possess the appropriate facilities with respect to premises, equipment, staff and expertise. Normally, before a licence is granted an inspection of the premises is made and the licensing authority has to take into account the premises, the equipment, the qualifications of the responsible individuals and the arrangements for securing and maintaining adequate records of those products manufactured or assembled.

The combined effect of the definitions of manufacture and assembly of a medicinal product is that a manufacturer's licence must be held for manufacturing processes that result in a medicinal product, but not for manufacturing a substance supplied to another manufacturer as an ingredient of a medicinal product.

A manufacturer's licence generally authorizes manufacture or assembly of a product only if the manufacturer also holds a product licence or is manufacturing or assembling it to the order of the product licence holder. As an exception, provision has been made for the manufacturer of products as a 'special dispensing service', i.e. the preparation of medicinal products in response to special orders received from retail pharmacists, hospitals, wholesalers and certain other persons or organizations. A person or company undertaking this service may be granted a special manufacturer's licence which, subject to various conditions, authorizes the manufacture of products in response to such orders without a product licence.

Wholesale dealers' licence

Wholesale dealing covers the sale of a product to a person who buys the product for the purpose of sale or supply to someone else; it also covers sale to a practitioner for administration to his patients. Licensing of wholesalers is concerned primarily with identification of the distributor, the suitability of the premises used for storage of products and adequate turnover of stock.

Clinical trial certificates

A clinical trial means an investigation or series of investigations consisting of the administration of one or more medicinal products, where there is evidence that they may be beneficial, to a patient or patients by one or more doctors or dentists for the purpose of ascertaining what effects, beneficial or harmful, the products have.

Most (> 95%) clinical trials are now conducted under the exemption scheme introduced in 1981. Otherwise clinical trials in patients must be covered by a product licence or clinical trial certificate. A product may not be imported for the purpose of such a trial unless it is authorized by a certificate or a product licence which expressly refers to the test. A manufacturer's licence is not required for the manufacture or assembly of a medicinal product for the sole purpose of a clinical trial.

Applications for clinical trial certificates are made to the licensing authority in the same way as applications for product licences. Supporting data on quality and safety are required and detailed guidelines on the data requirements are issued by the MCA. Applications are assessed in the same way as product licence applications. Efficacy is not an issue in determining applications for clinical trial certificates. The same legal rights regarding representations to advisory committees and the Medicines Commission apply to these applications as to product licences.

A clinical trial certificate is not required if there is in existence a product licence and if the product is to be made and used strictly in accordance with the licence. Even this latter requirement may be relaxed in certain circumstances at the discretion of the licensing authority. A new indication may not need a certificate if there is a licence in force (see MAL-32[3]).

Standard provisions

Standard provisions (conditions), laid down in regulations, are incorporated in all licences and certificates issued by the licensing authority. Exceptions and modifications may, however, be made at the request of the applicant or by the licensing authority, which may add other provisions. The most important provision in all licences and certificates is the requirement that the holder must inform the licensing authority of any data or information which casts doubt on the safety of the product.

Period of validity

Licences are granted for 5 years and may be renewed at the end of this period by application to the licensing authority. Clinical trial certificates are valid for only 2 years, but can also be renewed.

There are provisions in the Act under which the licensing authority may vary, suspend or revoke a licence. Such action is usually taken on grounds of safety. Ordinarily, any proposed action by the licensing authority to suspend, vary or revoke an existing product licence will allow the holder the right to make representations, in writing or orally, to the appropriate advisory committee before such action is taken. As in the case of applications for product licences and clinical trial certificates there is a further right to make representations to the Medicines Commission if the licensing authority still intends to take action against the licence. In the case of manufacturers' and wholesale dealers' licences representations against proposed actions by the licensing authority are made directly to the licensing authority since no advisory committees are involved.

If it appears to the licensing authority that in the interests of safety it is necessary to suspend a licence urgently, it may do so with immediate effect (i.e. without permitting the holder the right to make representations) for a period not exceeding 3 months in the first instance. This provision is invoked only when, in the judgement of the licensing authority, it would not be defensible in terms of patient safety to permit the delay involved in the standard procedure.

Variations

On the application of the holder the licensing authority may agree to vary the provision of any licence or certificate. This is the procedure normally adopted by a licence holder when he wishes, for example, to expand the indications on the licence or to alter the dosage in the stated indications. If the licensing authority does not agree with the proposed change the holder does not have the right to make representations to an advisory committee or to the licensing authority. The licensing authority itself may propose a variation as indicated in the last section; if the licence holder objects to the proposed change he does have the right to make representations in this case.

Transfer of licences

Product licences and clinical trial certificates are held by individuals named in the documents and cannot be transferred to other individuals. If an individual wishes to take over a licence or certificate from another individual he is obliged to apply himself for a new licence or certificate, referring to the supporting data in the application made previously. This referral will require the permission of the original licence or certificate holder and is a relatively rapid procedure. The procedure for the transfer of licences is one of several issues currently under review by the EC.

Legal status

In general the Act, and the appropriate orders, divides medicines for human use into three categories for the purpose of retail sale or supply: General Sale List (GSL), Pharmacy (P) and Prescription Only Medicines (POM). Substances were listed in the GSL and POM orders on the advice of committees set up by the Medicines Commission. These lists are available to the public; they are revised periodically:

1. *General Sales List*. The purpose of this list is to specify those medicinal products which can be sold with reasonable safety without the supervision of a pharmacist.
2. *Pharmacy*. Pharmacy medicines may be sold or supplied only in a registered pharmacy by or under the supervision of a pharmacist. There is no list of pharmacy medicines but all medicines fall automatically into the pharmacy category unless included in the GSL or POM orders.
3. *Prescription Only*. These medicines may be sold or supplied only from a registered pharmacy and in accordance with a prescription issued by a doctor or dentist. The substances so restricted are those whose use needs to be supervised by a practitioner because they may produce a toxic reaction or physical or psychological dependence, or may be a hazard to the health of the community.

New chemical entities are routinely included in the POM list. For licence applications containing established ingredients the legal status is automatically determined by the existing POM and GSL orders. To alter the legal status of any substance generally requires an amendment of the relevant order, a procedure which involves widespread consultations with appropriate outside bodies and organizations. The legal status of a medicinal product cannot be altered by making specific provisions in an individual product licence application.

Exemptions from licensing

The Act contains certain important exemptions from licensing and makes provision for further exemptions to be included in orders. The more important exemptions are outlined below.

Healthy volunteers

The term 'healthy volunteers' is not defined or mentioned in the Medicines Act. However, investigations in such individuals may be excluded by virtue of the provisions of section 130 of the Act. Substances to be administered to humans in the course of the business of the manufacturer or on his behalf, where he has no knowledge of any evidence that the administration is likely to be beneficial and where administration is solely by way of a test for ascertaining the effects of the substance, are not 'medicinal products' within the meaning of the Act. An investigation of the above nature is not therefore regarded as a clinical trial and a clinical trial certificate is not required to permit its execution.

Practitioners

Treatment of particular patients.
A doctor or dentist is not required to hold a product licence or clinical trial certificate for a product prepared to his prescription for administration to a particular patient. Nor are they required to hold a manufacturer's licence for this purpose. A doctor or dentist may also procure the manufacture or assembly without a product licence of stocks of a product for administration to patients, subject to a limit of 5 litres of fluid or 2.5 kg of solid of all such products. Similar exemptions apply in the case of veterinary practitioners.

This exemption reflects the important principle that UK legislation is not intended to interfere with the treatment of patients by their doctor. This freedom has now been enshrined in EC law. This exemption does not apply to other practitioners such as homoeopaths and naturopaths. Various special licences are available, however, to cover these latter activities.

Clinical trials
Doctors or dentists may be supplied with a stock of a medicinal product that is not covered by a licence or a certificate for the purpose of conducting a clinical trial. The essential requirements are that the trial is undertaken on the initiative of the doctor or dentist without the instigation of the manufacturer or any third party, and that the doctor or dentist is entirely responsible for the patients concerned. No supporting data on quality or safety need to be supplied to the licensing authority but the authority does have the power to object, on grounds of safety.

Nurses and midwives
Registered nurses or certified midwives do not require a manufacturer's licence in order to assemble medicinal products in the course of their professional activities.

Pharmacists
In certain circumstances products may be made up without the need for the manufacturer to hold a manufacturer's licence. This exemption applies to pharmacists preparing or dispensing products in accordance with a practitioner's prescription. It also applies to anyone assembling products under the supervision of a registered pharmacist provided that the products, which are not to be advertised, are for sale at that pharmacy. This exemption may also apply to prescriptions given by veterinary practitioners subject to certain restrictions in relation to vaccines, plasma or sera.

The pharmacist is also exempt from the need to hold licences where preparing or dispensing products for 'counter prescribing' in a registered pharmacy using personal judgment as to the treatment required for the person who is in the pharmacy at the time.

Clinical trial exemption scheme

Since 1981 pharmaceutical manufacturers and suppliers may supply medicinal products for the purpose of conducting clinical trials without holding clinical trial certificates or product licences under the provisions of this scheme. The Clinical Trial Exemption (CTX) scheme is now the principal route for conducting trials of medicinal products in the UK. It has proved to be a great success and is being copied by several other countries. The main requirements for this exemption are that the supplier notifies the licensing authority of their intention to supply investigators and supports this with a summary of the relevant pharmaceutical data and the preclinical safety data. The data requirements are the same as for clinical trial certificates but are submitted in summary form. The licensing authority has 35 days in which to consider and object to the notification, if it wishes; an additional 28 days may be invoked where necessary. If the licensing authority refuses the exemption then the applicant has no right to make representations – they will need to apply for a clinical trial certificate in the usual way.

Other conditions associated with this exemption scheme are that: (1) a doctor must certify the accuracy of the summary; (2) the supplier undertakes to inform the licensing authority of any refusal to permit the trial by an ethical committee; and (3) the supplier also undertakes to inform the licensing authority of any data or reports that affect the safety of the product.

Additional clinical trials may be conducted under this scheme by simply notifying the licensing authority of the intention to conduct such studies. At all times the licensing authority retains the power to terminate any exemption. In practice this particular exemption has rapidly replaced the former arrangements for clinical trial certificates.

Other exemptions involving foods, cosmetics, ingredients and special manufacture have been mentioned previously. The number of exemptions now permitted by the Act and associated statutory orders is considerable and in cases of doubt manufacturers and suppliers are advised to contact the MCA.

Review of medicinal products

When the *Medicines Act (1968)* came into effect, on 1 September 1971, provision was made for the granting of *product licences of right* (and clinical trial certificates of right) in respect of medicinal products that were already on the market in the UK. Such licences were granted automatically without consideration of quality, safety or efficacy. These licences in general had the same effect as full product licences.

In due course all such product licences will be scrutinized by reference to the same standards of quality, safety and efficacy as ordinary licences. Indeed all product licences for proprietary medicinal products must be in accordance with EC Directive 75/318 by 1990 at the latest (see below). New licences granted since November 1976 (the operative date of the directive) are in fact in accordance with the Directive.

The review of existing product licences began in 1975. The licensing authority is being advised by the CRM which has equivalent status to the CSM. The original systematic review of each therapeutic group of products has now been superseded by a more streamlined approach that is aimed at scrutiny of individual licences at the time of their renewal. Of course many of the older products are now of little commercial value and manufacturers have preferred in these cases to relinquish the licences rather than undertake the work necessary to establish their quality, safety and efficacy to modern standards.

Postmarketing surveillance

It is accepted that, in regulating the marketing of medicinal products, controls before marketing are not sufficient in themselves. However extensive the preclinical work in animals and in clinical trials, certain adverse effects may not be detected until a large number of patients have received the drug.

Adverse reaction (spontaneous) reports

Great importance is attached to the monitoring of possible adverse reactions to medicinal products. The advisory committees (particularly the CSM but also the CDSM) maintain a register of adverse reactions which consists of confidential reports about individual patients made on a voluntary basis by doctors and dentists. These reports are sent by post on specially designed prepaid 'yellow cards' which are issued to all doctors and dentists. Supplies of yellow cards are now to be found in prescription pads (FP-10s), British National Formulary, Association of the British Pharmaceutical Industry (ABPI)-Data Sheet Compendium and Medical Information Management System (MIMS). Summaries of information stored in the register are available to those who report suspected reactions and also for certain other authorized individuals. No information that would identify a patient is ever released without the written permission of the reporting doctor.

Epidemiological monitoring

Certain epidemiological monitoring programmes are also undertaken to identify hazards. The role of oral contraceptives in various forms of thromboembolic disease was investigated in this way. One programme investigated the drug histories of mothers of babies born with congenital abnormalities to detect any previously unidentified teratogenic risks.

Communication with the professions

Communication with the professions both to warn about adverse effects and to provide feedback of information is an important aspect of adverse reaction monitoring.

The chief ways in which communication is achieved are:

1. Through 'Current Problems' which is published approximately four times per year and brings to the attention of doctors various problems about drugs.
2. Urgent warnings may necessitate the issue of a letter to all doctors, dentists and pharmacists from the Chairman of the CSM or CDSM.
3. A doctor or dentist who submits an adverse reaction report is sent a copy of the relevant part of the printout of the register of adverse reactions.
4. Articles resulting from investigations are also published in the professional journals.

Defective products

Reports of defective products, fortunately very rare, usually relate to individual batches or groups of batches. Following consideration of a defect report, affected batches may need to be recalled. A recall may be needed for example in the case of serious mislabelling, microbial contamination or incorrect ingredients when it is considered that administration of the product would constitute a serious health hazard. Recall is then undertaken by the manufacturer, wholesale dealers, etc. in consultation with the MCA. Any country to which the product has been exported would also be informed.

References

1. *Medicines Act (1968)* and regulations, orders and copies of official EC publications. London: HMSO.
2. (1989) *The Rules Governing Medicinal Products in the European Community, Vol. II – Notice to Applicants.* Commission of the European Communities.
3. Medicines Act Leaflets (MAL documents). London: DoH. These provide accounts of the regulations and procedures operating in the UK. A complete list of these leaflets is available from the Medicines Control Agency, Market Towers, 1 Nine Elms Lane, London SW8 5NQ. These notes are written in simple non-legal prose, and should not be treated as an authoritative complete guide to the law.

8

The regulation of medicines in Europe
Don MacLean

Introduction

The regulation of medicines in Europe has been going on now for many years. Much of this has been via individual national member state legislation, with many of the principles being based on the UK Therapeutic Substances Act of 1925. Additionally, controls on early medicines occurred in Germany via the Paul Ehrlich Institute, and in France via the Institute Pasteur, who both introduced the concept of batch release, a process which is still used today for biological and biotechnology products.

Repercussions from the thalidomide disaster in the early 1960s were the main incentives for tightening national control of medicines in most European countries. In the UK this eventually led to the 1968 Medicines Act, in Germany the Bundesgesundheitsant (BGA; Federal Health Office) was set up along with the first German Drug Law of 1961 and in The Netherlands the 'College Ger Beoordeling van Geneesmiddelen' (Committee for the Evaluation of Medicines) was established in 1963.

From an EC perspective the impact of thalidomide prompted the then member states (six in all – France, Germany, Italy, Belgium, The Netherlands and Luxembourg) to introduce medicines legislation on an EC basis to provide a comprehensive framework for the regulation of medicines. The first pharmaceutical medicine directive was 65/65/EC[1] adopted by the Council of Ministers in January 1965. This directive had to be implemented into each member state's national legislation within 18 months and today is still the fundamental directive, although substantially expanded and clarified, on which medicines are regulated and approved for sale in the EC.

Background to the EC regulation of medicinal products

Since the introduction of Directive 65/65/EC over 25 years ago, the regulation of medicines in the EC has become widespread. EC Membership in 1992 includes 12 member states: the original six mentioned above plus the UK, Denmark and Ireland who joined in 1973, Greece in 1981 and Spain and Portugal in 1986.

There are a variety of different types of legislation originating within the EC upon which member states have to act.

Regulations:	binding for all member states; effective from the due data without having to be incorporated into national law
Directives:	binding for all member states; must be incorporated into national law within a defined period (e.g. 18 months)
	(This type of legislative route is the most common with pharmaceutical medicines.)
Recommendations:	not binding but advisory (e.g. guidelines)
Decisions:	binding for directed member states

The main directives on medicines in the EC

Directive 65/65/EC[1]
Introduced on 26 January 1965 on the approximation of provisions laid down by law, regulation or administrative action relating to proprietary medicinal products.

This is the main 'framework' setting directive and incorporates the concepts of a marketing authorization for medicines based on supportive evidence for: safety, quality and efficacy. Included in the directive are requirements concerning:

- Definition of a medicinal product
- Timings for health authority assessment
- Validity of a marketing authorization (5 years)
- Packaging and container labelling

Directive 75/318/EC[2]
Introduced on 20 May 1975 on the approximation of the laws of member states relating to analytical, pharmacotoxicological and clinical standards and protocols in respect of the testing of proprietary medicinal products.

Adopted in May 1975, this subsequent directive concerns documents and data requirements on:

- Physicochemical, biological or microbiological testing
- Toxicological and pharmacological testing
- Clinical testing

This is a particularly important directive for those concerned with the development of medicines in the pharmaceutical industry as it clearly spells out the basis on which health authorities in the EC expect to see the pharmaceutical industry develop and manufacture their medicines for eventual marketing authorization. The scientific and technical details around these requirements in Directive 75/318/EC are elaborated in numerous Guidelines prepared by advisory working parties.

Directive 83/570/EC[3]
Introduced on 26 October 1983 amending Directives 65/65/EC, 75/318/EC

and 75/319/EC on the approximation of provisions laid down by law, regulation or administrative action relating to proprietary medicinal products

Directive 75/318/EC has been amended and expanded over the last 17 years. First in October 1983 Directive 83/570/EC was adopted. This further elaborated on the risk/benefit concept, where data supporting a medicine must show that any potential risk is outweighed by demonstrated therapeutic efficacy. It also introduced the need for more information on areas like: development pharmaceutics (why/how did you choose and produce particular dose forms), and mutagenicity, carcinogenicity and bioavailability testing. A particularly important aspect of 83/570/EC was the need for an applicant to include a draft 'Summary of Product Characteristics' (SPC) in the supporting documentation for a marketing authorization. Once amended and approved by a member state this SPC forms the basis of eventual prescribing information for a physician, package leaflet for a patient or for advertising and promotion claims for the product. It is an extremely critical document in any application. The SPC covers information on product name, composition (active and excipients), dose form, pharmacological and pharmacokinetic properties, clinical information on (indications, contraindications, warnings or precautions) and pharmaceutical information on (shelf life or storage conditions).

Directive 91/507/EC[4]

Introduced on 19 July 1991 modifying the Annex to Council Directive 75/318/EC on the approximation of the laws of member states relating to analytical, pharmacotoxicological and clinical standards and protocols in respect of the testing of medicinal products

This directive was adopted in July 1991, with a couple of minor subsequent amendments. It contains revised and updated details of the information to be supplied in support of a marketing authorization. Primarily, this now includes and consolidates information from the following directives.

89/342/EC[5]:	on immunological medicinal products (e.g. vaccines for active immunity, diagnostic agents for determining the extent of immunity and agents producing passive immunity).
89/343/EC[6]:	on radiopharmaceuticals that contain one or more radioactive isotopes when ready for use.
89/381/EC[7]:	human blood products (e.g. immunoglobulins, albumin, coagulating factors).
89/341/EC[8]:	a general directive that extends the scope of earlier Directives to cover all medicinal products (generic and proprietary) and that also covers the requirements for having patient information.

Directive 91/507/EC also ratified the concepts of Good Clinical Practice (GCP) outlined in the guideline issued by the EC in July 1990.[9] Likewise, the directive also specifies that safety tests for medicines performed according to the requirements of 65/65/EC, as amended, have to be conducted according to Good Laboratory Practice (GLP). The concepts of GLP, to assure quality and validity of preclinical testing, were based on guidelines published by the OECD (Organization for Economic Cooperation and Development),[10] and established initially through Directive 75/318/EC and amended by Directive 87/18/EC.[11]

The third of these 'quality codes' – Good Manufacturing Practice (GMP) – has been functioning for many years. The basic requirements for the control of medicinal product manufacture appear in Directive 75/319/EC,[12] which discusses authorized manufacturers and the need for a 'qualified person' to release product for sale and record keeping. Guidelines on GMP were published in 1989[13] and additionally a Directive 91/356/EC[14] on GMP for human medicines was published in July 1991.

Directive 75/319/EC
Introduced on 20 May 1975 on the approximation of provisions laid down by law, regulation or administrative action relating to proprietary medicinal products.

This directive covers the legal and administrative framework for health authorities in the Community and was adopted in May 1975. Notably it established the formation of the Committee for Proprietary Medicinal Products (CPMP) who were to consider issues referred to it relating to marketing authorizations, i.e. approval, suspension, refusals or revocations.

A second key aspect to this directive was the establishment of the 'Multi-State' procedure, whose objective was to make it easier for a company which has already obtained a marketing authorization for a medicine in one country in the Community to obtain other authorizations in other member state countries by the principle of 'mutual recognition' of the original authorization. Time limits on how long member states involved have to raise objections (120 days) and the minimum number of member states which must be involved in such a procedure are discussed. The 'Multi-State' procedure was subsequently updated in Directive 83/570/EC. A full description of the operation of the Multi-State procedure can be found in *The Rules Governing Medicinal Products in the Community*, Vol. II, 1989.[15]

A third key aspect to this Directive was the introduction of 'Expert Reports'. Each of the three areas of an application for a marketing authorization:

- Chemical, pharmaceutical, biological testing
- Toxicological and pharmacological testing
- Clinical testing

All had to have a detailed report prepared by an appropriately qualified 'expert' in the area. Subsequently, in Directive 83/570/EC and in detailed guidelines published by an ad hoc CPMP working party entitled *Notice to Applicants for Marketing Authorisations for Medicinal Products for Human Use*, January 1989,[15] the requirements of such expert reports and the qualifications and experience of authors are discussed.

These three 'expert reports' are critical documents in any marketing authorization application. A great deal of effort needs to be spent on them as they are the primary documents examined by health authority staff and external reviewers. They have to be critical documents, evaluating the product from on a benefit/risk basis, and discuss why a particular development approach was taken on a medicinal product. With the 'Multi-State' procedure the country which initially authorized a product for marketing has to prepare an 'Assessment Report'. Good, well written and critically evaluating 'expert reports' should form the basis of such 'assessment reports'. It is thus important for pharmaceutical companies to prepare 'expert reports' which both meet the guideline and directive requirements properly and critically evaluate the product.

Directive 87/22/EC[16]

Introduced on 22 December 1986 on the approximation of national measures relating to the placing on the market of high technology medicinal products, particularly those derived from biotechnology.

The adoption of this Directive in December 1986 and its implementation from July 1987, were particularly important developments in the regulation of medicines in Europe. The directive concerned the mandatory procedure necessary to obtain approval of a marketing authorization for a 'biotechnology' medicinal product. In addition, it also introduced an optional procedure to obtain approval for highly innovative medicinal products.

The objective of introducing such a licensing procedure was to encourage the development of biotechnology and high technology medicinal products in the EC. The procedure would enable products approved through it to benefit from additional data protection from a second applicant for a period of 10 years (or 6 years in some member states). This concept is discussed in more detail below.

For biotechnology products – defined in the Directive under 'List A' products – it became mandatory for competent member states to discuss the application with each other before recommending approval. Likewise, companies wishing to obtain a marketing authorization in the EC had to use this procedure. For products of high technological innovation – defined in the Directive under 'List B products' – there became an option for companies to use this procedure to obtain marketing authorization approval, providing the concerned member states and the CPMP agreed.

The advantage of such a procedure to obtain a marketing authorization is that there is no need to obtain approval in one member state initially, before entering this European procedure; unlike the 'Multi-State' procedure discussed earlier.

The marketing authorization application is submitted to all participating member states simultaneously, with the assessment being carried out by a 'rapporteur' member state. Once all questions have been raised by member states and replied to by the applicant (all according to a predefined timetable), the CPMP provides an opinion on the application. If positive, member states have predefined time frames to act on this opinion. As the opinion is not legally binding for member states (neither is that from the CPMP in a 'Multi-State' procedure) they do not necessarily meet such time limits. However, overall this procedure is advantageous to companies using it as they generally obtain more marketing authorizations, in more member states, more quickly.

This procedure for the approval of marketing authorizations for medicinal products is often referred to as the 'Concertation' Procedure or the 'biotech/hightech' procedure.

Council Directive 87/21/EC[17]

Introduced on 22 December 1986 amending Directive 65/65/EC on the approximation of provisions laid down by law, regulation or administrative action relating to proprietary medicinal products.

This directive appeared concomitantly with the 'Concertation' Procedure directive for biotechnology and high-technology medicinal products (87/22/EC). It is primarily concerned with the protection of data contained in a marketing authorization application, protecting innovation and regulating when copy products can be produced. Generally, when an applicant applies for a marketing authorization they must supply the relevant supporting data, according to 65/65/EC, as amended, on chemical/pharmaceutical, pharmacological/toxicological and clinical aspects. However, for well established active ingredients, whose safety and efficacy are widely published, exceptions from supplying pharmacological, toxicological and clinical data are possible for a medicinal product which is 'essentially similar'. Directive 87/21/EC amends 65/65/EC and more clearly defines the conditions under which a 'second applicant', which generally refers to generic companies, may be exempt from supplying data.

Three exemptions are cited:

1. The authority of the first applicant is provided to refer to pharmacological, toxicological and clinical data,
2. Detailed references in the published literature are provided on pharmacological/toxicological and clinical data,
3. The product is 'essentially similar' to the first (originator's) product, authorized more than 10/6 years previously (6 years for Denmark, Ireland, Luxembourg; 6 years or patent term for Spain, Portugal and Greece; 10 years for any country via the Concertation Procedure).

This 'protection period' of 10/6 years was intended to supply protection of data for products, like biotechnology products, that might not have the normal intellectual property rights via patents. However, it does not provide any protection to a 'second applicant' who generates *all* the relevant supporting data, according to 65/65/EC as amended, including pharmacological, toxicological and clinical data on the product.

Other Directives

The above cited Directives supply the main basis for regulation of medicines on a European level. However, the following Directives also exist and have some impact on how medicines are regulated.

87/19/EC:[18]	introduces the regulatory committee procedure to help more rapid guideline updates and data needs due to technical progress.
78/25/EC:[19] and *81/464/EC:*[20]	concerns permitted colourings in medicines. (This will be updated soon taking into account the recently proposed directive on colourings in foods (Com (91) 44 – final – SYN 368[21]).
92/27/EC:[22]	covers labelling of medicinal products for human use and on package leaflets. (Implementation date 1 January 1994.)
92/28/EC:[23]	covers advertising of medicinal products for human use. (Implementation date 1 January 1993.)
92/26/EC:[24]	Classification of medicines – prescription only or 'over-the-counter'. (From 1 January 1993 member states have 2 years to produce lists).
92/25/EC:[25]	Wholesale distribution of medicinal products for human use. (Implementation date 1 January 1993.)
89/105/EC:[26]	Transparency of measures relating to the scope of national health insurance schemes. This came into force in 1990 and is currently under review (August 1992) with a revised draft (III/3749/91) under discussion. Nothing has been finalized but the trends indicate that the EC will leave pricing/reimbursement more in the hands of individual authorities for now. This Directive requires member states to make their pricing and reimbursement procedures 'transparent' and publish criteria upon which they make decisions.

Guidelines produced by the EC on the development of medicines

In addition to all the legislative pharmaceutical directives which regulate approval of marketing authorizations for medicinal products there are numerous, non-legally binding, guidelines.

In 1987, Directive 87/19/EC was introduced which allowed a rapid system for the modification of existing data requirements to keep up with the rapid changes in technology and science. A regulatory committee was established to do this, acting on proposals from the EC. The rapid introduction of Directive 91/507/EC, modifying and expanding Directive 75/318/EC is an example of how this process works well.

The original method of promulgating guidelines was via 'Recommendations' from the EC. For example, 83/571/EC[27] and 87/176/EC[28] were issued containing 19 guidelines which were annexed to Directive 75/318/EC. This procedure was overcomplicated and subsequently a less formal process for publishing guidelines was introduced. Guidelines are prepared by a series of CPMP working parties (e.g. quality, safety, efficacy, biotechnology, pharmacovigilance and operations) and go through a review period (1–2 years) with member state health authorities, pharmaceutical industry trade associations and pharmaceutical companies. At any given point in time there are thus both final and different stage draft guidelines available. All these provide useful advice for the pharmaceutical industry on 'what is needed to develop medicines now' and 'what the trends are for the future'. Finalized guidelines are periodically incorporated into *Rules Governing Medicinal Products in the EC*, vol III,[29] or published separately as they are ratified. Draft guidelines are published separately during their period of consultation.

Examples of the type of finalized guidelines available include:

Quality:	*References*
Chemistry of active ingredients	vol III, Jan 89
Analytical validation	vol III Addendum, July 90
Safety:	
Testing of medicinal products for their mutagenic potential	vol III, Jan 89
Efficacy:	
Anti-anginal drugs	vol III, Jan 89
Investigation of bioavailability and bioequivalence	III/54/89[30]
Biotechnology:	
Production and quality control of monoclonal antibodies of murine origin	vol III, Jan 89
Procedural:	
Abridged applications	III/3879/90[31]

Two useful sources of references for guidelines, both finalized and in draft are: *The Guide to the European Directives Concerning Human Medicines*,[32] published by the Association for the British Pharmaceutical Industry (ABPI), June 1992, and the *Regulatory Affairs Journal*, January 1992.[33]

Experiences of EC registration procedures

The Multi-State procedure

The 'Multi-State' procedure previously mentioned has been functioning since 1976 but has gone through two phases. Initially, Directive 75/319/EC restricted the procedure to instances where at least five member states had to be involved in receiving applications after the first initial member state approval. In Directive 83/570/EC, introduced in 1983, the minimum number of countries to receive an application was dropped to two.

The initial phase from 1976 to 1985 clearly showed that the procedure was not popular with the pharmaceutical industry; only 41 applications were used to initiate the process. The most common initiating marketing authorization for the process was from the UK (16:41) and the recipients were most frequently the Benelux countries (Belgium, The Netherlands, Luxembourg) and Italy.

Phase two of the Multi-State procedure (1985–July 1992) has proven to be much more favourable with industry; with 238 dossiers used to initiate the procedure. France and the UK were the most favourable first authorization countries. Reducing the threshold number of countries from five to two was the main factor producing this increased usage, along with the introduction of the 'assessment report' from the sponsoring member state and the rights for the applicant to have access to the CPMP via an oral hearing.

However, one can clearly see that the original intention to foster an environment of 'mutual recognition' has not worked. Every application which has gone through the 'Multi-State' procedure has required a CPMP opinion, i.e. in the 120-day review period there has always been at least one 'reasoned objection' raised by a recipient member state. Consequently, the system becomes overloaded and much of the focus of its operation is handling and dealing with the 'reasoned objections' and created responses. The pharmaceutical industry is today 'lukewarm' towards the Multi-State procedure; however, the procedure does offer some potential advantages for faster marketing authorization approvals in the slower reviewing member states, like Germany, who were the largest recipient country for Multi-State applications (122 from 1986 to March 1991). Similarly, Italy and Spain have also received many incoming applications.

Any CPMP opinion is not legally binding for member states and this also leads to the lack of 'mutual recognition', with individual member states' marketing authorizations differing in terms of approved labelling concerning indications, contraindications, warnings and precautions. In addition, little attention is paid by member states regarding the time limits within which they have to issue a marketing authorization after receipt of a positive CPMP opinion. Theoretically this is now 60 days, but in reality it can taken many months for all involved member states to issue a marketing authorization; 12 months is not uncommon.

The 'Concertation' Procedure

A total of 50 applications, up to July 1992, have been made since the introduction of this procedure in July 1987. The applicant can choose the 'rapporteur' member state for primary assessment and coordination of the application – countries most frequently used are the UK, The Netherlands and France. In addition, variations to an existing marketing authorization (before July 1987) for biotechnology products or for products approved by the 'Concertation' Procedure are required to go through this procedure, to try and maintain a 'harmonized' marketing authorization across the Community.

Experience to date indicates that the 'Concertation' Procedure is working better than the 'Multi-State' procedure and in general the pharmaceutical companies involved are positive towards it. The vast majority of products going through it are the compulsory 'List A' biotechnology products; only a few 'List B' high technology products have gone through. However, with the pending changes in European marketing authorization procedures (see below) it is likely that more 'List B' products will go through the 'Concertation' Procedure, with the support of member states, to allow both industry and health authorities to gain experience in handling them prior to setting up the new European Medicines Agency in January 1995.

Expansion of the EC

In 1992 the membership of the EC stands at 12 countries

Belgium	Denmark	France	Germany
Greece	Italy	Ireland	Luxembourg
The Netherlands	Portugal	Spain	UK

However, membership of the EC offers substantial economic benefits and other countries can be expected to join during the 1990s. Some have already applied, e.g. Sweden, Austria, and others like Switzerland are beginning discussions on the possibility of entry. This has led to many of these current non-EC countries (e.g. Sweden) to accept the format of an EC marketing authorization application and to be present as observers at some CPMP working party meetings. Currently of the Scandinavian or 'Nordic' countries (Denmark, Sweden, Norway, Finland and Iceland) only Denmark is a member of the EC. Some Nordic countries have now joined with the EC to form the European Economic Arena (EEA), which removes some of the trading barriers and is due to take effect from 1 January 1993. The EEA is basically made up of the EC and the EFTA (European Free Trade Association) countries (Austria, Finland, Iceland, Liechtenstein, Norway, Sweden and Switzerland). These developments can be seen as forerunners of eventual full EC membership by the majority of the EFTA countries.

Medicines regulation in Scandinavia

When one talks about the registration of medicines in Europe there is a tendency to focus on the EC; not unnaturally since this as a unit is a substantial pharmaceutical market. However, Scandinavian health authorities, notably those in Sweden, must not be forgotten because they provide high quality assessments of marketing authorization applications, often asking astute questions, and they are particularly good at the early identification of regulatory issues which often become a global concern. An example is the key issue of chirality and whether pharmaceutical companies should be developing drugs that are racemic mixtures of isomers or individual purified isomers. Sweden were the first to produce some guidelines in this area and now, in late 1992, both the EC and the US Food and Drug Administration (FDA) have draft guidelines out for comments.

The Nordic countries have published a series of guidelines for pharmaceutical companies developing medicines, under the umbrella of 'The

Nordic Council on Medicines'. This joint organization was set up in 1975 to promote the harmonization of legislation and administration of medicines in the Nordic countries. A series of guidelines by Nordiska Lakemedelsnamnden (NLN publications, numbers 1 to 24) are available covering areas like:

NLN 24:   Drug Applications – format and administration, March 1989[34]
NLN 18:   Bioavailability Studies in Man, October 1987[35]
NLN 11:   Clinical Trials of Drugs, June 1983[36]

When developing their guidelines the Nordic Council have taken steps to be consistent with the EC, with the view to making the eventual member-ship of the Community by any Nordic country easier as they would already have a similar marketing authorization application format and content. In 1989 the NLN decided to cease its activity on the preparation of guidelines with the view to adopting the EC guidlines. On 1 January 1993, when the Nordic countries form the EEA, the EC guidelines will be applicable in Scandinavia. As previously mentioned, Sweden have already indicated that marketing authorization applications are now acceptable in the EC format.

Clinical trials regulations in Europe

Unlike the active process of harmonizing the requirements for the regula-tion of medicines at the marketing authorization stage, there is no harmoni-zation today on the regulation of clinical trials in Europe. Each country has differing requirements ranging from almost nothing to comprehensive data summaries and approval procedures. The primary concern of any regula-tory authority in authorizing clinical trials to test a product in humans is patient 'safety'.

Although there is no harmonization of clinical trial requirements, the EC have published a paper on the need for a directive on clinical trials (III/3044/91).[37] This raised a number of issues such as: monitoring of clinical trials; harmonization of preclinical data; manufacture and GMP; inspection/audit of sites; labelling; archiving; and compliance. Nevertheless, industry has not been too keen on such a Directive and feels things are working fairly well at a national control level.

Some European countries control clinical trials via the 'deposition' of preclinical data and controls on the 'importation' of trial products. For example, in Germany the Bundesgesundheitsamt (BGA) require preclinical data to be deposited with them and the company can begin clinical studies once an acknowledgement letter has been received from the BGA, which usually takes about 1 month. In Belgium, there is no formal regulation and in The Netherlands an Import Licence is necessary which requires a rationale for the study, a protocol, the quantity of drug required, a statement from the medical monitor of the study, and that at study completion results will be made available to the health authorities;

obtaining an Import Licence takes about 2 weeks. In all these cases there is still a need to obtain 'Ethical Committee' approval, which is usually the rate-limiting factor in commencing any clinical study.

In the UK there is a very efficient scheme for obtaining clinical trial approvals in patients – the Clinical Trial Exemption (CTX) Scheme (studies in human volunteers are not controlled by the UK Health Authority). The CTX scheme allows a rapid assessment of comprehensively summarized chemistry/pharmacy, preclinical and any clinical data. Assessments take place within 35 days, with an option for a 28-day extension, after which the applicant is notified that there are 'no objections to the proposed trial' if the data are satisfactory (see Chapter 7).

In France a rationale for the study, a clinical protocol and ethical committee approval are required at the time of application. Again, the rate-limiting activity is obtaining ethical committee approval.

Clinical trial applications in the Nordic countries require summaries of the chemistry/pharmacy, preclinical and any clinical data. Approvals taken between 1 and 3 months.

Italy has a 'two-tiered' system, depending on whether previous clinical data are available. Where no previous clinical data are available, summaries of chemistry/pharmacy and preclinical data are needed and approvals can take between 6 and 9 months. If previous clinical data are available the approval process is generally quicker (1–3 months).

In Spain clinical trial applications can take up to 8 months for approval. However, continued interaction between the company and the Spanish authorities can speed this up.

The way forward – the European Medicines Agency and harmonization of standards

In November 1990 the European Commission issued a proposed Council Regulation discussing the setting up of a European Medicines Agency and amending the existing 'Multi-state' and 'Concertation' Procedures. The new procedures would be known as the 'decentralized' and 'centralized' procedures, respectively. The main differences would be that: the CPMP opinion would be legally binding for member states; with time the option for national marketing authorization applications in Europe would become obsolete and all new applications would be through either the 'centralized' or 'decentralized' procedure.

This proposal was widely discussed within the pharmaceutical industry, national health authorities and the CPMP, which led to some legal problems and a number of changes. All the major legal hurdles now appear to be resolved and the new European Medicines Agency and the introduction of both the 'centralized' and 'decentralized' processes for marketing authorization applications should be in place on 1 January 1995. Overall, the pharmaceutical industry should benefit from the introduction of these new procedures but until they begin and can be shown to be capable of handling the large predicted work load in a timely, effective manner there will be reservations. A principle concern is the gradual phasing out of multiple, simultaneous national applications. This would prevent repetition of the same application assessment by different health authorities, but in a 'decentralized' procedure, where it is necessary to wait for the initial approval before instigating the rest, approvals of a product in some countries could be delayed. However, if pharmaceutical companies concentrate on producing high quality marketing authorization applications, there ought to be fewer questions, and the time lines stated in the 'decentralized' and 'centralized' procedures should be adhered to. Combined with CPMP opinions that are legally binding for member states, this ought to result in more approvals, more quickly than today, with a much more consistent set of physician prescribing information and patient information, across all European countries.

For multinational pharmaceutical companies, there is a great deal of duplication of work necessary to meet the differing regulatory requirements of the major world markets. In November 1991, the first 'International Conference on Harmonization' (ICH1) took place in Brussels, Belgium. These conferences will take place every 2 years and they have as an objective to harmonize the regulatory requirements of the USA, EC and Japan for all areas of an application – chemistry/pharmacy, pharmacological/toxicological and clinical data. Some progress was made in the chemistry/pharmacy area on stability testing requirements and in the toxicology area on reproductive toxicology testing and long-term rodent studies. Little progress was made in the clinical area as this is where the widest differences occur and the greatest moves are needed by all to reach consensus. Hopefully, the 1993 conference in the USA will further develop the production of harmonized requirements, especially in the clinical area.

Summary

Medicines regulation in Europe has grown dramatically over the last two decades. Initially it was very much based nationally, with individual country health authorities working fairly autonomously in the assessment of marketing authorization applications. Today, however, there is a much greater awareness of the need for having medicines approved on a European basis, for striving to achieve harmonized physician and patient information based on consistent marketing authorization approvals across countries. The European approval processes, like the 'Multi-State' and 'Concertation' Procedures have made a start on this. During the 1990s the expansion of these procedures into the 'decentralized' and 'centralized' procedures will further develop the concepts of European medicines approval. Individual national health authority expertise should end up being more efficiently used across Europe and along with more harmonized, but comprehensive medicines legislation, effective and safe medicines should be available to the patient.

References

1. Council Directive 65/65/EC of 26 January 1965 on the approximation of provisions laid down by law, regulation or administrative action relating to proprietary medicinal products. *Official Journal of the European Communities* **22 (9.2.65)**.
2. Council Directive 75/318/EC of 20 May 1975 on the approximation of the laws of Member States relating to analytical, pharmacotoxicological and clinical standards and protocols in respect of the testing of proprietary medicinal products. *Official Journal of the European Communities* **147 (9.6.75)**.
3. Council Directive 83/570/EC of 26 October 1983 amending Directives 65/65/EC, 75/318/EC and 75/319/EC on the approximation of provisions laid down by law, regulation or administrative action relating to proprietary medicinal products. *Official Journal of the European Communities* **332 (28.11.83)**.
4. Commission Directive 91/507/EC of 19 July 1991 modifying the Annex to Council Directive 75/318/EC on the approximation of the laws of Member States relating to analytical, pharmacotoxicological and clinical standards and protocols in respect of the testing of medicinal products. *Official Journal of the European Communities* **270 (26.6.91)**.
5. Council Directive 89/342/EC of 3 May 1989 extending the scope of Directives 65/65/EC and 75/319/EC and laying down additional provisions for immunological medicinal products consisting of vaccines, toxins or serums and allergens.
6. Council Directive 89/343/EC of 3 May 1989 extending the scope of Directives 65/65/EC and 75/319/EC and laying down additional provisions for radiopharmaceuticals.
7. Council Directive 89/381/EC of 14 June 1989 extending the scope of Directives 65/65/EC and 75/319/EC on the approximation of provisions laid down by law, regulation or administrative action relating to proprietary medicinal products and laying down special provisions for medicinal products derived from human blood or human plasma. *Official Journal of the European Communities* **181 (28.6.89)**.
8. Council Directive 89/341/EC of 3 May 1989 amending Directives 65/65/EC, 75/318/EC and 75/319/EC on the approximation of provisions laid down by law, regulation or administrative action relating to proprietary medicinal products. *Official Journal of the European Communities* **142 (25.5.89)**.
9. *Good Clinical Practice for Trials on Medicinal Products in the EC, Rules Governing Medicinal Products in the EC.* July 1990, Vol. III, addendum.
10. *OECD Principles of Good Laboratory Practice.* Environment Monograph No. 45, Paris 1992.
11. Council Directive 87/18/EC of 18 December 1986 on the harmonization of laws, regulations or administrative provisions relating to the application of the principles of Good Laboratory Practice and the verification of their applications for tests on chemical substances. *Official Journal of the European Communities* **15 (17.1.87)**.
12 Council Directive 75/319/EC of 20 May 1975 on the approximation of provisions laid down by law, regulation or administrative action relating to proprietary medicinal products. *Official Journal of the European Communities* **147 (9.6.75)**.
13. *Guide to Good Manufacturing Practice, Rules Governing Medicinal Products in the EC.* January 1992, Vol. IV.
14. Commission Directive 91/356/EC of 13 June 1991 laying down the principles and guidelines of Good Manufacturing Practice for medicinal products for

human use. *Official Journal of the European Communities* **193 (17.7.91)**.

15. *Notice to applicants for marketing authorisations for medicinal products for human use in member states of the EC, Rules Governing Medicinal Products in the EC*, January 1989, Vol. II.

16. Council Directive 87/22/EC of 22 December 1986 on the approximation of national measures relating to the placing on the market of high technology medicinal products, particularly those derived from biotechnology. *Official Journal of the European Communities* **15 (17.1.87)**.

17. Council Directive 87/21/EC of 22 December 1986 amending Directive 65/65/EC on the approximation of provisions laid down by law, regulation or administrative action relating to proprietary medicinal products. *Official Journal of the European Communities* **15 (17.1.87)**.

18. Council Directive 87/19/EC of 22 December 1986 amending Directive 75/318/EC on the approximation of the laws of the Member States relating to analytical, pharmacotoxicological and clinical standards and protocols in respect of the testing of proprietary medicinal products. *Official Journal of the European Communities* **15 (17.1.87)**.

19. Council Directive 78/25/EC of 12 December 1977 on the approximation of the laws of the Member States relating to the colouring matters which may be added to medicinal products. *Official Journal of the European Communities* **11 (14.1.78)**.

20. Council Directive 81/464/EC of 1 October 1981 amending 78/25/EC on the approximation of the rules of the member states relating to the colouring matters which may be added to medicinal products. *Official Journal of the European Communities* **183 (24.6.81)**.

21. Proposal for a council directive on colours in foodstuffs, Com (91)-44-final-SYN 368. *Official Journal of the European Communities* **40 (11.2.89)**.

22. Council Directive 92/27/EC of 31 March 1992 on the labelling of medicinal products for human use and on package leaflets.

23. Council Directive 92/28/EC of 31 March 1992 on the advertising of medicinal products for human use.

24. Council Directive 92/26/EC of 31 March 1992 concerning the classification for the supply of medicinal products for human use.

25. Council Directive 92/25/EC of 31 March 1992 on the wholesale distribution of medicinal products for human use.

26. Council Directive 89/105/EC of 21 December 1988 relating to the transparency of measures regulating the pricing of medicinal products for human use and their inclusion within the scope of national health insurance systems. *Official Journal of the European Communities* **40 (11.2.89)**.

27. Council recommendation 83/571/EC on Guidelines for developing medicinal products, 1983. *Official Journal of the European Communities* **332 (11)**.

28. Council recommendation 87/176/EC on Guidelines for developing medicinal products, 1987. *Official Journal of the European Communities* **73 (1)**.

29. *Rules Governing Medicinal Products in the EC*, Vol. III, January 1989 and addendum July 1990.

30. *Note for Guidance on 'Investigation of Bioavailability and Bioequivalence'*, III/54/89, CPMP, Brussels, 1991.

31. *Note for Guidance on 'Abridged Applications'*, III/3879/90, CPMP, Brussels, 12.1991.

32. Charlesworth FA (1992). *The Guide to the European Directives Concerning Human Medicines*. London: ABPI.

33. Skeffington V (1992). EC legislation for human medicinal products *Regulatory Affairs Journal* **(4) January 1992**: 81–5.

34. NLN 24: Drug applications, Nordic Guidelines, Nordic Council of Medicines,

2nd edn, Uppsala, March 1989.
35. NLN 18: Bioavailability Studies in Man, Nordic Council of Medicines, Uppsala, October 1987.
36. NLN 11: Clinical Trials of Drugs, Nordic Council of Medicines, Uppsala, June 1983.
37. Discussion paper on the need for a directive on clinical trials, III/3044/91, EC Commisions, Brussels, 23.1.91.

9

The regulation of pharmaceutical products in the USA
Peter Barton Hutt

Introduction

The regulation of pharmaceutical products by the Food and Drug Administration (FDA) in the USA is extraordinarily detailed and complex, and has enormous public costs as well as public benefits. This chapter provides only a broad overview of this subject. Entire books, and thousands of articles, have been devoted both to a comprehensive review of the area and to specific aspects. Anyone who wishes to understand it in greater detail must consult the governing statutes, regulations, and guidelines, as well as the experience of experts who have spent their entire careers working in the field. Thus, this chapter presents a bare beginning, permitting a glimpse into this extremely important and fascinating area, but not a definitive analysis of any of its myriad aspects.

Regulatory framework

Federal regulatory requirements
In the USA regulatory policies are established by statutes enacted by Congress and signed by the President. These laws govern all regulatory requirements imposed upon pharmaceutical products. No additional or different requirements can be imposed by any administrative official, but the statutory requirements are continually subject to reinterpretation and thus expansion as they are implemented by administrative action.

Laws are usually written by Congress in relatively general terms. They are intended to be implemented and enforced by administrative officials, in this instance located in FDA. FDA is empowered to promulgate regulations implementing the governing statutes, in accordance with the procedural requirements established by the Administrative Procedure Act. These procedural requirements require that most regulations initially be published as proposals in the Federal Register, accompanied by a lengthy preamble explaining the purpose and meaning of the proposed regulations. Time is then given for public comment. After all public comment has been received it is reviewed by FDA, which makes a final decision on the regulations and promulgates the final regulations together with a preamble explaining the decision with respect to each comment received and the reasons for the final version of the regulation. The regulations are then codified in the Code of Federal Regulations, without the explanatory preambles.

Following the promulgation of a federal regulation, any interested person may challenge the legality of the regulation in the courts. The primary grounds for any such legal challenge are that the regulation exceeds FDA statutory authority or that the regulation is simply arbitrary or capricious. Any person who challenges an FDA regulation in this way has an extraordinarily heavy burden to demonstrate that the regulation is illegal, and in most instances FDA regulations are upheld by the courts.

Even though FDA regulations are more detailed than the governing statute, they nonetheless are still often worded in general terms and thus it becomes important to have more specific and detailed documents to guide daily decision making within the Agency. Such detailed policy comes in many forms, including written guidelines, letters, speeches and a host of other documents, as well as unwritten tradition and practice. It is this area that largely governs daily FDA action. Because the vast bulk of FDA policy is not set forth either in the statute or in the regulations, it is uniquely a field where experience and judgment play a very large role.

State regulatory requirements

Decades ago the states played an important part in the regulation of pharmaceutical products. As pharmaceutical science has become more complex and as FDA regulation of the pharmaceutical industry has become much more intense, however, the states have shifted their traditional regulatory responsibilities to concentrate more heavily on food products and other items that are more appropriate for local control. Thus, state regulation of pharmaceutical products is a relatively insignificant aspect of pharmaceutical regulation in the USA today.

The states have retained their statutes governing both non-prescription and prescription drugs, however, and on occasion will exercise their authority to regulate in these areas. In recent years this regulation has largely been limited to non-prescription drugs. For example, California established guidelines for slack fill in the packaging of non-prescription drugs. On occasion states have also switched a non-prescription drug to prescription status in order to address a local abuse problem, usually only for a short duration.

Product liability

The one aspect of state 'regulation' of pharmaceutical products that has increased is the area of product liability. Drawing upon common law precedent that extends back to mediaeval English origins, an individual harmed by a pharmaceutical product may bring a civil tort action under state law against the manufacturer or distributor of the drug for damages sustained. This can be a potent form of regulation. If a pharmaceutical product causes widespread damage to patients the resulting tort liability could endanger the future of the manufacturer. One example is the

Dalkon Shield, the damage actions from which resulted in the bankruptcy of R.H. Robbins. Further discussion of the field of product liability is beyond the scope of this chapter.

FDA history

The US Patent Office began its interest in agricultural matters in the 1830s. Eventually an Agricultural Division was established in the Patent Office, and a Chemical Laboratory was funded in that Division.

When Congress created the US Department of Agriculture (USDA) by statute in 1862, the Agricultural Division of the Patent Office, and its Chemical Laboratory, were transferred to form the nucleus of the new Department. A Chemical Division was immediately formed within the USDA. This became the Division of Chemistry in 1890, the Bureau of Chemistry in 1901, the Food, Drug, and Insecticide Administration in 1927, and FDA in 1930.

FDA remained a part of the USDA until it was transferred to the new Federal Security Agency in 1940. When the Department of Health, Education and Welfare (HEW) was established in 1953, as a successor to the Federal Security Agency, FDA became a part of HEW. HEW was renamed the Department of Health and Human Services (HHS) in 1979.

Throughout this entire period FDA (and its predecessor agencies) was created by administrative action, not by Congress. The governing statutes were all officially delegated for implementation and enforcement to the Secretary of Agriculture/HEW/HHS, not to the Commissioner of Food and Drugs. It was not until the Food and Drug Administration Act of 1988 that Congress officially established FDA as a governmental agency. To this day, however, the governing statutes delegate responsibility for implementation and enforcement to the Secretary of HHS.

Throughout this history the Commissioner of Food and Drugs and his predecessors have also occupied a position that was created solely by administrative action, not by Congress. The Food and Drug Administration Act of 1988 also officially created the position of Commissioner of Food and Drugs, and required that the Commissioner be appointed by the President by and with the advice and consent of the Senate.

The Secretary of HHS is a Cabinet position, appointed by the President with the advice and consent of the Senate. An Assistant Secretary for Health within the Department of HHS is responsible for the Public Health Service, of which FDA is a part. Thus, the Commissioner of Food and Drugs reports to the Assistant Secretary for Health, who in turn reports to the Secretary of HHS.

Within FDA there is an Office of the Commissioner and five product-oriented centres located in Washington, DC. The Center for Drug Evaluation and Research, the Center for Biologics Evaluation and Research, and the Center for Devices and Radiological Health, are responsible for regulation of pharmaceutical products. Outside of Washington, DC, FDA has an extensive field force located in regions and districts throughout the USA, where FDA employees inspect pharmaceutical establishments and conduct enforcement activities. The FDA field force is also responsible for inspection of foreign pharmaceutical establishments located throughout the world.

Historical overview of drug regulation

Government concern about the adulteration and misbranding of pharmaceutical products extends back to ancient times. Pliny the Elder, for example, criticized 'the fashionable druggists' shops which spoil everything with fraudulent adulterations' in the first century AD. As a result, various forms of government control to prevent the adulteration and misbranding of food and drugs can be found in virtually every recorded civilization. These regulatory controls were brought to the American colonies by early settlers, were enacted into state law following the American Revolution, and eventually were adopted by Congress as nationwide requirements in a series of federal statutes.

During most of the 19th century regulation of food and drug products was thought to be a matter of state and local concern, not appropriate for federal legislation, under the United States Constitution. During this period most federal laws governing food and drugs therefore related to foreign commerce rather than to domestic commerce. It is only since 1900 that regulation of food and drugs in the USA has been concluded to be a matter of national concern that justifies the enactment of federal statutes. The following paragraphs present a brief chronology of the major federal regulatory statutes governing non-prescription and prescription drug products in the USA.

The Vaccine Act of 1813
Following Edward Jenner's discovery of a smallpox vaccine in 1798, and the demonstration by Benjamin Waterhouse in the USA in 1800 that the vaccine was effective, fraudulent versions of the vaccine were marketed throughout the country. A Baltimore physician, John Smith, initially convinced the Maryland legislature to enact a statute designed to assure the availability of an effective smallpox vaccine supply, and then persuaded Congress to enact the Vaccine Act of 1813 for the same purpose. This statute authorized the President to appoint a federal agent to 'preserve the genuine vaccine matter and to furnish the same to any citizen' who requested it.

The President promptly appointed Dr Smith as the first and, as it turned out, only federal vaccine agent. Following an outbreak of smallpox in North Carolina in 1821 that was thought to be caused by a contaminated lot of vaccine supplied by Dr Smith under the 1813 statute, the matter was investigated by two committees of the House of Representatives. The second committee concluded that regulation of smallpox vaccine should be undertaken by state and local officials rather than by the federal government, and as a result the 1813 Act was repealed in 1822. As will be discussed below, 80 years later another drug tragedy led to enactment of a new statute in 1902 under which vaccines are currently regulated by FDA.

The Import Drug Act of 1848

A congressional investigation in 1848 discovered that a wide variety of drugs imported into the USA for use by American troops in Mexico were adulterated. Congress therefore enacted a statute dealing solely with imported drugs. The 1848 Act required that all imported drugs be labelled with the name of the manufacturer and the place of preparation, and be examined and appraised by the US Customs Service for 'quality, purity, and fitness for medical purposes'. The Customs Service was directed to deny entry into the USA any drug determined to be so adulterated or deteriorated as to be 'improper, unsafe, or dangerous to be used for medical purposes'. This law remained in effect until it was replaced by another statute in 1922.

The Biologics Act of 1902

As the result of a series of problems with biological drugs during the late 1890s, cumulating in the death of several children in St Louis from a tetanus-infected diphtheria antitoxin, Congress enacted the Biologics Act of 1902. This statute is the first known regulatory law in any country that required premarket approval. The 1902 Act required approval of both a product license application (PLA) and establishment license application (ELA) before any biological product could be marketed in interstate commerce. Although it was recodified in 1944, it has remained in effect without significant change since 1902. It was initially implemented by the Public Health Service, but was transferred to FDA in 1972. Today it is implemented by the Center for Biologics Evaluation and Review (CBER) within FDA, which is located in buildings on the campus of the National Institutes of Health where it had been located prior to the 1972 transfer to FDA.

The Federal Food and Drugs Act of 1906

The first legislation to establish comprehensive nationwide regulation of all food and drugs was introduced in Congress in 1879. Largely because regulation of food and drugs was at that time thought to be a matter for state and local control, Congress debated this legislation for 27 years, ultimately enacting the Federal Food and Drugs Act in 1906. This law broadly prohibited any adulteration or misbranding of drugs marketed in interstate commerce. Although it was quite short, and very broad and general in nature, it was extremely progressive for its time and included sufficient authority to permit FDA to take strong enforcement action against unsafe, ineffective, and mislabelled products that flooded the US marketplace in the late 1800s. Unlike the Biologics Act of 1902, however, it contained no provisions requiring premarket testing or approval for new drug products. An attempt by FDA to obtain this type of authority in 1912 was unsuccessful. Thus, Congress initially provided premarket approval authority for biological drugs but not for chemical drugs.

The Federal Food, Drug, and Cosmetic Act of 1938

Shortly after President Franklin D. Roosevelt took office in 1933 the Commissioner of Food and Drugs persuaded the new administration to propose legislation to modernize the Food and Drugs Act of 1906. The legislation introduced in 1933, and ultimately enacted as the Federal Food, Drug, and Cosmetic Act of 1938 (the FD&C Act), was debated by Congress for 5 years. Initially, it was intended primarily to add cosmetics and medical devices to the 1906 Act and to require additional affirmative labelling for food and drug products. In September 1937, however, more than 100 people died of diethylene glycol poisoning following use of Elixir Sulfanilamide, which used this chemical as the solvent without any form of safety testing. As a result Congress added a premarket notification requirement for new drugs to the pending legislation and enacted the new law in June 1938. Under this statute a 'new drug' was defined as a drug that was not generally recognized as safe (GRAS) for its intended use. Before a new drug could be marketed it was required to be tested on humans in accordance with investigational new drug (IND) regulations promulgated by FDA. When sufficient data were obtained under a notice of claimed exemption for an investigational new drug (commonly referred to as an IND application) to demonstrate the safety of the drug, the manufacturer was required to submit a new drug application (NDA) for the drug to FDA. If FDA did not disapprove the NDA within 60 days after filing the NDA became effective and the drug could be marketed.

The Insulin and Antibiotics Amendments

Following enactment of the FD&C Act in 1938 insulin, penicillin and other antibiotic drugs were developed and marketed. Because of the unique production processes for these new pharmaceutical products, Congress enacted special provisions in the law requiring both that FDA approve each of them as safe and that FDA have the authority to require that each batch be certified by FDA as conforming to standards established for them by the agency. Thus, insulin and antibiotics have been regulated by FDA under provisions that were similar to, but nonetheless different from, those established both for biologics and for chemical drugs.

The Drug Amendments of 1962

Although thalidomide was marketed throughout Europe the NDA for this drug did not become effective in the USA. When it was learned in mid 1962 that thalidomide was a potent human teratogen, Congress immediately enacted the Drug Amendments of 1962 to strengthen the new drug regulatory system to make certain that there was adequate statutory authority in FDA to assure that any such drug could not be marketed in the future. The 1962 Amendments made a number of important changes. First, and most important, the amended law requires FDA explicitly to approve an NDA, rather than simply allowing the NDA to become effective through FDA inaction. Thus, the new drug provisions of the law were converted in 1962 from premarket notification to premarket approval, making them parallel with the Biologics Act of 1902. Second, a new drug was required to be shown to be effective as well as safe. Third, FDA was given additional authority to require compliance with Good Manufacturing Practice (GMP) regulations, to control the advertising of prescription drugs, to register drug establishments and to implement other regulatory requirements. Finally, FDA was required to review all NDAs that became effective during the period 1938 to 1962 to determine whether these drugs were effective as well as safe. Although the IND provisions of the FD&C Act were not significantly changed, FDA promulgated new regulations for the first time requiring submission to FDA of a notice of claimed exemption for an investigational new drug (commonly referred to as an IND) before clinical testing of an investigational new drug may begin.

The Controlled Substances Act of 1970

Beginning in the early 1900s Congress enacted a series of laws to control narcotic drugs and other drugs subject to abuse. All of these laws were repealed in 1970 and replaced by the Controlled Substances Act. Responsibility for enforcement rests with the Drug Enforcement Administration (DEA) of the Department of Justice. FDA may approve an NDA for any controlled substance that has a legitimate medical use, but DEA may impose upon any new drug that is also a controlled substance additional regulatory requirements to prevent abuse and misuse.

The Poison Prevention Packaging Act of 1970

In response to concern about household poisoning of children with hazardous household products Congress enacted the Poison Prevention Packaging Act to require the use of special child-resistant packaging. In accordance with regulations established by the Consumer Product Safety Commission, this type of packaging is now common for virtually all prescription drugs and for most non-prescription drugs.

The Drug Listing Act of 1972

The Drug Amendments of 1962 included a requirement that every owner of a US drug establishment register that establishment with FDA. Congress enacted the Drug Listing Act of 1972 to add the requirement that every person who registers an establishment shall include a list of all drugs manufactured at that establishment.

The Orphan Drug Act of 1983

An orphan drug is a drug that is intended for use for rare diseases and thus for which there is not a sufficient market to justify the investment needed to demonstrate safety and effectiveness in order to obtain approval of an NDA. For more than 20 years FDA had permitted orphan drugs to be distributed through a permanent IND, with little or no thought that it would ever progress to an approved NDA. In 1983 Congress enacted the Orphan Drug Act to provide economic incentives for industry to make the investment necessary to develop this category of drugs. When that proved insufficient the Act was amended in 1985 to expand its coverage substantially; by providing that any drug with a use that has a target patient population of fewer than 200 000 people is automatically classified as an orphan drug. Although the Orphan Drug Act does not provide for any different regulatory requirements from those applied to non-orphan drugs, the tax incentives and, in particular, a 7-year period of market exclusivity during which no competing NDA may be approved by FDA, combined with the extraordinary expansion in 1985 of the number of drugs covered by this statute, has had a major impact on drug development in the USA.

The Drug Price Competition and Patent Term Restoration Act of 1984

Under the new drug provisions as initially enacted in 1938 and as amended in 1962, all information in an IND and NDA were regarded as confidential proprietary business information that could not be revealed by FDA to any competitor and could not be used as the basis for any subsequent approval of a generic version of the pioneer new drug. Even after the patent for a pioneer new drug expired competitors were unable to obtain an approved NDA for a generic version without duplicating all the animal and human testing needed to demonstrate safety and effectiveness. Congress therefore enacted the Drug Price Competition and Patent Term Restoration Act of 1984, which authorized FDA to approve an abbreviated NDA for a generic version of a pioneer drug after the patent and the statutory period of market exclusivity for the pioneer drug have expired. The result has been a substantial increase in the number of generic drugs available in the USA.

At the same time Congress recognized that the effective patent term of pioneer drugs was reduced dramatically because of the time required for drug development by the FDA IND/NDA requirements prior to marketing. On average the effective patent life for a pioneer drug was less than half the 17-year period specified by Congress under the patent law, as of the time of NDA approval. For some drugs no patent could be obtained. As part of the 1984 legislation Congress therefore directed the Patent Office to extend the patent for a pioneer drug for up to 5 years in order to compensate for the lost patent life resulting from FDA regulatory review requirements. Congress also specified a minimum period of 3 or 5 years of market exclusivity during which no generic version could be approved by FDA even if there were no patent protection.

The Drug Export Amendments Act of 1986

Under the FD&C Act as enacted in 1938 adulterated and misbranded drugs could lawfully be exported but an unapproved new drug could not. This was a drafting error, but it was nonetheless enforced by FDA.

Congress therefore enacted the Drug Export Amendments Act of 1986, which authorizes the limited export of unapproved new human drugs and biological products where FDA has approved an export application. An export application may be approved only if there is an active IND; approval of an NDA is actively being pursued in the USA; the product is exported to one or more of 21 listed countries with sophisticated regulatory systems; the product is currently approved and marketed in the receiving country; FDA has not disapproved the product; the product is manufactured in conformity with GMP and is not adulterated; the product's labelling lists the countries to which FDA has permitted it to be exported; FDA has not determined that domestic manufacture of the drug for export is contrary to the public health and safety of the USA; the product is properly labelled for export. Not surprisingly these restrictions are so tight that most US companies prefer to move their manufacturing facilities overseas, and thus source the drug from abroad, rather than to make it in the USA and attempt to obtain FDA approval of an export application.

The Prescription Drug Marketing Act of 1987
Congressional investigations in the mid 1980s demonstrated that pharmaceutical products were being exported from the USA and later imported back into the country without adequate assurance that they had not become adulterated or misbranded while abroad. Congress responded by enacting the Prescription Drug Marketing Act of 1987, which makes the importation of American drugs by anyone other than the manufacturer illegal. It also prohibits the sale of drug samples and the resale of drug products initially sold to health care institutions. Distribution of drug samples by pharmaceutical manufacturers is permitted only in response to a written request for which a receipt is obtained. The provisions requiring state licensure of wholesale distributors of prescription drugs were subsequently clarified in the Prescription Drug Amendments of 1992.

The Generic Drug Enforcement Act of 1992
Following enactment of the Drug Price Competition and Patent Term Restoration Act of 1984 FDA embarked on a major campaign to expedite approval of abbreviated NDAs for generic versions of important pioneer drugs for which the patents had expired. Because of the enormous economic profit that could be made by the generic drug company that marketed the first generic version of an important pioneer drug, a number of generic drug manufacturers submitted fraudulent data to FDA as part of abbreviated NDAs and even paid illegal bribes to FDA officials in an attempt to obtain preferential handling of their applications. When this scandal came to light, in addition to the criminal prosecution of the individuals and companies involved, Congress enacted the Generic Drug Enforcement Act of 1992 to increase the penalties for such illegal behaviour. These new penalties include mandatory and permissive debarment of corporations

and individuals, suspension and withdrawal of approval of abbreviated NDAs, and civil money penalties. Although the 1992 Act applies primarily to generic drugs, it also provides mandatory and permissive debarment for *individuals* who engage in wrongdoing with respect to *any* drug, whether a generic or a pioneer drug. All of the provisions of the Act apply to both non-prescription and prescription drugs.

The Prescription Drug User Fee Act of 1992

Following enactment of the Drug Amendments of 1962 the time needed to develop the data and information to demonstrate the safety and effectiveness of a new drug, and to obtain FDA approval of an NDA, escalated. As a result a 'drug lag' developed between the pharmaceutical products available in the rest of the world and those available in the USA. FDA on many occasions pointed out that the time needed for FDA review of an IND or an NDA was at least in part a function of the resources available to the agency. Although both FDA and the pharmaceutical industry initially opposed the imposition on the industry of 'user fees' that would generate additional revenue to permit FDA to hire additional people to review INDs and NDAs, both abruptly reversed their earlier positions and agreed to the enactment of the Prescription Drug User Fee Act of 1992. Under this new statute FDA will collect user fees of more than $325 million over 5 years based on annual fees levied for each pioneer prescription drug and each pioneer prescription drug establishment as well as a one-time fee for each NDA for a pioneer new drug. The fees do not apply to generic drugs or to pioneer drugs after they become subject to generic competition. All of the revenue from these user fees is required to be an addition to the existing FDA budget and must be used solely for the IND/NDA review system.

Other pharmaceutical products

In addition to biological and chemical drugs, two other categories of pharmaceutical products deserve brief mention: animal drugs and human medical devices. Both are beyond the scope of the present chapter.

Animal drugs

Animal feed and drugs were regulated under the same provisions as human food and drugs under the Food and Drugs Act of 1906 and the FD&C Act of 1938. A separate statute, the Animal Virus, Serum, and Toxin Act of 1913, was enacted by Congress to authorize the USDA to regulate biological drugs intended for use in animals, and the USDA retains jurisdiction over that statute to this day. To simplify FDA regulation of animal feed and drugs Congress enacted the Animal Drug Amendments of 1968. Following the approach of the 1984 statute authorizing FDA approval of generic versions of human new drugs, Congress also enacted the Generic Animal Drug and Patent Term Restoration Act of 1988.

Medical devices

Medical devices were first made subject to FDA regulation under the FD&C Act of 1938. At that time the statute included no requirement for premarket testing or approval. Congress enacted the Medical Device Amendments of 1976 to require premarket notification for all medical devices and premarket approval for some old and new devices for which there is no adequate assurance of safety and effectiveness. The 1976 Amendments established a broad new array of statutory requirements and enforcement provisions. This new regulatory approach was supplemented by the Safe Medical Devices Act of 1990 and further refined by the Medical Device Amendments of 1992.

Two classes of drug products

There are two classes of drugs under the FD&C Act in the USA: non-prescription drugs and prescription drugs. Neither the Food and Drugs Act of 1906 nor the FD&C Act of 1938 distinguished between non-prescription and prescription drugs or established a class of mandatory prescription drugs. Shortly after the FD&C Act was enacted in 1938, however, FDA promulgated a regulation establishing criteria for a class of drugs that could only lawfully be sold by prescription. That regulation was later codified into law by Congress in the Durham–Humphrey Amendments of 1951. Under this statute prescription status is mandatory for 17 specific drugs listed in the law, drugs that are not safe for use except under a practitioner's supervision and drugs limited to prescription sale under an NDA. The statutory criteria for determining prescription status are toxicity, other potentiality for harmful effect and the method of use and collateral measures necessary to use the drug. In all instances today the prescription or non-prescription status of a new drug is determined by the NDA.

A drug may be switched from prescription to non-prescription status. Prior to 1970 this was most often accomplished by FDA promulgation of a regulation. During the last 20 years a switch from prescription to non-prescription has most frequently been accomplished as part of the FDA OTC (Over-The-Counter) Drug Review, discussed in detail below. Now that the OTC Drug Review is largely complete, and with the availability of market exclusivity under the Drug Price Competition and Patent Term Restoration Act of 1984, a switch from prescription to non-prescription status is accomplished primarily through a supplemental NDA.

Non-prescription drugs may be sold at any kind of retail store in the USA, ranging from a pharmacy to a grocery store to a gasoline filling station. There are, in short, no criteria or limitations upon the method of distribution and sale for non-prescription drugs. Pharmacy groups have contended that FDA should establish a 'third class' of drugs that would be available only through a pharmacy, and have used as one example of the need for such a new class those prescription drugs that are in the process of being switched to non-prescription status. FDA has declined to establish such a third class of drugs, on both policy and legal grounds. First, FDA has stated that any drug switched by the agency from prescription to non-prescription status is sufficiently safe for sale in any retail establishment, and that a requirement limiting sale to a pharmacy would provide an unjustified monopoly to pharmacists. Second, FDA has stated that the FD&C Act provides no authority for FDA to restrict distribution of non-prescription drug to pharmacies.

Regulation of non-prescription drugs

Adulteration and misbranding

Since 1906 the adulteration or misbranding of a non-prescription drug has been illegal in the USA. Both 'adulteration' and 'misbranding' are defined in the statute. Adulteration includes such acts as the failure to comply with GMP; the use of a container that may render the contents injurious to health; the use of an illegal colour additive; failure to comply with United States Pharmacopeia requirements; failure to meet labelled strength or purity; and related prohibited acts. Misbranding includes such labelling violations as any false or misleading labelling; the failure to include mandatory information relating to the name and address of the manufacturer and the net quantity of contents; the failure to bear adequate directions for use and warnings against unsafe use; the failure to meet packaging and labelling requirements established by the United States Pharmacopeia; the failure to use packaging and labelling to reduce product deterioration; danger to health when used as recommended in the labelling; the failure to obtain batch certification for an antibiotic for which such certification is required; and the failure to comply with a large number of other statutory requirements including drug estab- lishment, registration and product listing, and poison prevention and tamper-resistant packaging. The adulteration and misbranding provisions of the statute itself are continually expanded by FDA regulations that impose additional requirement either for all non-prescription drugs or for specific categories. Accordingly, current requirements can be deter- mined only by consulting FDA regulations and other policy statements as well as the statute itself.

The IND/NDA system

Since 1938 non-prescription drugs have been subject to the new drug provisions of the Act as well as the adulteration and misbranding provi- sions. As a practical matter, however, the new drug provisions cover an extremely small segment of the non-prescription drug market and thus are relatively unimportant to the non-prescription drug industry. Most new drugs are restricted by FDA to prescription status. Only a handful of new chemical entity drugs that require an NDA – fewer than one per year – are marketed initially with non-prescription status. For those non-prescription drugs that do go through the IND/NDA system, the requirements are no different than for a prescription drug. These requirements are discussed in detail below.

The OTC Drug Review

During the period beginning with enactment of the new drug provisions in the FD&C Act in 1938 and ending with enactment of the Drug Amendments of 1962, there were approximately 420 NDAs for non-prescription drugs. Many of these NDAs were for long established ingredients for which no NDA was truly required, but it was so simple to obtain an effective NDA during that time that many were submitted simply to obtain a perceived marketing advantage. As part of the Drug Amendments of 1962 FDA was required to review these 420 NDAs and to determine whether the drugs were effective as well as safe. Rather than limit its inquiry to these 420 specific non-prescription drug products, FDA concluded instead to broaden the scope of its review to all active ingredients used in all non-prescription drugs on the market at that time. The agency also concluded to review the labelling as well as the active ingredients in these products.

In 1972 FDA announced the beginning of its massive OTC Drug Review – undoubtedly the largest and most extensive review of the safety, effectiveness and labelling of non-prescription drugs ever undertaken. FDA established panels of experts to review individual categories of non-prescription drugs and to prepare reports on their conclusions and recommendations. Those reports were published as proposed monographs establishing the conditions for safe, effective and properly labelled non-prescription drugs within each category. Following public comment FDA published a tentative final monograph. Following additional public comment and a public hearing before the Commissioner FDA established the final monograph. The documents that comprise these public proceedings represent an extremely important record of the status of non-prescription drug active ingredients and finished products in the USA.

By the early 1980s all of the FDA panels had completed their deliberations and issued their reports. Because the industry largely followed the conclusions and recommendations of these reports, most of the impact of the OTC Drug Review has already been reflected in the marketplace. Nonetheless, a number of monographs remain to be completed and it will be some years before the OTC Drug Review is totally finished.

An OTC drug monograph establishes those conditions under which an OTC drug is generally recognized as safe and effective (GRAS and GRAE) and is properly labelled, and thus may be lawfully marketed in the USA without the need for an NDA or any other type of FDA approval. Any person may market a non-prescription drug in the USA today in compliance with one of these monographs (or, where no final monograph has been issued, in accordance with a tentative final monograph or proposed monograph). One of the major purposes behind the OTC Drug Review was to establish, by regulations, the criteria under which an NDA is not required. Where a product is marketed with any deviation from an OTC drug monograph, however, some form of NDA is required in order to justify that deviation before marketing will be permitted. In short, complete compliance with an OTC drug monograph guarantees immediate marketing without any form of premarket approval. Of course, all non-prescription drugs must comply with the general adulteration and misbranding provisions of the law, including GMP, establishment registration and drug listing.

Tamper-resistant packaging
In September 1982 it was discovered that several people living in Chicago had died from cyanide poisoning after taking Extra-Strength Tylenol capsules. FDA promptly promulgated regulations requiring tamper-resistant packaging for most non-prescription drug products. Congress followed by enacting the Federal Anti-Tampering Act of 1983, which makes it a crime to tamper with a consumer product with reckless disregard for the risk of persons or with intent to cause injury to a business. A number of individuals have in fact been prosecuted for illegal tampering under this statute.

Industry self-regulation
The Nonprescription Drug Manufacturers Association (NDMA), the US trade association representing the non-prescription drug industry, has established a number of voluntary codes and guidelines to supplement FDA regulation of non-prescription drugs. Among those guidelines are recommended package sizes for certain non-prescription drug categories; label 'flags' to bring the attention of consumers to significant product changes; label disclosure of inactive ingredients; mail sampling of non-prescription drugs; expiration dating of non-prescription drugs; product identification of solid dosage non-prescription drugs; and label readability for non-prescription drugs. Although these are not legal requirements, they are widely followed in the non-prescription drug industry.

Regulation of prescription drugs

It is particularly difficult to summarize FDA regulation of prescription drugs. The statutory provisions are long and complex, the regulations consume hundreds of pages in the Code of Federal Regulations, the preambles cover thousands of pages in the Federal Register, and the guidelines and policy directives are so numerous and diverse that they have never been collected in one place or even listed in a comprehensive way. The discussion will therefore begin with a historical overview of the development of FDA regulation of prescription drugs. This is followed by a brief analysis of how the current system works.

This section is limited to drugs regulated under the FD&C Act. Biological drugs are considered in the next section.

Historical overview
As enacted in 1938, the FD&C Act defined a 'new drug' as any drug that was not GRAS. Section 505 of the 1938 Act provided that an NDA must be submitted for every new drug, and authorized FDA to permit an NDA to become effective or to disapprove the NDA, but not affirmatively to approve an NDA. If FDA took no action within 60 days after the filing of

an NDA, the NDA automatically became effective and the drug could lawfully be marketed.

The pharmaceutical industry submitted thousands of NDAs within the first few years after 1938. Because FDA was unprepared to deal with this large number of NDAs, FDA advised drug manufacturers that NDAs were not required for 'old drugs' that were GRAS, and in fact refused to accept NDAs for these drugs. This substantially reduced the numbers of NDAs that were submitted to and accepted by FDA. For example, more than 4000 NDAs were submitted by 1941, but by 1962 NDAs for only 9457 individual drug products had become effective. Most prescription drugs were marketed on the conclusion of FDA or the manufacturer that they were GRAS and thus old drugs that did not require an NDA.

Following enactment of the Drug Amendments of 1962 FDA immediately encountered two problems. First, the pharmaceutical industry submitted a substantially increased number of INDs and NDAs, which again overwhelmed the resources of FDA to deal with these submissions. Second, the 1962 Amendments required FDA to review all of the NDAs that had become effective between 1938 and 1962 on the basis of a demonstration of safety, and to determine whether these drugs were also effective. Because of the overwhelming number of current INDs and NDAs for new products, FDA had no resources to devote to this requirement. Accordingly, in June 1966 FDA contracted with the National Academy of Sciences (NAS) to conduct the review of 1938–1962 NDAs.

The NAS review was conducted by panels of experts in specific drug categories. The NAS rated each drug as one of the following six categories: (1) effective; (2) probably effective; (3) possibly effective; (4) ineffective; (5) effective but other drugs are preferable; or (6) ineffective as a fixed combination. Because roughly half of the drugs were no longer marketed, the NAS ultimately reviewed approximately 4000 different drug formulations. Brief reports, many consisting only of a single sentence, were transmitted to FDA by the NAS between 1967 and 1968. FDA then undertook to implement these reports in the form of notices published in the Federal Register as part of what the agency called the Drug Efficacy Study Implementation (DESI) programme.

In order to implement the NAS reports, FDA found that it must first address a number of important policy issues. First, FDA was required to determine whether the NAS findings would apply only to the pioneer drug which submitted the NDA, or also to all subsequently marketed generic versions of the drug. FDA determined that the latter approach was required, which led to extensive litigation. FDA policy on this matter was ultimately upheld by the Supreme Court in June 1973.

Second, FDA had to confront the fact that it had issued hundreds of 'old drug' opinion letters prior to the 1962 Amendments for generic versions of pioneer new drugs. It therefore issued a statement of policy in May 1968 revoking all of those opinions.

Third, FDA was confronted with the potential of thousands of requests for formal trial-type administrative hearings for pre-1962 new drugs which were found to be less than effective. The requirement of formal administrative hearings would have effectively precluded implementation of the

1962 Amendments. FDA resolved this by publishing in the Federal Register regulations defining the new statutory requirement of adequate and
well controlled clinical investigations, and issuing summary judgment
notices withdrawing approval of new drugs that failed to submit clinical
studies that on the face of it the requirements of the new regulations. The
regulations defining adequate and well controlled clinical investigations
were upheld in the courts, and the summary judgment procedure was
also upheld. Thus, the number of drugs for which formal administrative
hearings were required was substantially reduced.

Fourth, FDA established a new procedure for regulating generic versions
of pre-1962 pioneer drugs that were found under the DESI programme
to be safe and effective. FDA established the 'abbreviated' NDA that
required submission of information to FDA only on bioequivalence and
manufacturing controls, and not on basic safety and effectiveness. Any
manufacturer who wished to market a generic version of a pre-1962 pioneer
found to be safe and effective under the NAS review could obtain FDA
approval for marketing through an abbreviated NDA.

In 1972, 10 years after the 1962 Amendments were enacted, three lower
court rulings threatened to destroy the FDA approach to these matters.
The agency successfully took all three cases, as well as a fourth in
which FDA had prevailed, to the US Supreme Court, and in June 1973
the Supreme Court sustained FDA on all of the legal issues involved.
From then on the basic approach to FDA implementation of the 1962
Amendments was established and strengthened.

The FDA pace of implementation of the 1962 Amendment was, however,
necessarily slow. The American Public Health Association therefore
brought a lawsuit to require FDA to complete its DESI programme for
pre-1962 new drugs, and the federal district court entered an order
requiring completion within 4 years. Although FDA to this day has still
not completed this programme, the court order did impose a greater sense
of urgency and has led FDA to devote greater resources to this matter.

Throughout this time FDA was groping for a consistent approach to
the handling of generic drugs. Initially it revoked all 'old drug' opinion
letters. Later it proposed a procedure for determining old drug status for
products. Following that, it concluded that an abbreviated NDA should
be submitted for all generic versions of pre-1962 new drugs. In 1975 it
again reversed itself and decided to develop old drug monographs, similar
to the non-prescription drug monographs, for which an NDA would not
be required. Still later it abandoned that approach and again stated that
an abbreviated NDA would be required for all generic versions of pre-1962
new drugs. That position was challenged in the courts, but was upheld by
the Supreme Court.

An attempt was made between 1977 and 1980 to resolve all of these
issues through a comprehensive revision of the new drug provisions of
the FD&C Act. Because the legislation was so detailed and complex,
however, it never came close to enactment.

By 1980 a new problem had emerged. FDA had administratively created
the concept of an abbreviated NDA to handle generic versions of pre-1962
pioneer new drugs, but there was no similar mechanism for approval of

generic versions of post-1962 new drugs. As time went by, more and more post-1962 pioneer new drugs lost patent protection, but retained an equivalent protection under the FD&C Act because FDA had no authority to approve any form of an abbreviated NDA for generic versions of these drugs. FDA therefore began to search for a solution to this problem. In 1978 FDA announced it would approve a 'paper' NDA for a generic copy of a post-1962 pioneer new drug based upon the published scientific data for the drug. This policy was upheld in the courts, but it had relatively little impact because there was insufficient published animal and human data to approve generic versions of most post-1962 new drugs. Thus, relatively few paper NDAs were approved by FDA.

Another drug tragedy in early 1984 focused FDA on yet another aspect of regulating prescription new drugs. An intravenous vitamin E product marketed without an NDA produced serious adverse reactions that required a nationwide recall. FDA concluded that there were approximately 5000 prescription drugs marketed without an approved NDA of any kind. Some 1800 would eventually be subject to the requirement for an abbreviated NDA when the DESI programme was fully implemented, but another 2400 were never subject to the NAS review because they were on the market prior to the FD&C Act of 1938 or were otherwise grandfathered. FDA was forced to concede that these products could remain on the market until the agency could find the resources to review them and consider appropriate regulation. Indeed, new versions of these products can still be marketed as long as they are identical to the previously marketed versions. FDA did promulgate a regulation requiring adverse drug reaction (ADR) reports for all prescription drugs marketed without an approved NDA, in order to track any potential public health problem.

In the past decade FDA has slowly but surely marched ahead with the DESI programme, implementing the NAS review of pre-1962 new drugs. Where a drug has been found ineffective, most have been taken off the market using the summary judgment procedure. A few manufacturers have succeeded in requiring an administrative hearing, but none has prevailed before an administrative law judge, the Commissioner or the courts.

In a surprisingly large number of instances manufacturers have decided to market new drugs without any NDA, and thus to market new drugs outside the 1984 FDA policy permitting such products if identical to old products that never had an NDA, solely on the basis that they are old drugs because they are generally recognized as safe and effective (GRAS and GRAE) and therefore do not require an approved NDA. FDA has brought enforcement actions against dozens of these products, and has prevailed in every case.

As indicated above, the status of generic versions of both pre-1962 and post-1962 new drugs was settled by Congress in the Drug Price Competition and Patent Term Restoration Act of 1984. That statute will be discussed in greater detail below.

Accordingly, most of the large conceptual issues that confronted FDA following enactment of the Drug Amendments of 1962 have now been resolved, and most of the large categories of prescription drug products on the market have been brought under regulatory control. The major category of products that remains without any form of NDA approval are the approximately 2400 pre-1962 new drugs that were never the subject of an NDA and for which FDA has not yet conducted some form of regulatory review.

Regulatory categories of prescription drugs

There are two primary categories of prescription drugs: those not currently subject to any form of NDA approval, and those subject to some form of NDA approval.

No NDA

Those not subject to any form of NDA approval consist only of products for which an NDA has never been required or obtained, and which thus were not subject to the NAS review of 1938–1962 new drugs. This is a limited category.

In its 1984 policy statement FDA stated that new versions of one of these drugs could be marketed, until FDA institutes some form of regulatory control, only if the new version is in all significant respects identical to the old version. The life of one of these products is, of course, uncertain. FDA could at any time conclude to regulate any or all of these products in a more comprehensive way. The precise status of any of these drugs can be determined only by a detailed review of all of the facts available for the specific product involved.

Three forms of NDA

The vast bulk of prescription drugs on the market today are subject to the requirement for some form of an approved NDA. Following enactment of the Drug Price Competition and Patent Term Restoration Act of 1984, there are now three clearly established types of NDA: a full NDA; a paper NDA (now called a Section 505(b) (2) NDA); and an abbreviated NDA. Each of these types of NDA is discussed in the sections that follow.

The full NDA

For any new chemical entity, whether or not it has been marketed abroad, and whether or not it is chemically related to some other approved new drug, FDA requires compliance with the full IND/NDA process.

The IND

Before submitting an NDA to FDA, the sponsor of a drug must conduct, or arrange to be conducted, various types of non-clinical (*in vitro* and animal) tests and clinical (human) studies designed to demonstrate that the drug is safe and effective for its intended use.

For non-human studies no IND is required. Companies may perform *in vitro* testing to obtain, for example, chemical information necessary to set exact specifications for the active ingredient or to obtain stability data. The company may also conduct animal toxicology tests to establish an adequate margin of human safety. Animal toxicology testing must be conducted in accordance with the FDA Good Laboratory Practice (GLP) regulations, but no IND or any other type of notice to FDA is required for any type of non-human studies. FDA also has both formal and informal guidelines to govern animal toxicity testing.

After adequate preclinical testing has been completed, an IND must be submitted to FDA to justify clinical investigation in humans. The content and format of an IND are set out in detail in the FDA regulations, and therefore need not be repeated here. The IND must contain all relevant information about the safety and effectiveness of the new drug, the protocols intended to be used in the investigations, the chemistry, manufacturing, and control information, pharmacology and toxicology information, previous human experience, and other pertinent information. In all respects the FDA IND regulations must be followed in detail.

After submission FDA has 30 days within which to evaluate the IND. By the end of 30 days one of several things will have occurred. First, FDA may approve the IND, in which case testing can begin. Second, FDA may place the IND on formal clinical hold, in which case testing cannot begin. Third, FDA may say nothing, or may raise questions, or may offer suggestions, or may say virtually anything in response to the IND. The sponsor must then determine whether to proceed in light of these developments or whether to delay testing until the matter is clarified. Many sponsors conclude that the only reasonable thing to do is to delay testing until all issues are fully resolved, but others proceed in the face of open questions.

Once the initial 30-day period has expired the IND may be amended and updated periodically. For example, additional protocols may be added. There is no 30-day delay for any subsequent amendment. Once again, however, sponsors must determine whether to delay testing until FDA is consulted and any issues are fully resolved.

An essential element of the IND is approval of the investigation by an institutional review board (IRB), usually in the institution in which the drug will be tested. The IRB is charged with reviewing both the ethical and moral dimensions of the study as well as the scientific merit. IRB approval does not guarantee FDA approval, nor does FDA approval guarantee IRB approval. They are separate and independent requirements, and both must be fulfilled before testing may begin under an IND.

Adherence to the IND by the sponsor is essential. Variations from any aspect of the IND are not permitted. Before there can be any change in any aspect of the IND – including the specifications of the drug, the nature of the manufacturing process, the protocol for the investigation, and the identity of the investigators, to name just a few – the IND must be amended.

No investigational new drug may be promoted or otherwise commercialized. No charge may be made for an investigational new drug without the prior approval of FDA.

The FDA IND regulations contain requirements for various types of records and reports that must be adhered to without exception. Immediate reports are required by FDA for any serious and unexpected adverse experience associated with the drug. Annual reports are required for every IND. Records must be kept to document all aspects of the IND.

Clinical testing under an IND is usually regarded as proceeding through three phases. Phase I includes the initial introduction of an investigational new drug into humans under closely monitored conditions, usually in a teaching hospital. This phase involves a relatively small number of subjects and is intended to obtain basic information on the pharmacology of the drug. Phase II includes controlled clinical studies conducted to evaluate the effectiveness of the drug and to determine common side effects and other risks. It involves a greater number of subjects, but is not a large-scale trial. Phase III involves expanded controlled and uncontrolled trials to gather additional information about safety and effectiveness that is needed to evaluate the overall benefit/risk relationship, and may involve up to several thousand subjects. In recent years these three phases have tended to overlap substantially, and approval has been obtained on the basis of Phase II or Phase II/III studies for a number of important drugs.

Three types of unusual IND situations deserve special mention. First, the regulations contain a provision governing emergency use of an investigational new drug, where FDA will permit such use by telephone or other rapid communication means. In these situations the IND must subsequently be amended to reflect the new situation. Second, FDA will approve specific treatment protocols for compassionate use of an investigational new drug where the drug is intended to treat a serious or immediately life-threatening disease, where there is no satisfactory alternative, where the drug is under clinical investigation pursuant to an IND and where marketing approval is actively being pursued with due diligence. After a treatment IND has been approved the sponsor may provide the drug to any patient who meets the criteria in the treatment IND and may charge in order to recoup the cost of the drug. Third, FDA will approve 'parallel track' protocols for AIDS where there is no therapeutic alternative and individuals cannot participate in the controlled clinical trials, in order to assure widespread use of the most promising drugs at the earliest possible stage. As a practical matter it is difficult, if not impossible, to distinguish between a parallel track IND and a treatment IND.

Compassionate use of investigational new drugs has been permitted by FDA since the 1950s in order to assure that individual patients, who have no other alternative, are not denied any promising treatment. The more recent terminology of 'treatment IND' and 'parallel track' are therefore simply a continuation of this longstanding policy, with no significant substantive change. In addition to these new forms of compassionate use INDs, the pharmaceutical industry continues to use the traditional form of compassionate use protocol as well.

The NDA

After the sponsor has completed all non-clinical and clinical testing necessary to demonstrate the safety and effectiveness of the drug, the test results must be compiled in an NDA for submission to FDA. Like the IND the content and format of the NDA are set forth in the FDA regulations and must be followed in detail. The NDA must begin with a summary, to be followed by technical sections relating to: (1) chemistry, manufacturing, and controls; (2) non-clinical pharmacology and toxicology; (3) human pharmacalcanetics and bioavailability; (4) microbiology; (5) clinical data; and (6) statistics. Proposed labelling must also be included. The typical NDA comprises tens of thousands or even hundreds of thousands of pages.

The statute requires that a new drug be shown to be both safe and effective. Because no drug has ever been shown to be completely safe or effective, in all cases this has been interpreted to mean that the benefits of the drug outweigh its risks under the labelled conditions of use for a significant identified patient population. The statute is very broadly worded with respect to the required proof for safety and effectiveness, and FDA has exercised substantial discretion in applying these requirements. New drugs have been approved on the basis of only one study, on the basis of Phase II studies that have never progressed to Phase III, on the basis of foreign studies alone, and with results that could not be regarded as definitive from a scientific standpoint. In most instances, however, FDA requires more than one adequate and well controlled clinical trial.

Under the statute FDA must evaluate the NDA and approve or disapprove it within 180 days. This almost never occurs. The average time for approval of an NDA is between 2 and 3 years. This period has remained largely unchanged for the past 20 years, in spite of repeated promises and attempts by FDA to speed up the process. FDA is able to avoid the 180-day statutory time deadline in several ways. First, FDA starts the clock when it accepts the NDA for filing, not when it is submitted. Second, FDA stops the clock whenever new submissions are made. Third, FDA will request an extension of time from the applicant, who has no choice but to agree. Fourth, FDA will simply ignore the 180-day deadline, and there is nothing that the applicant can do about it anyway.

During the NDA evaluation by FDA there are no guidelines or rules that require open communication between FDA and the applicant. It is impossible to generalize about the relationship between drug applicants and FDA reviewers. The Center for Drug Evaluation and Research (CDER) review divisions have quite varied reputations for openness, promptness and cordiality. Thus, discussion between an FDA review division and the applicant varies all the way from virtually no communication to constant discussion. Relations range from friendliness to near hostility. The NDA review process is, in short, entirely an *ad hoc* and informal process of negotiation that may go very well or very poorly, and over which the applicant has virtually no control. Attempts to obtain resolution of disputes through the FDA ombudsman or by appealing issues to higher officials are almost never successful and often worsen relations with the NDA reviewers. Pharmaceutical companies uniformly fear retaliation unless they cooperate fully with every request from the NDA reviewers.

For every NDA some clinical study is almost certain to remain in progress at the time that the NDA is submitted. Safety update reports are therefore required to be submitted to FDA by the applicant while the NDA is pending, and particularly following receipt of an approvable letter. Detailed systems and procedures are required to ensure that the data in the NDA and the safety updates are accurate and complete, and the failure to meet these requirements is regarded by FDA as a serious deficiency.

It is customary for FDA to submit one or more letters of disapproval as part of the NDA review process. These frequently lead to submission of new information, a revision of labelling and further negotiation. In a relatively small number of cases FDA will issue a definitive disapproval letter determining that there is no additional information on the basis of which the drug could be approved. The applicant then has available various administrative and judicial appeals that can be taken. In no instance since 1938, however, has any applicant successfully challenged FDA denial of approval of an NDA. For that reason it is generally understood that there is no practical way to challenge whatever FDA requires during the NDA process, and that the only realistic alternative is to negotiate the best possible approach with FDA in a cooperative spirit.

Confidentiality of information

Under the Freedom of Information Act, all information in government files is subject to public disclosure unless it falls within a specified exemption. FDA has promulgated detailed regulations governing the status of general categories of data and information in its files, and particularly data and information submitted as part of an IND or NDA. In general no data or information submitted to FDA as part of an IND or NDA will be made public prior to FDA approval or disapproval of the NDA. Even the existence of an IND or NDA will be kept confidential by FDA if it has not been disclosed by the sponsor. Upon approval FDA issues a summary of the basis for the agency approval of the product, which describes the safety and effectiveness data on which the agency replied. Whether FDA will also release the reports and data relating to the testing for safety and effectiveness will depend upon whether the company can convince FDA that this data retains value as 'confidential commercial information'. In general FDA will release the full data and information on safety and effectiveness after a drug becomes subject to generic competition, but not before. Agency regulations spell out FDA's confidentiality policies in great detail, but there still are often disputes about their application to any particular set of facts.

Advisory committees

There is no statutory requirement that FDA review the approval of an NDA with an advisory committee before final action is taken. Since 1970, however, this has been the customary practice, particularly with important new drugs.

The review of an NDA by an advisory committee is an extremely important step in the approval process. It represents the best opportunity that the applicant has to address the FDA and the public about the evidence of safety and effectiveness and the importance of the drug to public health. In the vast majority of cases FDA accepts the recommendation of the advisory committee for approval, further testing or outright disapproval. Where the advisory committee recommends approval and FDA disagrees, however, the agency will almost always take a long time to implement the advisory committee recommendations or may even add additional testing requirements before approval is eventually obtained. The importance of advisory committee review is widely recognized in the pharmaceutical industry, and it is common for a company to engage in extensive preparation for the company presentation and to seek supportive statements from independent outside experts as well.

Postapproval requirements
Following approval of an NDA FDA requires the submission of three different types of reports by the owner of the NDA. First, serious and unexpected adverse drug reactions (ADRs) must be immediately reported to FDA regardless whether the company believes they are causally related to the drug. Second, ADRs as well as other safety and effectiveness information must be reported periodically to FDA, at intervals specified in the FDA regulations. Third, information relating to all other aspects of the drug must be reported immediately to FDA if it represents a potential problem, but otherwise may be included in an annual report. Foreign as well as domestic ADRs and other information must be included in these reports.

Changes in the NDA after approval
Any significant change from the detailed terms and conditions specified in the approved NDA must be the subject of a supplemental NDA submitted to FDA, and cannot be put into effect until the supplemental NDA has been approved by FDA. The only changes in an approved NDA that may be made without approval of a supplemental NDA are set forth in FDA regulations, and those exceptions must be reflected in the annual report submitted to FDA. Where FDA finds that changes have been made from an approved NDA beyond those permitted without a supplemental NDA, very stringent regulatory action can be taken, including recall of the product and the inability to manufacture any more product until the unapproved changes are eliminated. Accordingly, it is essential that all aspects of an approved NDA be followed in detail unless a clear exception is created in the FDA regulations.

Summary suspension of approval
The statute provides that the Secretary of HHS may summarily suspend approval of an NDA upon a finding that the drug represents an imminent hazard to public health. This authority is delegated to the Secretary of HHS alone, and cannot be exercised by FDA or anyone else. It has been used only once, and was upheld in the courts.

Antibiotic drugs
New antibiotic drugs are subject to the same IND and NDA requirements contained in the FDA regulations as other new drugs. Although the statute provides that FDA may require batch certification for antibiotics, in 1982 FDA exempted all classes of antibiotic drugs from this requirement because of the high level of manufacturer compliance with antibiotic standards.

Thus, antibiotics today are regulated in a manner that is virtually indistinguishable from other new drugs.

User fees

Under the Prescription Drug User Fee Act of 1992 FDA has authority to collect user fees of more than $325 million during fiscal years 1993–1997. These user fees apply only to pioneer drugs, and only until such time as generic competition is approved. The fees include: (1) a one-time NDA fee; (2) an annual product fee; and (3) an annual establishment fee. The precise amount of each fee escalates each year and is subject to modification according to detailed provisions in the statute. The funds obtained from these fees must be in addition to the existing resources for the IND/NDA system, as adjusted for cost-of-living increases, and must be used solely for the IND/NDA process. In return for receiving user fees FDA has committed to specific goals for improving the drug review process, by reducing the backlog of applications and meeting specified time deadlines. The extent to which these commitments can be kept will become apparent only in the coming years.

The paper NDA

When Congress enacted the Drug Price Competition and Patent Term Restoration Act of 1984 it included a provision based upon the concept of a paper NDA but one which in fact expanded that concept significantly. The former paper NDA is therefore now often called a Section 505(b) (2) NDA. As currently interpreted, it applies to those situations where an applicant is unable to submit an abbreviated NDA because the modified drug differs in some substantial way from the pioneer drug. A Section 505(b) (2) paper NDA relies upon the pioneer NDA for all information except the data needed to support the one element of substantial difference. Thus, the new paper NDA need not include any data relating to the basic safety and effectiveness of the drug except insofar as the difference between the pioneer drug and the applicant's modification of that drug bears upon safety or effectiveness.

As will be discussed below, minor differences between a pioneer drug and a generic version of that drug may be approved by FDA as appropriate for an abbreviated NDA pursuant to a 'suitability petition'. Where those differences become substantial, however, FDA will deny the suitability petition and will require the approval of a more complete NDA. In these circumstances the Section 505(b) (2) paper NDA will be sufficient, and a full NDA will not be required. Thus, the new paper NDA is midway between a full NDA and an abbreviated NDA. The same regulations and requirements apply to a Section 505(b) (2) paper NDA under the 1984 Act as apply to a full NDA.

The abbreviated NDA

All of the regulations and requirements for an abbreviated NDA developed by FDA in the late 1960s as part of the implementation of the Drug Amendments of 1962, and all of the proposed changes that FDA considered to adapt those requirements to post-1962 new drugs, were eliminated when Congress enacted the Drug Price Competition and Patent Term Restoration Act of 1984. The 1984 Act established detailed requirements that supersede everything that went before.

Under the 1984 Act an abbreviated NDA may be approved by FDA for a pioneer new drug after: (1) all relevant product and use patents have expired; and (2) all relevant periods of market exclusivity have also expired. The statute contains detailed and complex rules for determining precisely how this system works. No attempt will be made here to discuss the specific provisions, but they are extremely important in determining the commercial value of a pioneer new drug because they govern when the drug will become subject to generic competition.

There are basically two types of situations where an abbreviated NDA may be submitted. The first situation is where the generic version is the same as the pioneer version in all material respects. Where this is true the applicant for the generic product simply submits the abbreviated NDA and FDA may approve it without further consideration about the basic safety and effectiveness of the drug. The second circumstance is where the generic version is different from the pioneer drug in any significant respect (e.g., a different active ingredient, route of administration, dosage form, or strength). In these circumstances the generic applicant must first submit to FDA a 'suitability petition' demonstrating that the difference between the drugs is not sufficient to preclude an abbreviated NDA and that additional studies to show safety and effectiveness are not needed. If FDA grants the suitability petition an abbreviated NDA may be submitted. If the suitability petition is denied the applicant must submit either a Section 505(b) (2) paper NDA or a full NDA. In all other respects the regulations and requirements for an abbreviated NDA are the same as those for a full NDA.

The fraud policy

As a result of the generic drug scandal described above, where generic drug manufacturers submitted fraudulent data and bribed FDA officials, FDA adopted a 'fraud policy' in September 1991 to cover situations where FDA concluded that an applicant who had engaged in a wrongful act would need to take corrective action to establish the reliability of data submitted to FDA in support of pending applications and to support the integrity of products already on the market. Under the fraud policy FDA issues a formal letter invoking the policy and requiring the applicant to cooperate fully with the FDA investigation. The applicant is required to identify all individuals associated with the wrongful act and to ensure that they are removed from any substantive authority on matters under FDA jurisdiction. A credible internal review must be conducted to identify all instances of wrongful acts, to supplement FDA's own investigation. The internal review should involve an outside consultant or team qualified by training and experience to conduct such a review. Finally, the applicant must commit in writing to developing and implementing a corrective action operating plan. Although the fraud policy was developed in response to the generic drug scandal, it also applies to pioneer drug companies and to data in full NDAs.

Labelling and advertising

The labelling for a new drug must be included as part of the NDA and must be approved explicitly by FDA. No significant change may be made in the labelling without prior FDA approval through a supplemental NDA. Because this rule is so clear and so stringent, the pharmaceutical industry seldom takes chances with deviations in product labelling that could result in FDA enforcement action.

The Drug Amendments of 1962 gave FDA authority to regulate advertising for prescription drugs, as well as labelling. The FD&C Act was not amended, however, to give FDA premarket approval over advertising similar to its premarket approval over labelling. Accordingly, FDA must reply upon general policing of prescription drug advertising to determine whether it is false or misleading.

In accordance with its statutory authority, FDA has promulgated regulations that illustrate ways in which prescription drug advertising may be false, lacking in fair balance or otherwise misleading. As the pharmaceutical industry has expanded its promotional activities, FDA has also issued a variety of policy statements on various types of advertising practices that do not fall within the existing regulations. These policy statements deal with such issues as press conferences, medical seminars, journal supplements, tv and radio talk shows and a wide variety of other means of communication. It is essential that anyone engaging in prescription drug marketing be fully familiar with the latest FDA policy in these areas.

A recent innovation has been direct-to-consumer prescription drug promotion. Because current FDA regulations require a summary of the entire approved package insert to appear with any prescription drug advertisement, it is extremely difficult to use radio or tv advertising for this purpose. Most consumer advertising for prescription drugs is therefore limited to the print media. FDA reviews these advertisements very carefully, and thus caution must be used in preparing them. It is sound practice to review proposed advertising of this type with FDA prior to its use.

Good manufacturing practices (GMP)

One of the most important parts of an NDA is the description of the manufacturing procedures and controls. FDA has traditionally placed substantial reliance on this part of the NDA in assuring the safety and effectiveness of the drug. One study conducted a decade ago found that more questions were raised by FDA reviewers about this section of the NDA than about the safety and effectiveness of the drug itself.

Beginning in 1991, moreover, FDA announced a new enforcement technique designed to assure adequate GMP compliance before approval of an NDA. Prior to FDA approval of an NDA the FDA field force now inspects the drug establishment where the new drug is to be manufactured. If the manufacturing facility deviates in any way from either the description in the NDA or the general requirements for GMP in the FDA regulations, the NDA will not be approved until full compliance is achieved. Pursuant to this policy, the approval of numerous NDAs has been substantially delayed. Compliance with GMP is therefore essential to any NDA approval.

After approval of an NDA FDA periodically inspects a drug establishment for two purposes. First, FDA determines whether any unapproved changes have been made in the manufacturing process from those set forth in the approved NDA. If any such changes are made beyond those permitted without a supplemental NDA FDA may well bring stringent enforcement action. Second, FDA routinely inspects all establishments to determine compliance with GMP. Although FDA has not changed its GMP regulations, the interpretation and application of those regulations by FDA inspectors are thought by the pharmaceutical industry to have been substantially tightened and made more strict in the past few years.

Where FDA determines any deviation from GMP the inspector leaves a Form 483 specifying the manufacturing deficiencies. It is essential in these circumstances that the company immediately make all corrections and respond to FDA in writing about them. It can be expected that FDA will reinspect the establishment and look both for what has been done to correct the prior deficiencies and for any new deficiencies that can be found. The pharmaceutical industry believes that FDA often lists insignificant matters, that establishments which have passed without observed deficiencies in the past will suddenly be the subject of major deficiencies because of a change of interpretation, and that the requirements vary widely from individual inspector to individual inspector and from FDA district to FDA district. The industry has found, however, that its complaints fall on deaf ears, and thus that it must comply with whatever is required by the individual inspector or face the threat of serious regulatory action.

Distribution controls

On one occasion FDA sought to limit the distribution of a new drug to hospital-based pharmacies and to prohibit it through community pharmacies. When challenged by the pharmacy profession the courts ruled that this was an illegal restriction that was not authorized by the FD&C Act. Since then FDA has approved the labelling for new drugs under which the sponsor has voluntarily included restrictions on distribution, but the agency has not itself imposed distribution controls on any new drug.

Import and export

Import

In general a prescription drug may lawfully be imported into the USA only in full compliance with all of the laws and regulations applicable to domestic drugs. There is, however, one exception. Since 1977 FDA has stated that the agency will not detain unapproved new drugs imported for personal use. This became important when patients suffering from AIDS began to import drugs not available in the USA. Subsequently, AIDS organizations established buying-clubs to import drugs for all of its members. FDA has not sought to prohibit this activity except where it is done for commercial profit or involves unsafe or fraudulent products for which the agency has issued an import alert (such as RU-486). Where FDA has considered cracking down on such imports public pressure has forced the agency to back off from enforcement action.

Export

The Drug Export Amendments Act of 1986, described above, places such stringent limitations on the export of unapproved drugs from the USA that it raises enormous commercial potential for foreign countries. Many US pharmaceutical companies can reasonably anticipate that their drugs will receive approval for use outside the USA before they are approved by FDA, and cannot take the risk that they will be able to obtain and maintain FDA approval of an export application. Under these circumstances, they have no option other than to build their manufacturing facilities abroad rather than in the USA. For this reason foreign countries compete in attempting to attract these pharmaceutical factories. No other country in the world controls exports in the same way as the USA, and thus a pharmaceutical establishment may be located anywhere other than the USA without fear of unreasonable limitations on international trade. Accordingly, it is essential for any US company to be able to source its drugs abroad, rather than in the USA, if it is to be assured of the ability to market throughout the world.

Orphan drugs

Under the Orphan Drug Act of 1983 and its numerous amendments an orphan drug is eligible for two types of benefit. The first type, which is often of minor significance, consists of tax credits. The second type, which has proved to be of enormous importance, is the market exclusivity provided by the prohibition against any form of FDA approval of the same drug for another company for 7 years. The company that obtains FDA approval of an NDA for an orphan drug is thus assured of greater protection under the Orphan Drug Act than under any other statute, including the patent laws.

As enacted in 1983 the Orphan Drug Act had relatively little impact because the scope of the term 'orphan drug' was considered by FDA to be relatively narrow. When Congress amended the law in 1985 to define an orphan drug as any drug, or any single indication for a drug, for a condition afflicting fewer than 200 000 patients in the USA, however, the impact of the law changed dramatically. Some orphan drugs are now blockbusters on which entire companies can be founded. Although Congress has considered legislation to cut back some of the provisions of the Orphan Drug Act, one bill was vetoed by the President and no other bill has since come close to enactment. Even if the benefits available from the Orphan Drug Act are changed they are likely to remain important to drug companies for the foreseeable future.

Physician prescribing
The FD&C Act has been interpreted by FDA as applying only to the labelling, advertising and marketing of a new drug, and not to the practice of medicine as reflected in the physician's prescription of the drug for a particular patient. In a policy first published in 1972 and reiterated many times FDA has stated that the physician may, within the practice of medicine, lawfully prescribe an approved drug for an unapproved use. Because the Drug Price Competition and Patent Term Restoration Act of 1984 provides no significant market protection for companies that obtain FDA approval of new uses for previously approved new drugs, companies rarely submit supplemental NDAs to request FDA approval of an unapproved use for an approved drug. As unapproved use has expanded the prescription drug package insert approved by FDA has become substantially outdated. In many areas the unapproved uses of a new drug overwhelm the approved uses. Although FDA has deplored this fact, it has thus far done little to find an adequate resolution.

Patient freedom of choice
Beginning with enactment of the Drug Amendments of 1962, organized patient groups have argued strenuously that they should have the freedom to purchase whatever drugs they may wish to use, regardless of their FDA status, particularly where individuals are suffering from life-threatening disease. Cancer patients argued for use of Krebiozen and Laetrile, but FDA sought to prohibit those drugs through every means available, and the courts ultimately upheld the agency.

With the dramatic rise in AIDS, however, a larger, more vocal, and more politically active interest group has again challenged the authority of FDA to deny experimental and unapproved drugs to any patient who wishes to use them. This time the activists have had a greater impact. FDA has declined to take enforcement action in many instances where it would have done so in the past. The agency has also expedited the approval of AIDS drugs on the basis of scientific information that would not have been accepted as sufficient for any other disease area. Thus, FDA has bent its rules for putative AIDS treatments but has refused to expand its flexibility into other disease areas as well. The result is an inconsistent series of decisions approving drugs for one disease on the basis of preliminary information and withholding approval of more extensively tested drugs for other diseases.

The costs and benefits of the IND/NDA system
There have been hundreds of investigations and reports on the IND/NDA system. Numerous analyses have been done of the costs and benefits, and

hundreds of recommendations have been made about ways to improve the system. Feelings run deep on these subjects, and the philosophical and emotional element often dwarfs the factual and analytical element.

A recent study has demonstrated that the average NDA requires an investment of about $231 million. In the last year of NDA approval the average carrying cost (cost of capital) alone was $31 million. Critics argue that this is largely the result of unrealistic regulatory requirements, that it results in higher drug prices, that the delay in drugs reaching the market substantially harms public health, and that the high cost of drug development discourages drug research and development and directly hinders the development of life-saving drugs for the future. Supporters of the system point to drug tragedies of the past, argue that any relaxation of regulatory controls will dramatically increase drug risks and reduce drug effectiveness, and state that the only sound way to protect public health is to continue and indeed strengthen the present system. Supporters of biotechnology charge that the present system is destroying the opportunity presented by this new technology, and critics of biotechnology applaud that result.

Biological drugs

For 90 years biological drugs have been regulated under the Biologics Act of 1902, in accordance with statutory requirements that have not significantly changed. When FDA was delegated the responsibility for regulating biologics in 1972, however, the agency promulgated regulations adding a number of the drug regulatory provisions under the FD&C Act to those already available under the Biologics Act. Present regulation of biologics therefore incorporates requirements from both statutes and is the responsibility of the CBER.

The ELA

Before a company may manufacture any biological product an ELA must be submitted to and approved by FDA for the product involved. To obtain approval of an ELA the applicant must demonstrate full compliance with FDA GMP regulations for prescription drugs. Thus, FDA approval of an ELA is comparable to the new policy of FDA to require inspection of the proposed manufacturing site for a new drug before approving the NDA. FDA inspection relating to an ELA is comprehensive and detailed, and only full compliance with GMP will result in approval.

The PLA

The product approval system for a biological drug is the same as for a chemical drug. Non-clinical studies may be conducted without FDA knowledge or approval. Clinical investigation in humans must be preceded by the submission of an IND, and all the IND regulations discussed above for chemical drugs apply equally to a biological drug. It is only the PLA that has a different name and a somewhat different focus.

A basic premise of the regulation of biological drugs is that, because they come from natural sources, they cannot adequately be characterized by chemical specifications and must instead be regulated very rigidly by rigorous adherence to detailed manufacturing procedures. For this reason approval of a PLA depends on the specific establishment specified in that PLA and approved in the ELA. If the owner of an approved PLA wishes to manufacture all or part of the biological drug in a new establishment, it has long been standard policy under the Biologics Act to require not just that the new biological product be shown to be the same as the old, but also that new clinical studies independently demonstrate the safety and effectiveness of the new product as manufactured in the new establishment. This goes beyond the requirements that FDA has applied to chemical drugs.

With modern biotechnology, however, this rigid requirement by FDA is undergoing re-evaluation. Some biological products can be characterized by chemical or biological specifications as easily as can chemical drugs. It is therefore likely that, in the future, FDA will adopt a more flexible policy on this matter.

With the advent of biotechnology the work in the CBER has changed dramatically. For decades the only biological products regulated under the Biologics Act of 1902 were vaccines, blood, allergenic extracts and other related products that did not pose the difficult problems of balancing benefits against risks that were faced daily by the CDER. As a result the CBER was able to review and approve ELAs and PLAs rapidly, in a fraction of the time that it took the CDER to do the same job. Now the two are indistinguishable. In the past few years the time required for review and approval of a biologics application has become comparable to that for an NDA and is now a full year longer. The backlog at the CBER has risen dramatically. Critics have suggested that review and approval of new pharmaceutical products by the CBER is actually now slower and more difficult than by the CDER.

Enforcement

FDA has available to it a wide variety of enforcement authorities under the FD&C Act. They apply equally to all products regulated by FDA. For generic drugs FDA can rely also on the provisions of the recently enacted Generic Drug Enforcement Act of 1992. The following sections summarize some of the more important enforcement provisions utilized by FDA for regulating all pharmaceutical products.

Factory inspection

For purposes of enforcing the law FDA inspectors may at any time inspect any non-prescription or prescription drug establishment. For a non-prescription drug establishment FDA is not authorized to require access to any records or documents. For a prescription drug establishment FDA inspectors may see all records and documents except those that relate to financial data, sales data other than shipment data, pricing data, personnel data and research data. An FDA inspector may spend whatever amount of time is necessary to complete such an inspection, even weeks or months. Where significant enforcement issues have been found FDA inspectors have been known to spend more than a year at a single establishment.

Seizure

FDA has statutory authority to request the Department of Justice to 'seize' any illegal product. If FDA asserts that the drug is dangerous to health or the labelling is fradulent or misleading in a material respect the statute authorizes multiple seizures throughout the country. FDA must demonstrate interstate commerce, but this can readily be shown for virtually all drug products.

Injunction

FDA also has statutory authority to request the Department of Justice to seek a court injunction against continued violations of the law by a prescription drug manufacturer or distributor. FDA has had mixed results in attempting to obtain injunctions from the courts, who realize that an injunction can shut down a company entirely or subject it to arbitrary demands by FDA. FDA has therefore sought to obtain the equivalent in the form of stipulated agreements with companies that are filed as consent orders and thus fully enforceable as a requirement of law.

Criminal penalties

All violations of the FD&C Act are automatically criminal violations of law. On two occasions the US Supreme Court has held that any person standing in a responsible relationship to a violation of the FD&C Act is criminally liable, regardless of the lack of knowledge or intent. The nature of the offence is the failure of an individual to take action to prevent a violation and to assure compliance with the law.

This is an extremely harsh statute. As a practical matter FDA exercises its prosecutorial discretion only to bring cases for continuing violations of law, violations of an obvious and flagrant nature and intentionally false or fraudulent violations. Although there have been attempts to change the criminal liability standard under the FD&C Act by legislation, none has been successful thus far.

Section 305 Hearing

The FD&C Act provides that, before any violation is reported by FDA for institution of a criminal proceeding, the person against whom the proceeding is contemplated shall be given appropriate notice and an opportunity to present views. In accordance with this provision it is the custom of FDA to provide an informal hearing to individuals, to show cause why they should not be prosecuted. Where a grand jury is convened, however, FDA usually does not provide this type of hearing. Where such a hearing is given it is obviously important for the individual to demonstrate good faith in attempting to comply with the law and an intent to correct and prevent any deficiencies in the future.

Other criminal statutes

The United States Code contains a number of criminal provisions related to enforcement of the FD&C Act. These laws prohibit any criminal conspiracy, false reports to the government, mail fraud, bribery, perjury or other similar illegal activity. FDA has in fact used these provisions on a number of occasions to bring criminal prosecution against individuals and companies who have violated the FD&C Act.

Civil money penalties

The Prescription Drug Marketing Act of 1987 includes civil penalties for violation of the drug sample provisions of the FD&C Act. The law provides that a manufacturer or distributor who violates these provisions is subject to a civil penalty of not more than $50 000 for each of the first two violations resulting in a conviction in any 10-year period and for not more than $1 million for each violation resulting in a conviction after the second conviction in any 10-year period. These penalties may be imposed only by a federal district court. FDA has no administrative authority to impose any civil penalties under these provisions.

Restitution

The courts have interpreted the FD&C Act not to authorize FDA to require restitution by a manufacturer to purchasers of a product that has been found to violate the Act. In contrast, the Medical Device Amendments of 1976 explicitly provide such authority for medical devices.

Recall

For decades FDA has worked with product manufacturers to request, and to help carry out, the recall of illegal products from the market. Two courts have split on whether the FD&C Act authorizes an injunction that includes a requirement for product recall. As a practical matter, however, the precise legal authority of FDA on this matter is irrelevant. Manufacturers routinely cooperate with FDA on the recall of any dangerous product. FDA has established detailed administrative policy governing recall procedures.

Informal enforcement

The FD&C Act authorizes FDA to decline to institute formal enforcement proceedings for minor violations whenever FDA believes that public interest will be adequately served by a suitable written notice or warning. In accordance with this provision, in the early 1970s FDA began to issue a 'regulatory letter' in lieu of bringing formal court enforcement action. This permitted more rapid, less costly and more efficient enforcement of the law. Regulatory letters were recently renamed 'warning letters', but otherwise remain unchanged. Any warning letter must be given immediate attention in order to avoid more serious formal enforcement action in the courts.

Publicity

FDA has explicit statutory authority to issue information to the public. The courts have upheld the right of FDA to publicize illegal activity and to issue publicity about products and practices that it concludes to be harmful to public health. This is regarded by many as the most potent enforcement tool available to FDA.

Enforcement statistics

In the first few decades of the 1900s FDA brought hundreds of seizure and criminal actions to enforce the FD&C Act. Gradually the formal court enforcement actions have been replaced in two ways. First, FDA has promulgated hundreds of regulations that establish the precise requirements of the law, thus reducing the need for many court enforcement actions. Second, formal court enforcement actions have been replaced by informal administrative enforcement actions such as recalls and regulatory (warning) letters. FDA statistics demonstrate that the increase in administrative enforcement actions has been greater than the decrease in formal court enforcement actions, and thus that overall FDA enforcement activity has continued to increase.

Conclusion

This brief survey of the FDA regulation of pharmaceutical products demonstrates the breadth and depth of FDA activity in this field. Although there are repeated calls for reform of the IND/NDA system, it appears unlikely that any substantial change will occur in the near future. It is therefore important that any person who enters the prescription drug industry in the USA be fully informed about the requirements, understand the regulatory risks involved, and comply adequately with all of the FDA requirements.

Further reading

The Federal Food, Drug, and Cosmetic Act, 21 U.S.C. § 301 *et seq.*
The Biologics Act, 42 U.S.C. § 262.
Title 21 of the United States Code of Federal Regulations.
PB Hutt, RA Merrill (1991). *Food and Drug Law: Cases and Materials*, 2nd edn. Foundation Press.

10

Issues in the economics of the pharmaceutical industry
Klaus von Grebmer

The scope of the problem

Economics of health: three basic questions

The economics of health care and the economics of pharmaceuticals deal with three basic questions:[1]

1. *The allocation of resources*: What share of resources should be spent on health care and how should these resources be divided among the various types of care?
2. *Optimal production*: How can health care be produced efficiently in both ethical and economic terms?
3. *Distribution*: How should health care be distributed among the population?

The specific solution a country chooses is not only an economic question but rather depends on value judgements and political decisions. Consequently health economics must be seen within the framework of political goal-setting and goal-achieving processes as even different political systems today are confronted with similar problems, some examples of which are noted below.

- What percentage of the Gross National Product do we spend on health care? How much health care do we want? How much health care can we afford?
- Should we invest our health care money in prevention, cure, rehabilitation, basic research . . .?
- Should inpatient treatment, outpatient treatment or drug treatment be favoured?
- Should physicians be paid on a fee for service system, a per case system or a salary system? How does the payment system influence the medical decisions and the utilization of services?
- Does cost sharing influence the demand for health care?
- How should an insurance system be structured in order to optimize results from a medical and economic point of view?

Pharmaceuticals can fulfil four different functions, namely:

1. Prevent diseases (e.g. polio vaccination).
2. Cure diseases (e.g. antibiotics).
3. Improve the quality of life for people suffering from a disease for which there is still no curative treatment (e.g. reduce inflammation and pain in rheumatic disease).
4. Influence biological processes (e.g. contraceptives).

Pharmaceutical drug therapy therefore is one way of producing a healthier population. But economics does not say which of competing goals should be adopted and economic analysis only helps to determine whether a particular measure contributes to stated goals and at what cost.[2] Thus, the question of how a pharmaceutical market should best be organized to contribute to the production of health care in an efficient way cannot be given a general answer. Nevertheless, recent research has shown that among the various methods of producing a healthier population (e.g. hospital care, physicians' services, drug therapy), the highest increases in productivity have originated and will continue to originate from advances in drug therapy.[3] Hence an environment with public policy providing an innovative climate and workable competition within the pharmaceutical market is desirable both from the standpoint of improving a nation's health and strengthening its industry.

The current status of the research-based pharmaceutical industry

The origin of the pharmaceutical industry lies in the production and processing of bulk chemicals. Product efficiency was important, but rapid product obsolescence, patent and trademark protection and government regulation were not.[4] The modern pharmaceutical industry is largely based on the discovery and development of specific synthetic pharmaceutical chemicals.

However, the introduction of sulphonamides in 1935 changed the nature of the industry. Advances in chemotherapy drew together the strands of earlier origins and brought about an acceleration of development to create the pharmaceutical industry structure with which we are familiar today.[5] Despite the significant innovations with drug therapies such as β-blockers, contraceptives and steroids, none are ideal and there are still several less tractable illnesses such as cancer and multiple sclerosis for which no cure exists to date. As Fig. 10.1 illustrates, there is a need for further research.

The pharmaceutical industry endeavours to find drug therapies to cure such illnesses. Thus pharmaceutical innovation – the discovery of new medical therapies – is the highest social function of the pharmaceutical industry.[6] But pharmaceutical research entails a large degree of both technical and commercial uncertainty. In 1970, the USA performed pharmacological tests on 703 900 substances; this compares with only 1013 substances that were clinically tested and only 16 new chemical entities which reached the market that year.[7] Pharmaceutical sales and

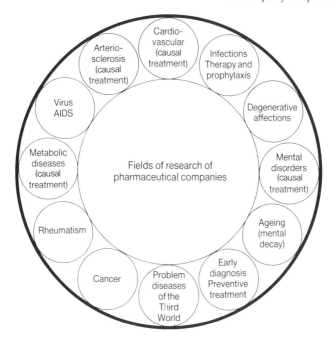

Fig. 10.1   Illustration of the necessity for further pharmaceutical research.

consumption levels have grown at lower rates since 1975 in practically all industrialized countries. Industry experts and health economists are not sure whether this slowing down is a consequence of political intervention or market saturation, a phase which virtually every fast growing industry enters at some stage. Saturation may also be the result of a combination of both effects. Fig. 10.2 shows the typical development pattern of an industry, the possible causes of saturation and its consequences. The introduction of new technologies can of course overcome a phase of temporary saturation as in the watch, camera and calculator industries. An analogous development may be likely in the pharmaceutical industry with breakthroughs in biotechnology.

An industry under siege
Few industries generate more criticism in the media than the pharmaceutical industry. This is partly due to an emotional 'political' belief that it is wrong to make a profit out of ill health. As can be seen from Fig. 10.3, the pharmaceutical industry is the only supplier of health care goods and services that actually earns a return on investment. Other suppliers merely earn their personal income from the difference between payment for services and costs incurred.

However, some of these criticisms against the pharmaceutical industry stem from misconceptions, as revealed by results of public opinion polls indicating that the public overestimated the cost of medicines in total

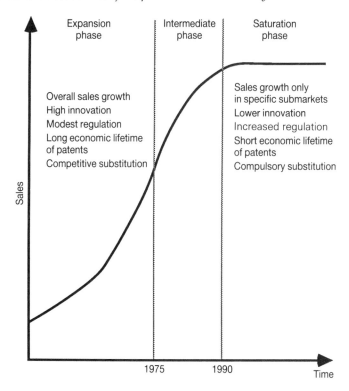

Fig. 10.2 Demonstration of the typical development pattern of an industry.

health care expenditure. In the UK, for example, people estimated the share of drugs in the total National Health Service (NHS) budget at about 35 per cent. The actual share however is less than 10 per cent (Fig. 10.4).

A breakdown of health care expenditure reveals that drugs in most industrialized countries account for no more than 15 per cent of expenditure, a share which has been declining over the past years. After deducting the pharmacist's share, the wholesaler's share and the value added tax (VAT) the industry's share amounted to 7 per cent. Assuming that profits before tax of the pharmaceutical industry amounted to 15 per cent of sales the maximum savings that could be achieved by eliminating all profits made by drug manufacturers would be less than 1 per cent, and this would of course destroy the industry.

However, due to chronic budget stringency politicians striving to cut health care costs find drug expenditure the easiest target. Drugs seem to be the best way whereby they can demonstrate devotion to fiscal responsibility while minimizing their risks at the polls.[8] In most countries there has been no single coherent policy towards the pharmaceutical industry. The role of the industry varies according to the context in which it is seen, and the differences are mirrored in the attitudes of the administrative organs with which it is concerned. For example, to a Department of Health it is important that drugs are effective, safe and readily available; to a

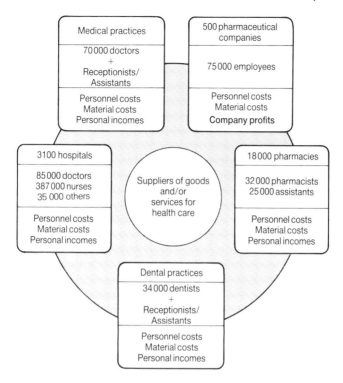

Fig. 10.3 The pharmaceutical industry is the only supplier of health care goods and services which actually earns a return on investment (West German data). (Data reproduced with permission from *Basisdaten des Gesundheitswesens*, BPI, Frankfurt/M, 1988/89.)

Treasury that they are cheap. A Department of Industry may foster the pharmaceutical sector as a source of wealth, a Department of Labour to relieve unemployment.

Consequently the actions which result from these different perceptions and goals may and sometimes do have contradictory effects, thus subjecting the pharmaceutical industry to a variety of diverse uncoordinated interventions. This diversity, already existing at a national level, multiplies for an internationally active company.[9]

Market structure and competition

Market structure
World pharmaceutical consumption amounted to $190 000 million in 1991 (Fig. 10.5). Of this, the industrialized countries in Western Europe, North America, Japan, Australia, South Africa and New Zealand consumed about 75 per cent of world drug production; only one-fifth was consumed in developing countries.

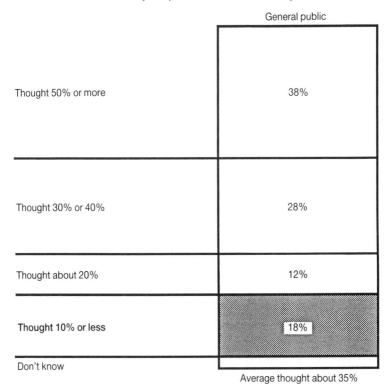

General public

Thought 50% or more | 38%

Thought 30% or 40% | 28%

Thought about 20% | 12%

Thought 10% or less | 18%

Don't know

Average thought about 35%

Fig. 10.4   The public's estimate of the costs of prescribed drugs as a percentage of all NHS costs. (Reproduced with permission from the Association of the British Pharmaceutical Industry.)

Pharmaceutical research is concentrated in a few highly industrialized countries, with a small number of companies active in each. The leading 20 research-based companies are located in only five countries and the leading 50 companies in only six countries. The research-based pharmaceutical companies are usually larger companies or multinational as they have the financial strength to afford the high investment required for the large-scale research and development activities. Estimates place the average costs of developing and introducing a product at Swiss Francs 311 million (approximately £100 million), with about 15 per cent being accounted for by the synthesis of the active substance and the remaining 85 per cent by developmental work, i.e. animal and clinical testing.

In addition, new products are introduced on a worldwide basis in order to obtain quicker returns on heavy research investment. With increasing regulatory requirements, limited patent protection time and increased product registration time, the effective patent life is reduced considerably. No therapeutic group in any national market offers the volume of sale necessary to recover the high research and development expenditures as well as the marketing costs and provide an adequate return on investment within the patent life of a major product.[10]

The present rate of new product innovation is too low for small compa-

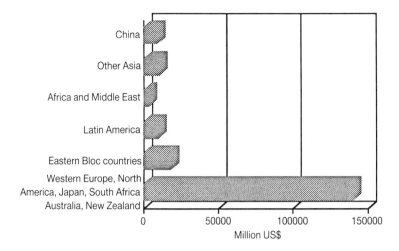

Fig. 10.5 World pharmaceutical consumption in 1991: Total, US$190 000 million (manufacturers prices). Source: author's own estimates.

nies to receive an adequate return on pharmaceutical research and development. Hence, one of the distinguishing features of the pharmaceutical industry is the high degree of internationalism in national markets (Table 10.1), a result of the large number of internationally active companies (multinational corporations).

There are very few industries in which a market can be lost as quickly as in pharmaceuticals. In the drug industry 'the place at the top is a very slippery place'. As Table 10.2 illustrates, over the past 6 years, American Home Products has fallen from rank 2 to rank 6, Pfizer (rank 4 in 1986) has fallen from the top 10 companies worldwide, while Glaxo has reached rank 3 within only 4 years.

Despite the existence of multinationals in the pharmaceutical industry the overall degree of market concentration is not very high either on a national or international level (Fig. 10.6).

Table 10.1 Market structure by nationality (1987)

| Market | Nationality (market share in %) | | | | | |
	National companies	Other EC	Total EC	US	Swiss	Other
Germany	56	14	70	18	8	4
France	49	20	69	23	7	1
Italy	43	25	68	22	9	1
UK	39	19	58	33	7	2
Belgium	10	43	53	34	11	2
USA	76	15	15	76	8	1
Japan	80	7	7	10	3	–

Based on total pharmacy purchases

Table 10.2   Ranking order of the leading international pharmaceutical companies

Rank	1986	1987	1988	1989	1990	1991
1	MSD	MSD	MSD	MSD	MSD	MSD
2	Am. Home	Am. Home	Ciba-Geigy	Ciba-Geigy	Glaxo	Bristol-M.
3	Ciba-Geigy	Ciba-Geigy	Am. Home	Glaxo	Ciba-Geigy	Glaxo
4	Pfizer	SKB	SKB	Hoechst	Am. Home	SKB
5	SKB	Pfizer	Hoechst	Am. Home	Hoechst	Ciba-Geigy
6	Hoechst	J & J	Pfizer	SKB	J & J	Am. Home
7	Eli Lilly	Hoechst	Glaxo	Pfizer	Bayer	J & J
8	J & J	Eli Lilly	J & J	J & J	SKB	Hoechst
9	Bristol-M.	Bristol-M.	Eli Lilly	Sandoz	Pfizer	Eli Lilly
10	Roche	Roche	Sandoz	Bayer	Sandoz	Bayer

Table 10.3 illustrates that over the past 5 years there has been a decrease in market dominance.

However, in selected therapeutic markets, companies can be in a very strong position for a limited period of time due to the introduction of a new, highly innovative product, e.g. Roche with Librium and Valium in the tranquillizer market.

Hence, according to the nature of the pharmaceutical industry changes in the rank of companies often go hand in hand with changes in the rank amongst leading products. New innovative products can become best sellers very soon after introduction, e.g. Zantac and Renitec (Table 10.4) But such cases are rare. As Fig. 10.7 illustrates, in many countries a majority of the leading 15 products are those introduced about a decade ago.

In no other industry does one encounter a similar degree of concentration in the range of products. Of the 10 major research-based pharmaceutical companies in the former Federal Republic of Germany, 50 per cent

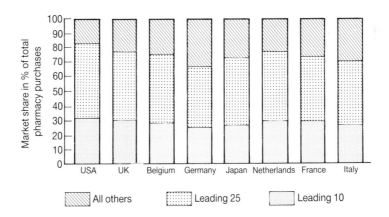

Fig. 10.6   Market shares of the leading 10 and leading 25 companies.

Table 10.3   Changes in market shares of the leading 10 and leading 25 companies

	Leading 10 companies	Leading 25 companies
USA	−5.0%	−2.7%
UK	−0.8%	−4.8%
Belgium	−1.0%	−0.9%
Germany	−5.1%	−4.7%
Japan	+0.9%	−0.5%
The Netherlands	−0.6%	−2.6%
France	−1.5%	±0.0%
Italy	+0.6%	+2.8%

Based on total pharmacy purchases

of the sales were achieved by 5 per cent of the products.

For some firms a single product accounts for up to 60 per cent of its turnover. Consequently patent expiry accompanied by generic substitution or exclusion of such a product from the reimbursement lists can place the company in a dire financial situation.

At a national level the market share of the leading products varies considerably, with the top 100 products accounting for almost three-fifths of the British market but hardly a third of the German market.

Another feature of the pharmaceutical industry is the high export/production ratio in most major markets except for Japan (Fig. 10.8).

The high export orientation of the pharmaceutical industry makes the issue of transfer pricing all the more crucial. The Japanese companies have so far only concentrated on consolidating their hold on the lucrative national market. However, with pressure from the domestic front to keep drug expenditure down, they are looking for new markets and are already making inroads into foreign markets. The question worrying most of the western world is whether the Japanese can and will have the same impact on the pharmaceutical industry that they have had so far on the automobile, computer, camera and electronics industries.

Table 10.4   Ranking order of the leading products in the world market

Rank	1986	1987	1988	1989	1990	1991
1	Tagamet	Tagamet	Tagamet	Zantac	Zantac	Zantac
2	Inderal	Zantac	Zantac	Tagamet	Tagamet	Renitec
3	Zantac	Feldene	Adalat	Adalat	Renitec	Capoten
4	Feldene	Inderal	Tenormin	Capoten	Adalat	Tagamet
5	Naprosyn	Naprosyn	Feldene	Renitec	Capoten	Voltaren
6	Keflex	Tenormin	Naprosyn	Tenormin	Tenormin	Adalat
7	Valium	Keflex	Capoten	Naprosyn	Naprosyn	Naprosyn
8	Tenormin	Adalat	Voltaren	Voltaren	Voltaren	Tenormin
9	Aldomet	Valium	Keflex	Feldene	Feldene	Cardizen
10	Adalat	Voltaren	Kefral	Kefral	Cardizen	Mevacor

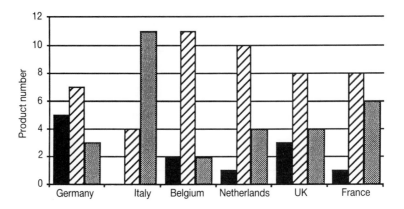

Fig. 10.7   The 15 leading products in 1987 by period of introduction: ■, before 1970; ▨, 1970–1979; ▩, 1980–1987.

Pharmaceuticals: normal consumer goods?

The pharmaceutical market is not a single entity, rather a series of submarkets in which varying companies position their products for an indication or a group of indications. Consequently competition generally takes place on a submarket level and not on the market level.

Both the intensity of competition as well as the price trends and pricing vary from one submarket to another depending on the phase of that market (i.e. phase of experimentation, expansion or maturity). Competing drug treatments within the same submarket are generally of a hetero-

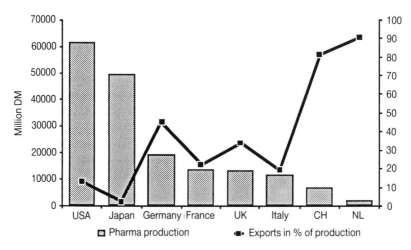

Fig. 10.8   The relation between pharma and pharma exports (1984).

geneous kind and not homogeneous.[11] The marketing of a drug by no means implies an end of the development phase as is generally the case with consumer goods. Drugs, unlike consumer goods, never reach the 'no problems stage' but remain in the 'more information needed' stage for all of their effective life. Valium, for example, was medically documented as appropriate for only two indications in the year of its introduction in 1963, but by 1974 as a result of continuous research and development the number of applications had increased to 18 (Fig. 10.9). An expansion in the range of indications of a drug necessitates the dissemination of this new information amongst the medical profession.

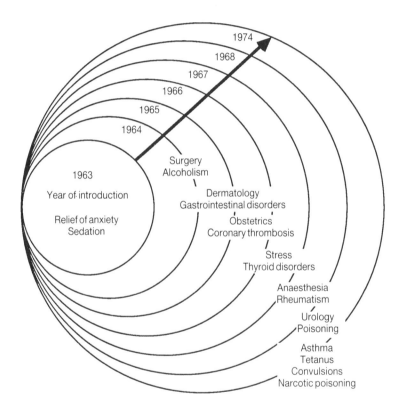

Fig. 10.9 The expansion of a drug's range of indications between 1963 and 1974. Example of a minor tranquillizer.(Reproduced with permission from F. Hoffmann La Roche, Basel.)

The competitive process
The degree of pricing freedom of a research-based company is limited to a large extent by the existence of or the potential of competitors and heterogeneous competition. This ensures that high price differentials for small amounts of innovation will be rejected by the market.[12,13] However,

if with the introduction of innovation in certain fields a company earns high profits, its competitors will divert resources to these same fields, thereby eroding the profits of the company that pioneered the innovation. Even during the patent protection period companies will try to compete by introducing substitute products.

On patent expiry products are no longer exclusive to their original innovator and the licensed competitors who pay royalties to the patentee. Any manufacturer can enter the market, produce and sell 'look-alike' products, i.e. chemical equivalents. Such products, usually referred to as 'generics', are sold without a number of services which are offered for original products by research-based companies, such as drug monitoring, research, medical information, etc.

Consequently there are major differences in the cost structure of research-based and non-research-based companies due to fundamental differences between the two. Empirical evidence shows that an imitator can undercut an innovator's price by 40 to 60 per cent with no research and development and by not dispensing scientific information and make an even higher profit on a lower capital investment. Generally the response of research-based companies to new manufacturers who undercut their price is to let themselves be priced out of the market after patent expiration.[11] Thus, high price differentials exist between the original product and the generic product, leading to a substantial decrease in sales for the innovator. Some research-based companies however defend their market position by price reductions. For example, Upjohn's price for Neomycin[4] went down from 60 cents per tablet in 1952 to less than 20 cents in 1963 due to 18 new entrants to the market. This however weakened their competitive abilities in the innovative market due to the allocation of increased resources to compete in the imitative market. According to Telser, prices tend to fall in response to entry. Entry itself is an increasing function of sales growth, market size and promotional intensity. There is a statistically significant and inverse relationship between the rate of change of prices and industry entry.[12]

The three basic options open to research-based pharmaceutical companies are:

1. Ignore the generics market and concentrate exclusively on innovative business.
2. Go generic worldwide.
3. Pursue a differentiated policy adapted to country-specific market situations.

The first option has the advantage of being a clearly demarcated business policy (i.e. no two-tiered product policy, price differentials, etc.) but risks losing out on potential business ventures. The second variant could jeopardize the subsequent existence of the company due to a decrease in resources available for research, and thus change it into a run-of-the mill chemical company: this could be advantageous and successful only in the short run. Implicit in the last variant are problems with a two-tier pricing system and stimulation of further trading in generics. However, it would be a good business reaction towards defending a market position and satisfying consumer needs.

Generics are not just a passing fashion but represent a trend which will probably become more marked in times of economic recession. Generic competition is not a pharmaceutical specific problem but is common to other highly technological industries such as cameras and computers. It fulfils a legal and social obligation by creating price erosion of innovative products upon patent expiry and by forcing new innovations from research-based companies to defend their market position. The two competitive dimensions of heterogeneous and homogeneous competition regulate drug prices in the pharmaceutical market, ensure that the market stays dynamic and that prices are kept in line, and thus protect consumers against excessive prices.

However the competitive process can become biased in favour of imitative companies by state intervention via:

1. Pressure on physicians to prescribe the cheapest drug.
2. Pressure on the pharmacist to substitute generics for original products.
3. Direct government purchasing (Third World countries).
4. Restrictive lists forbidding or limiting the introduction of new drugs.

Fig. 10.10 shows the effect of a restrictive list in the UK which excluded product groups like minor tranquillizers, antacids, vitamins, etc. from reimbursement by the NHS.

The impact of such lists is far more drastic than the effect of competitive substitution. Thus direct government intervention on market forces could distort competition by favouring imitative products and thus in the long run hamper progress in drug therapy. This could have negative repercussions on society from both a health and an economic point of view.

Pricing issues

Pricing and cost structure

The pharmaceutical industry is characterized by a low ratio of direct or variable costs to total costs. Variable costs tend mainly to be in the area of production, distribution and promotion, while research and development costs are substantial and fixed, cannot be allocated with any accuracy to individual products and are more correctly viewed as overheads. Therefore prices set at marginal costs in the pharmaceutical industry would not cover total costs (Table 10.5). A similar situation exists in other industries characterized by a low ratio of variable costs, such as airlines, railways and utilities.[13]

Research-based companies can allocate only a small fraction of their costs directly to individual products. Empirical evidence places this

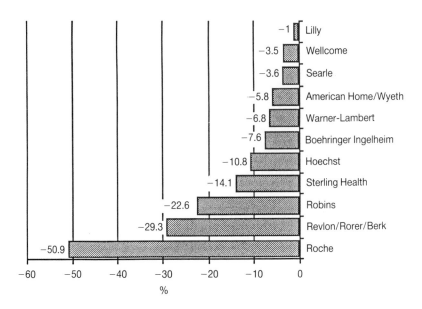

Fig. 10.10   Reduction of company sales between 1984 and 1985 after introduction of the 'black list' in the UK which excluded six product categories from reimbursement by the NHS.

estimate at no more than 30 per cent of total costs. The remaining costs and profit margin must be covered by contribution (the difference between the selling price and the directly attributable costs) of the total product range of companies. Production costs for research-based companies constitute about 40 per cent of the selling price on a consolidated average; for individual products, however, it may account for 10 per cent or less.

Thus, price competition takes place among manufacturers in their competitive striving on all dimensions of the product's quality, since changes in the quality change the actual price.[14]

Pricing in a competitive market
The drug market is a unique one, with its tripartite division whereby the doctor prescribes the drug, the patient consumes it and the state

Table 10.5   Dimensions involved in the pricing of pharmaceutical products

Quality information	= efficacy + safety + clinical evidence + experience communicated to doctors and other professionals + reputation of manufacturer based on performance of prior products
Nominal price	= price to wholesaler − discount to wholesaler − discounts and rebates to hospital or other distribution outlets
(Actual) price	= nominal price − quality

or insurance finances it. This phenomenon apparently could lead to a doctor's indifference to drug prices. According to this argument, as the patient needs the drug immediately, demand is practically inelastic. Consequently, the manufacturer can charge any price without negative impact on his sales. Following this chain of thought, the maxim found in the economic textbook[15] to the effect that demand falls as price rises and vice versa does not apply to the pharmaceutical market. Demand can be regarded as an unvarying factor that must be satisfied at any price. However an inelastic demand for drugs may not even be realistic for selected drugs. Generally each drug is in competition with others for a particular type of treatment. Thus, companies with pricing policies based on the assumption of an inelastic demand for drugs will soon learn better.

The pricing policy adopted by a pharmaceutical firm under a system of free competition varies widely due to a number of factors: the perceived therapeutic value of a new drug; the degree of novelty which the drug embodies over existing products; the degree of product substitution; the level of acceptability of a new drug in the market place; physician prescribing habits; the investment costs throughout the development cycle; the complexity and costs of manufacture; prevailing and competitive prices for alternative therapies at both daily dosage costs and total treatment costs; potential new competitors; the anticipated volume of sales; government price controls, local taxation and the remittance of profits; royalty payments on patents and processes; patent coverage; promotional expenditure; and internal company return on investment criteria.[10]

Profits, particularly high profits, are the driving force behind a competitive market system. In principle, there are about three pricing strategies open to a manufacturer.

The first strategy is to market the product initially at a comparatively high price and then gradually reduce this price during the useful life of the product. This *skimming price strategy* is favoured when the product enjoys patent protection and consequently precludes competitors from entering the market quickly. However, a high skimming price must be weighed against the reaction it causes amongst competitors to hasten their market entry plans. Sales volume may initially be slow under this method.

An optional strategy is to adapt the new product price to those already on the market, establish brand loyalty and keep two steps ahead of the competition. This *penetration pricing strategy* may be instituted at product launch or may follow a skimming period.[13] The total sales and profits might be identical with either strategy adopted when calculated in terms of the effective life of the product. Both strategies are potentially defensible in a free competition system.

A pricing possibility which has not yet been thoroughly investigated is the *competition oriented pricing*. This is a pricing strategy whereby companies price their products in line with the existing products on the market. Under this system, due to the lack of a full cost calculation, the prime relation is not between price and cost or demand but is based on the price the competition charges. Firms assume quite logically that the average price level represents a reasonable one.[16] If this is the main strategy followed, government intervention in the prices of single drugs could start price wars. In the long run this would hurt all but the strongest companies.

The demand curve for products under patent protection also eventually develops a sag (i.e. kinky demand curve). The company has the freedom to manoeuvre its prices within certain limits, this being subject to economic laws governing competition. However, if the price exceeds the upper limit it might have a detrimental effect on the sales as doctors or consumers may switch to rival products.

A decline in sales leads to a decrease in the product's contribution in actual terms. Price reductions lead to the same end if the reduction is not appreciable enough to cause an increase in sales. When the time factor is taken into consideration, even price variations within certain limits will cause some reaction in the market in the long run.

Pricing in regulated markets

Practically all the EC member states, with the exception of Denmark, have instituted formal controls for drug pricing. The mechanisms employed to regulate drug prices vary considerably amongst member states, ranging from direct state control of individual product prices to indirect control via price comparisons or reference prices. Only in Denmark are prices allowed to find their own level according to market forces (Fig. 10.11).

Direct and indirect controls on products are exercised at the outset of

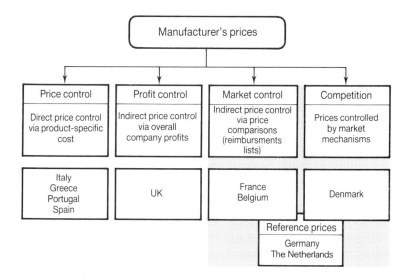

Fig. 10.11 The approaches to pricing of new pharmaceutical products in the European Community.

marketing unlike the retro-active British system. In a system of reimburse-ment list, admittance to such a list is essential for the commercial success of a product. Prices are consequently negotiated on the basis of a costing formula calculating the cost of the raw materials through to the public price. Italy, Belgium and Greece have individual product price negotia-tions, which has led to weakening of the financial situation of both national and international companies active in the market. This can be seen by the number of mergers and liquidations.[11]

In the UK controls are imposed on companies by controlling their level of profitability. Under this system, termed the Pharmaceutical Price Regulation Scheme (PPRS), the business operations of a pharmaceutical company are analysed in their entirety, taking into consideration their investment in research as well as their contribution to the economy. The distribution of the allowed total return amongst a given company's products is of no interest to the authorities. The PPRS constitutes a lesser evil than regulation of a company's products. However, if the controls are too strict capital will be diverted into more attractive fields of business; if they are too lax the industry will receive intervention subsidies, which are paid for by the consumer.

Additional controls are emerging in the area of monitoring of the products that physicians prescribe and of the quantity involved. In most of the EC countries drug price comparisons of similar products are circulated to increase the cost consciousness of physicians and to reduce overprescribing.

All these controls are having and will continue to have direct financial repercussions for the pharmaceutical industry. Eventually adverse effects on both current and future profit levels will lead to a liquidity squeeze on the investment level of research and development. This could also force a number of the less financially sound companies to merge, thus producing a higher level of concentration, or to pursue a diversification policy away from the pharmaceutical industry.

The pharmaceutical industry will prove less attractive to diversifica-tion or investment if the sociopolitical environment, with its increasing state controls on the industry and the short-term lack of cash surpluses, continues to persist.[10]

International transfer prices

International transfer pricing is a necessity for internationally active industries, particularly chemicals, oil and electronics, where the basic ingredients, components or other raw materials are produced in one country and sold to a subsidiary or third party in another country. In addition the nature of the pharmaceutical industry, with its high level of research concentrated in a few selected countries, makes the export orientation of the industry inevitable. Hence the transfer pricing technique is an exceedingly critical and political issue influencing the structure, conduct and performance of the industry to a high degree.

The appropriateness of the transfer price has three methods of assessment: 'market price method'; 'market minus method'; and 'cost plus method'.

If the goods or service in question has a market price, the prevailing price can serve as a yardstick to judge the appropriateness of the transfer price. The Organization for Economic Cooperation and Development (OECD)[9] refers to this principle as the 'comparable uncontrolled price method' and it offers the most direct way of determining an arm's length principle. But this method has a number of pitfalls, such as determining economic comparability, comparable market levels and comparability of goods. Moreover, this method is hardly applicable to research-based pharmaceutical companies as exchanges comprise both goods and services.

In cases where a market price cannot be established the 'market minus method' is used. The customary gross profit margin can be deducted from the resale price charged by the purchasing company (Fig. 10.12) with the resultant amount then considered as an appropriate delivery price. This method would be appropriate in cases where companies can charge market prices for their products. However, in many countries pharmaceutical prices are regulated either at product launch or at a later stage when price increases come into the question.

If it were feasible to establish a customary profit margin for the branch

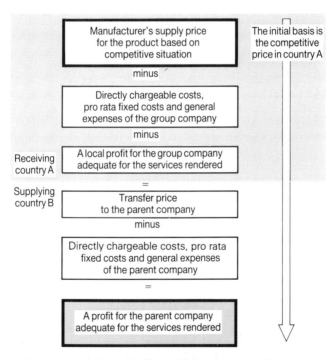

The group profit (national and central) is a 'residual amount', the adequacy of which is regulated by the market conditions, independently of the group costs.

Fig. 10.12   The 'market minus method'.

of industry concerned the 'market minus method' would be suitable in all cases where market prices prevail. But the 'market price method' is inappropriate in cases where prices are fixed below market prices by government authorities. The appropriateness of the transfer price would be judged by a process of circular reasoning on the basis of a final selling price which is itself controlled. In such cases, with controlled final prices and predetermined appropriate profit margin, it would be coincidence if the sum that remained was sufficient to cover central costs as well as an appropriate rate of interest on centrally invested capital. Even if this sum were appropriate at the time of product introduction, local inflation and currency depreciation, coupled with the freezing of final prices, would bring it increasingly below the required level. These limitations are not mentioned in the OECD report but are the typical scenario of a pharmaceutical market.

The essence of the last variant, the 'cost plus method' of pricing, is that it allows the supplying company both primary cost coverage as well as an appropriate profit margin. The primary costs are, namely, those of *production* (material, labour, general expenses), *marketing* (advertising, promotion, sales force), and contribution to the central company's *overhead expenses* (medical information, research and development, central administration). However, a major problem inherent in this system is the appropriate allocation of costs and the determination of an appropriate profit margin (Fig. 10.13).

Future prospects and conclusions

Trends in research and development

The pharmaceutical industry today is maturing in terms of manufacturing efficiency, drug licensing and diversification, and is growing with respect to its marketing and development skills. Yet the key growth factor in this industry has traditionally been research. However, the number of new drug applications (NDAs) and new chemical entities (NCEs) approved by Food and Drug Administration (FDA) has declined substantially over the past three decades. The reasons for this decline are complex and difficult to disentangle but certainly involve economics (both costs of research and expected return on investment), regulation and the scientific demands of the state of the art.[6] The level of maturity also has considerable impact on the industry:

1. The average research and development costs per project increase considerably.
2. The average timespan for successfully achieving research and development projects increases considerably.
3. The number of breakthroughs decreases over time.

One explanation for the decline offered by the industry is the severe scientific and political pressure exerted in the mid 1970s on the industry's preclinical research, plus a significant increase in requirements and costs

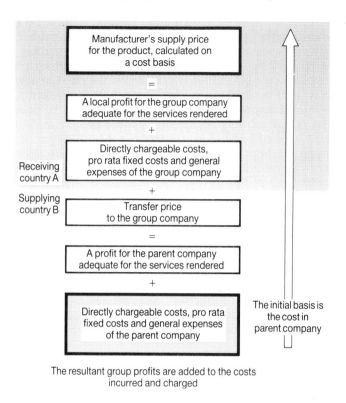

Manufacturer's supply price
for the product, calculated on
a cost basis

=

A local profit for the group company
adequate for the services rendered

+

Directly chargeable costs,
pro rata fixed costs and general
expenses of the group company

Receiving
country A

+

Supplying
country B

Transfer price
to the group company

=

A profit for the parent company
adequate for the services rendered

+

Directly chargeable costs, pro rata
fixed costs and general expenses
of the parent company

The initial basis is
the cost in
parent company

The resultant group profits are added to the costs
incurred and charged

Fig. 10.13   The 'cost plus method'.

at all stages. As Fig. 10.14 illustrates, the total development time has nearly doubled over the past 18 years.[17]

Research and development will continue to represent the primary catalyst to growth in the pharmaceutical industry and its extent and success will be the determining factor of the future of both the industry and the individual companies. One of the main areas of future development will be the improvement of certain product characteristics for which existing products fall short, such as freedom from side effects, desirable onset and duration of action, broad efficacy and targeted delivery.

Biotechnology represents another field of great potential. Development in biotechnology will not only lead to specific new agents that may have higher purity and more effectiveness, but also to increased yields of products that hitherto have been derived from animal and/or human sources of which there is a limited supply.

An area where further competitive advantages can be derived will be from innovations in advanced drug delivery system. They provide an opportunity not only to extend product lines but also to recycle a product back into a protected position. The latter aspect will gain importance due to increasing generic competition, stimulated in certain countries by cost containment pressure coupled with important patent expiration.

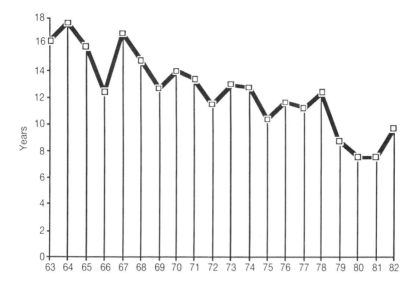

Fig. 10.14 Average effective patent life of new drug products 1963–1982. Pharmaceutical Manufacturers Association (PMA) Survey of member companies.

Drug productivity

Drug therapy has produced huge benefits in the form of both lower costs for health care and simultaneous improvement of its quality. Some of these economic benefits have been direct: savings as cheaper drug therapies are substituted for more expensive forms of intervention, and reduction in the need for surgery or hospitalization. Indirect savings have been achieved by a reduction in absenteeism etc. However, criticisms of drugs must also be mentioned, such as excessive prescribing, overconsumption, social abuse and misuse.

Many of today's illnesses, such as cancer and circulatory diseases, require intensive treatment involving hospitalization. Reduction in morbidity and mortality rates with the aid of drug therapy would result in considerable savings to society.

In the 1960s it was still possible to achieve increases in efficiency in the provision of health care of over 100 units, given a total rise in the health care costs of 100 units. However, in the future the situation looks more dismal, since 100 unit increases in costs will bring additional benefits far below 100. This unfavourable cost/benefit ratio will only be altered by continuous progress in productivity. This progress is unlikely to be achieved in the service sector of the health system. Consequently improvements in drug technologies will be the decisive factor. Unfortunately until now research-based pharmaceutical companies have put little emphasis on cost/benefit studies showing the 'productivity' of drug therapy.

Entrepreneurial duty of the pharmaceutical industry

Empirical proof of progress in 'productivity' of medical care with the use of pharmaceuticals is difficult. The main emphasis for such studies should come from the pharmaceutical industry but so far research-based pharmaceutical companies have been more concerned with conducting efficient research and production and selling drugs profitably. This however will change.

Some institutions in Europe have already started to deal professionally with these issues: The Office of Health Economics in London, the Institute of Health Economics in Lund (Sweden) and HealthEcon, a private consulting company for all interdisciplinary questions concerning health care in Switzerland.

The pharmaceutical industry is currently facing a relatively hostile environment so its growth must inevitably be inhibited. We see extensions of government regulations surrounding the testing and marketing of new medicines; controls on prices and profits; restrictions on sales promotion; erosion of patent life; weakening of brand name protection and increased pressure for generic medicines; and finally general consumerist pressure against pharmaceutical expansion. All of these adverse influences threaten to stifle future innovation, sending it into a decline.

The question facing the industry, government and consumerist bodies is quite simply this: will today's diseases be conquered in the next 30 years; or will society instead be left only with yesterdays' innovations as the generic drugs of tomorrow?

An innovative climate is a prerequisite for progress in productivity and better drug therapy. Such a climate can only be created and maintained through better public awareness of the services provided by the pharmaceutical industry. This would improve the competitive position of individual companies, leading to an increase in productivity for society as a whole. The public has tended to regard the pharmaceutical industry as an industry making money out of illness, and has considerably underestimated its positive contribution to the health of the nation, the national economy and to employment.

Such a gross misunderstanding represents an entrepreneurial challenge which, if accepted by the pharmaceutical industry, could provide it with the innovative environment it desperately needs for future progress and productivity.

References

1   Feldstein PJ (1979). *Health Care Economics*. New York: Wiley Medical Publication: 4–10.
2   Lipsey RG, Steiner PO (1978). *Economics*, 5th edn. New York: Harper & Row: 34–48.
3   Stahl I, von Grebmer K (1980). Drugs and health care; a productivity approach. *The Pharmaceutical Journal* **225**: 144.
4   Bureau of Consumer Protection (1979). *Drug Product Selection*. Washington DC: Staff Report to the Federal Trade Commission: 15.
5   Teeling-Smith G (1980). *Medicines 50 Years of Progress 1930–1980*. London:

Office of Health Economics.

6 Wardell W (1982). Personal communication.

7 Schwartzmann D (1979). The regulation of drug prices. In Teeling-Smith G (ed.) *Medicines For the Year 2000*. London: Office of Health Economics: 43.

8 Engmann L (1982). *The Second Pharmaceutical Revolution*. London: Office of Health Economics: 23–4.

9 OECD Report (1979). *Transfer Pricing and Multinational Enterprises*. Paris: OECD Committee on Fiscal Affairs: 34–44.

10 James BG (1977). *The Future of the Multinational Pharmaceutical Industry to 1990*. London: Associated Business Programmes Ltd.

11 Kearny AT (1979). *A Survey and Synthesis of Literature on the Economics of the Prescription Pharmaceutical Industry*. Alexandria, VI: AT Kearny, Inc.

12 Reekie DW (1979). Economic competition in pharmaceuticals. In Teeling-Smith G (ed.) *Medicines for the Year 2000*. London: Office of Health Economics.

13 Weston JF (1979). *Pricing in the Pharmaceutical Industry, Issues in Pharmaceutical Economics*. Lexington, MA: Lexington Books.

14 von Grebmer K (1983). *Drug Therapy and its Price*. Montreal: Medicöpea: 56–8.

15 Dorfman R (1972). *Prices and Markets*, 2nd edn. Englewood Cliffs, NJ: Prentice-Hall Inc.

16 Rosenberg LJ (1977). *Marketing*. Englewood Cliffs, NJ: Prentice-Hall: 361–7.

17 Pharmaceutical Manufacturers' Association (1986). *Statistical Fact Book*. Washington DC: PMA: 3–25.

11

Ethics of clinical research
Brian T. Marsh

Introduction

The last 30 years have seen an enormous expansion of clinical research in humans which, to a great extent, has coincided with a corresponding increase in the number of new therapeutic discoveries from the pharmaceutical industry. The demand for ethical monitoring of clinical research was less dramatic at the beginning of this period, but is now of such great importance that Food and Drug Administration (FDA) in the USA will only accept data from clinical studies that have met the ethical standards described in the Declaration of Helsinki or the laws of the country of origin.

Guidelines on the supervision of the ethics of clinical research have been published from time to time since the Nuremberg Code in 1947.[1] However it was not until the Tokyo meeting in 1975 of the World Medical Association (WMA)[2] that the following principle was explicitly stated: 'the design and performance of each experimental procedure involving human subjects should be clearly formulated in an experimental protocol which should be transmitted to a specially appointed independent committee for consideration, comment and guidance.'[3]

We are in an era characterized by scientific and technological advances in all spheres of life. Morals and ethics are integral to the acceptance of these advances by the general public. It is essential, therefore, that the morals and ethics relating to clinical research are continually assessed and reassessed in times of rapid change.

The assessment of moral and ethical dilemmas by the scientific community should accurately reflect the prevailing mood of the general population in and on whom the research is to be performed. Much of the clinical research undertaken will contribute to the benefit of the individual patient, but other research will be solely for the purpose of contributing to medical knowledge and will not be designed to benefit the particular individual on whom it is performed. The recognition of these dilemmas and the difficulty for one individual, who may personally be closely involved in the research project, in resolving them have led to the acceptance that ethics committees are the only means of clearly showing that a research project has been subjected to independent ethical scrutiny.

Historical perspectives

In this section some of the more important publications relating to the development of ethics committees are mentioned. Those readers particularly interested in this subject are recommended to read the original papers.

The first internationally registered code of ethics relating to medical experiments on human subjects was set out in the reports on the Trials of War Criminals before the Nuremberg Military Tribunals in 1949 and is known as the Nuremberg Code.[1] It is salutary to remember, however, that it was the German Ministry of the Interior who, in 1931, issued some of the first national guidelines for new forms of medical treatment that were clearer, more concrete and more far-reaching than either the Nuremberg Code or the Helsinki Declaration.[4]

The WMA drew up a code of ethics on human experimentation in 1962. This was confirmed at the WMA meeting in Helsinki in 1964 and became the Declaration of Helsinki.[5] In the same year the Medical Research Council (MRC) in the UK issued a statement on the 'Responsibility in Investigations on Human Subjects'.[6]

In 1966 the US FDA, in association with the National Institutes of Health, issued guidelines governing the use of human subjects and, in the same year, the Royal College of Physicians of London (RCP) set up a committee whose report on the 'Supervision of the Ethics of Clinical Investigations in Institutions' was published in 1967.[7] This report was distributed to hospital authorities in May 1968 by the then Ministry of Health with the suggestion that the RCP recommendations on setting up ethical committees should be put into effect.

The first World Health Organization (WHO) pronouncement on ethics committees appeared in a report by the WHO Scientific Group on the 'Principles for the Clinical Evaluation of Drugs' where a section was devoted to ethical and legal aspects.[8]

In 1973 the RCP updated its 1967 report[9] and this too, together with notes on the use of foetuses and foetal material for research, was circulated to hospitals in 1975 by the Department of Health and Social Security (DHSS).[10] Also in 1975, in Tokyo, the WMA revised its Helsinki recommendations on biomedical research involving human subjects and this is known as the Declaration of Tokyo.[2] In 1983 in Venice further revisions were made and this document comprises Appendix B.

As there is always concern relating to research in children, in 1978 the British Paediatric Association set up a working party on the ethics of research in children. In 1980 its report 'Guidelines to Aid Ethical Committees Considering Research Involving Children' was published in the *British Medical Journal*.[11]

Following discussions between the British Medical Association (BMA) and the Association of the British Pharmaceutical Industry (ABPI) it became apparent that there was no accepted definition of what was a properly constituted ethics committee. The BMA investigated the constitution of ethical committees throughout England and Wales and found not only that they varied enormously, but also that only about 35 per cent had general practitioner representatives. It was suggested that the present hospital-based ethics committees should be reconstituted to cover all clinical research in an area and that members from both general practice and hospital medicine should be represented on these so-called local ethical committees.[12]

The structure and functioning of ethical review committees was examined at the XVth CIOMS (Council of International Organizations of Medical Science) Round Table Conference on Human Experimentation and Medical Ethics in Manila in 1981 under the auspices of WHO. A summary of this meeting gives a general survey of the principal issues to be taken into account in the establishment and operation of ethical committees, together with advice on the setting up of such committees and the procedures to be followed.[13]

In 1990 two reports were published by the RCP of London. The first one deals with research involving patients[14] and the second one gives guidelines for ethical committees.[15] Both are summarized in Appendix A.

Ethics committees

The 1973 report of the RCP of London[9] on the supervision of the ethics of clinical research investigations in institutions has three important statements which are listed below. The report also made the point that the term 'clinical research investigation' was to be regarded as covering all forms of investigation in humans and did not just apply to those involving drug therapy.

1. The object of ethical committees is to safeguard patients, healthy volunteers and the reputation of the profession and its institutions in matters of clinical research investigations.
2. To function efficiently ethical committees should be small and they must not be so constituted as to cause an unreasonable hindrance to the advancement of medical knowledge.
3. Supervision of ethics should normally be the sole function of an ethical committee.

These three statements succinctly described the rationale, constitution and function of an ethics committee, but due to the way in which the stimulus for such committees has developed in the UK there is no example of an 'official' ethics committee, although a suggestion has been made in a statement on local ethical committees by the BMA.[12] Ethics committees vary in constitution from one institution to another, and there is little cohesive action between committees, although there are occasional meetings of the chairmen of ethics committees convened by the RCP.

The variability in composition and methods of working of ethics committees is enormous. A survey of research committees in Scotland revealed that of the 34 committees replying to a questionnaire: the size varied from one to 73 members; 10 committees had no nurse representative;

only three committees had lay members without direct National Health Service (NHS) connections; 16 saw their role as advisory rather than supervisory; and 13 committees had not met in the past 12 months. Of the 370 proposals submitted, only seven were rejected outright. The authors concluded that the ethics committees in this survey seemed to provide only limited safeguards for patients and research workers.[16]

Other papers by O'Brien and Mahadevan,[17] Allen and Waters[18] and Denham *et al.*[19] have outlined the workings of ethics committees in Durham, Southampton and Northwick Park Hospital, and the activities of the Ethical Committee, University College Hospital, were reported in 1981.[20] All have evolved their own structure, function and methodology, and all seem to have found general acceptance within the community they serve. This last point is of supreme importance in commenting on the value of ethics committees. No committee can or will function efficiently if it is not accepted by the community in which it works, both scientific and lay, or where it is deliberately bypassed. It is interesting, therefore, to read in this context of a European ethical review committee that was founded in 1977 with the purpose of reviewing protocols of drug trials submitted by pharmaceutical companies. The committee has 31 members from nine European countries and at least 10 members attend each meeting. No member of the committee is employed in the pharmaceutical industry and no outside agency has any role in selecting members. So far, 294 protocols have been reviewed.[21]

There is one area of research in which there has been rather less comment in regard to ethics committees and that is in the pharmaceutical industry itself. Many pharmaceutical companies conduct clinical pharmacology studies 'in-house' on volunteer subjects who are usually employees of the company, but who occasionally may come from the local community. In this situation submission of the research protocol to an independent ethics committee is desirable, particularly as the research is usually being conducted on normal volunteers who may also be paid for their services. There seems to be no good reason why studies conducted by the pharmaceutical industry should be exempt from ethical review. Such a review by an independent body reduces the vulnerability of the company and its employees in addition to protecting the volunteer subjects.[22]

The only firm guidance as to the constitution of an ethics committee has been provided by the BMA.[12] They suggest that the membership should consist of two senior hospital doctors, one junior hospital doctor, two general practitioners, one representative of community medicine, one nurse and one lay member, a total of eight members. The RCP recommend in their Guidelines on the Practice of Ethics Committees that the committee should be of a manageable size, for example less than 12 members.[23] The ABPI considers that a core of five members is necessary.[24]

A further area of contention that has become apparent is in regard to the possible extension of the role of ethics committees into patient management.[25] Ethical issues on the provision of treatment, e.g. organ transplantation, kidney dialysis and assisted ventilation, have been suggested as ones in which a judgment by a committee may be better or fairer than that by an individual. Such a wider role may become necessary, but it will cause an inevitable increase in workload.[26] The USA is at the forefront in this development and it is pertinent to point out here a potential confusion regarding nomenclature. In the UK and Europe ethics committees usually only concern themselves with the review of research projects. In the USA Institutional Review Boards are required by law to scrutinize federally funded research and ethics committees or, as they are sometimes called, bioethics committees, concern themselves with the review of patient management and other such decisions.[27]

There are dangers with such committees in that pressures to reach agreement may lead to ethically questionable recommendations such as the criteria of social worth when providing life-prolonging dialysis.[28] In certain circumstances these committees may be regarded as alternatives to the courts.[29]

It is clear that, as yet, there is no generally accepted constitution for ethics committees in the UK or much of Europe. This is in direct contrast to the USA where the constitution, functions and activities of the comparable Institutional Review Boards were published in the Federal Register in 1981.[30] It remains to be seen which is the most acceptable and efficient method of developing ethics committees for clinical research and it will be interesting to see how they develop over the next 30 years.

Patient consent

Few patients or volunteers can ever claim to fully understand or be acquainted with all the facts relating to a particular study in which they have been asked to participate. If the ideal could be achieved, then probably there would be no need for ethics committees.

Thus patient consent, often called informed consent, is a key area in the debate on ethics in biomedical research. As few, if any, patients can be expected fully to understand all the complex issues, the ethics committee acts for the patient, the committee then taking on the responsibility for examining the experimental design, the procedures to be employed, the expertise of the investigators and any other points that it deems of importance in protecting the patient or volunteer. Of particular importance to the committee will be the way in which consent is to be obtained, the information to be given to the patient and how the patient will signify consent, such as in writing or verbally.

By performing the above role an ethics committee tacitly accepts that there can never be true informed consent. In spite of this, however, no human experiment normally should be performed without the consent of the patient. It is the duty of the ethics committee to decide on the degree and breadth of the explanation given to the patient and to ensure, as far as possible, that this explanation can and will be understood. Such explanation will of course vary according to the nature and complexity of the study and to the education and intelligence of the patient.

The concern about the definition of informed consent could, perhaps, be reduced if it was described as 'valid consent'. There are situations where no one can be fully aware of all the risks, such as at the first administration to human of a new drug. This might also take into account the patient who does not want any explanation but simply says 'I leave it to you doctor'. There are many patients who do not want to take part in the decision making process yet wish to help in clinical research. Should they be excluded from a clinical trial simply because they do not wish to have a full and detailed explanation of the study? As Fost[31] has pointed out, among the justifications for limiting or waiving informed consent is the patient's expressed wish not to be informed of the detailed choices before him.

An important distinction is whether the research will directly benefit the patient or whether it is simply a general study with no direct benefit. Special emphasis must be given to the latter type of study, both in the overall examination of the rationale and procedures and in the manner of obtaining the consent.

The requirement to obtain consent for a medical or surgical procedure is not new and has not arisen solely as a result of the vast increase in human experimentation. It arises out of two medicolegal principles – that of a fiduciary relationship between doctor and patient, and that of patient self-determination. Under the concept of fiduciary relationship a person in whom another has placed a special trust or confidence (as a result of his special training or expertise) is required to act in good faith and in the interests of the person reposing the trust or confidence. Such a relationship imposes on the doctor a duty to disclose to the patient all pertinent facts regarding the patient's condition and the treatment recommended. In regard to self-determination, a legally competent person has the right to decide what is to be done to their body and cannot be compelled to accept treatment that they do not want. There have been certain exceptions in the past, notably the force feeding of hunger strikers and blood transfusions to members of certain religious sects. The current reasoning is that even in these two examples legally competent persons have the right to refuse treatment. Such rights do not, however, automatically apply to parents or legal guardians, but this is a much more complex issue, and not suitable for discussion here.

The principle of patient consent was enunciated in the Nuremberg Code in 1947 and has become progressively refined over the succeeding 30 years. In 1975, when the WMA revised the Declaration of Helsinki in Tokyo,[2] it firmly restated this principle:

'In any research on human beings, each potential subject must be adequately informed of the aims, methods, anticipated benefits and potential hazards of the study and the discomfort it may entail. He or she should be informed that he or she is at liberty to abstain from participation in the study and that he or she is free to withdraw his or her consent to participation at any time. The doctor should obtain the subject's freely-given informed consent, preferably in writing.'

It is only in the USA that federal regulations have been published to try and ensure protection for human subjects taking part in clinical investigations. These regulations have been published in the Federal Register and were updated in January 1981. There are seven basic conditions regarding patient consent that can be highlighted from these requirements of Institutional Review Boards (the bodies responsible in the USA for making ethical decisions) before approval for a study can be given. These conditions must be explained to the patient or his legal adviser:

1. The procedure to be followed in the study.
2. The discomforts and risks that are to be 'reasonably expected'.
3. The anticipated benefits for the individual.
4. The alternative methods of therapy.
5. If more than minimal risk is expected, an explanation of compensatory procedures in case of injury.
6. The willingness of the investigator to answer enquiries.
7. The right to refuse or withdraw from the study without prejudice.

There is no such legislation in the UK, yet common sense dictates that the majority, if not all, of these basic conditions should be followed when patient consent is obtained. One condition that is often not sufficiently emphasized to the patient is the right to refuse or withdraw from the study without prejudice. In a clinical trial the need to carefully assess response to treatment often gives the feeling that the patient in a trial receives better treatment than the normal patient. Hence the need to explain to the patient that this refusal to enter a trial or decision to withdraw during the course of a trial will not result in receiving inferior treatment.

Furthermore, it is essential that the patient be told if the treatment in the clinical trial is to be randomized. As Scarman[32] has pointed out, there is danger for the doctor who does not give such a warning to the patient if something goes wrong.

Having decided on the basic information to be given to a patient, the next difficulty is to ensure that it is given correctly and understood. One way of doing this is to explain the position in the presence of a third party, who is able to appreciate and understand what is being said but who is not part of the research team. This person can then identify themself entirely with the patient's interests.[33] This has been described by Vere[34] as the 'subject's friend' concept. During this process it is easy to forget that the informed consent procedure itself may bias the result of a clinical trial.[35] It has been shown also that the consent form is a possible cause of increased side effects from drug therapy.[36]

As in all medicine, good record keeping is essential. Whenever patient consent for an experimental procedure is obtained it should be noted in the patient's file together with a short summary of what was said (or a copy of the printed information if given in this manner), who was also present (the subject's friend) and, if possible, the patient's signature. This last point is not always possible. In such cases it is wise to insist on a third party being present when the procedure is explained and for the third party to sign and acknowledge that verbal consent was obtained.

Special circumstances arise in studies involving children, the mentally handicapped and in institutions such as prisons and the armed forces. If research is performed with prisoners or members of the armed forces the ethics committee will need to examine in even more detail the procedures to be used in obtaining consent to ensure no undue pressure is brought to bear or expectation of benefit promised.

In paediatric clinical research great emphasis is placed on whether the research is therapeutic and therefore of direct benefit to the child or non-therapeutic and hence of no direct benefit. In particular there has been doubt as to whether anyone could give legally effective consent for non-therapeutic research in a child. This view has been challenged by Skegg[37] and Dworkin,[38] who argue that consent is possible provided the research is for the common good and involves no or minimal risk to the child. However, in all cases of non-therapeutic research in children, the benefit/risk ratio will have to be much greater than that required for an equivalent therapeutic research procedure.

Further argument has arisen as to the age at which a child is to be regarded as capable of giving consent on their own account. The age of 12 has been suggested by many authorities. Skegg[37] has pointed out, however, that there is no absolute age of consent, since the capacity to consent depends upon whether a person is capable of understanding and coming to a decision on what is involved; age is simply one factor to be taken into account.

Therefore, when considering consent for a proposed non-therapeutic research procedure on a child the following considerations should be taken into account:

1.   There is no, or minimal, risk from the procedure.
2.   If a child is capable of giving voluntary consent, the child must be asked for this consent.
3.   Even if the child can consent on its own behalf it is politic to obtain the parents' agreement as well.
4.   If the child is unable to give consent then, in certain circumstances, a parent may do so provided he or she acts as a 'reasonable parent' in the eyes of the law.

Similar considerations must, of course, be taken into account when a therapeutic research project is proposed, the only differences being the degree of acceptable risk and perhaps the type of procedure allowed. Examples of the types and degree of risk and benefit that might be considered acceptable have been given in the report of the Working Party on Ethics of Research in Children.[11]

Much of what has been said about consent in children can be said to apply to the mentally ill or handicapped. Here, however, it may involve rather more consideration of obtaining consent from parents, relatives or legal guardians. The fact that a patient has been admitted to a mental hospital does not necessarily indicate their ability to give or withhold consent. The question is whether the patient is able to appreciate the reasons for the nature and the possible complications of the proposed treatment. Similar questions need to be asked when considering the elderly patient and informed consent. The elderly are a large segment of the population and the drug regulatory authorities often require specific studies in this group. Studies have shown that the elderly exhibit significantly poorer comprehension of consent information than younger age groups. The provision of special instructions for elderly patients participating in a clinical trial may be necessary.[39]

Few clinical studies are approved by ethics committees without provision for patient consent. In instances where informed consent is not required by an ethics committee, such as in studies of chemotherapy in terminally ill cancer patients, there is always a risk that failure to ask for consent will be misconstrued and regarded as against the patient's interest. An example of this occurred in 1982[40] and the discussion is still continuing. A decision not to ask for patient consent must always involve the most careful and full discussion beforehand. The whole problem of informed consent and its need has been aired by Baum,[41] who argues that double standards are used when comparing controlled clinical trials and routine treatment by individual doctors. He suggests that many people would consider the former to be unethical for a variety of reasons or would impose restrictions on them, yet allow the individual doctor to make his own, perhaps poorly controlled, comparison in the course of routine treatment. His fear is that ill-formed and hostile criticism of clinical experimentation will lead to ill-judged governmental legislation that will frighten away both doctors and patients from participation in clinical trials.

The following list of requirements for a proposed consent is used by the ethics committee of an Australian group of hospitals[42] and incorporates most of the basic conditions required by Institutional Review Boards in the USA.

1. A statement of the general purpose of the trial.
2. An invitation to participate.
3. A statement as to why the patient was selected.
4. A description of the procedures to be followed, including their purpose, how long they will take, and their frequency.
5. Use of placebos should be disclosed.
6. A description of the discomforts and inconveniences that might reasonably be expected.
7. An estimate of the total amount of the subject's time likely to be required.
8. A description of any risks of involvement.
9. Any benefits to the subject that can be reasonably expected should be described.
10. Any withholding of standard treatment should be disclosed.
11. If any data to be obtained from the study are to be made available to any person or organization, the purpose of the disclosure and the nature of the information should be described.

12. Any provision for payment to the participant should be stated.
13. It should clearly indicate that the subject is free to decide not to participate or later to withdraw their consent and discontinue participation without prejudice.
14. It should contain an offer to answer any enquiries concerning the procedures of the study and the name and address of an investigator who can be contacted.

Research on healthy volunteers

The past decade has seen an increase in the number of studies performed on normal healthy volunteers, particularly as Phase I human volunteer studies have now become part of the normal development of new medicines.[43] However, these studies are not without risk and both the increase in number of studies and the death of two volunteers resulted in the Medicines Commission requesting the RCP to set up a working party to consider this aspect of medical research.[44] Its report was published in 1986 and provides a comprehensive set of recommendations including the suggestion that laboratories performing human studies should be inspected and registered.[45]

To safeguard the volunteers the working party recommends that all preclinical and toxicological data to support such studies be assessed by an independent body with the expertise that may be lacking in a local ethics committee. There are, in addition, many worthwhile and detailed recommendations on ethics, recruitment and financial considerations, safeguards, design of the study and patient consent, and compensation and insurance.

The difficulties associated with the use of so-called normal volunteers were highlighted by the sudden death of a volunteer in a Phase I tolerance study.[46] Here, the volunteer failed to report his attendance at a psychiatric clinic during the study and that he had received a depot injection of a neuroleptic drug. Soon after receiving the test drug he collapsed and died despite emergency life-support procedures. An example of the difficulties in assessing causality arose in a different drug study when three healthy volunteers developed a rash whilst receiving the drug.[47] The study was suspended until a colleague of the volunteers suffered a similar illness four weeks later and viral studies in the volunteers indicated a recent infection with parovirus. The study then continued.

A survey of normal volunteer studies performed by or on behalf of 43 pharmaceutical companies over a period of 1 to 6 years provides a reasonably favourable perspective of the situation.[48] There were no deaths or life-threatening reactions in a total of 18 671 in-house subject exposures and there were five serious suspected reactions – a rate of 0.27 per 1000 subject exposures. With external studies there was one death, no life-threatening reactions and eight serious suspected reactions (0.91 per 1000) in 8753 subject exposures.

Many of the recommendations of the working party of the RCP are already being followed by ethics committees and investigators. It remains to be seen whether, in the UK, legislation is used to enforce these recommendations.

General practice trials

In the UK a large number of pharmaceutical companies sponsor clinical trials in general practice and in some companies there are groups within the medical department specializing only in this field of clinical research.

As the numbers of general practitioner trials increased, concern was expressed about the methods of conducting such trials and their lack of ethical review. A few companies produced individual Codes of Conduct for general practice clinical trials that were handed out to each investigator and some also instigated the setting up of independent ethics committees to review their protocols for these clinical trials. This resulted in more specific suggestions being put forward to regularize this area of research.[49]

These suggestions involved two aspects – a code of practice and the setting up of local ethics committees. Discussions took place between the ABPI, the BMA and the RCGP (Royal College of General Practitioners) to develop and draw up a Code of Practice for the Assessment of Licensed Medicines in General Practice. All three parties agreed on the requirements and content of the code.[50]

The code covers the main requirements of any clinical trial together with comments on company monitoring, patient confidentiality and methods of inviting general practitioners to participate in a study. An important clause is one stating that the protocol must be submitted to and approved by an independent and properly constituted ethics committee.

In 1981 the BMA published a report on Local Ethical Committees,[12] with particular emphasis on general practitioner participation, and a model constitution was recommended for consideration. Some progress has been made towards setting up these local ethical committees which are to be based on district hospitals. At the present time there are 192 Health Districts in England and Wales, each one eventually needing a local ethics committee. However, the BMA stated in its report that there was no justification for changing existing ethics committees if they were working satisfactorily, even if they did not exactly conform to the model. This comment also applies to those ethics committees set up by individual pharmaceutical companies and which can also show themselves to be independent and working satisfactorily.

One of the problems inherent in general practice trials is the need for large numbers of general practitioners to participate if large numbers of patients are required. It is rare that one general practitioner can supply more than 10–20 patients, yet many studies need several hundreds of patients to ensure that the results can reach statistical significance. This raises the problem of reciprocity of ethical approval by different ethics committees. The two extremes are clear – approval by one ethics committee can be accepted countrywide or every general practitioner must submit each protocol to his local ethics committee. A compromise is suggested in the Code of Practice. Approval by a recognized ethics committee will be sought before every clinical trial conducted in general practice. All participating doctors will be informed that ethical approval has been granted by a named and designated ethics committee. It is then up to the participating doctor either to accept this statement or, if he is still in doubt, to submit the protocol to his own local ethics committee. It is likely that general acceptance will be the rule, although there is the freedom to obtain a second opinion. A further possibility is for the general practitioner or pharmaceutical company to submit the protocol to a central ethics committee, such as the one that has been set up by the RCGP. However, the sponsor of a multicentre clinical trial should be prepared for surprising differences to exist in the constitution and working practices of ethics committees.[51] A multicentre research project submitted to 25 largely Health Authority based ethics committees resulted in 18 committees granting approval and three refusing. The four remaining committees failed to give an answer for a variety of reasons. Many approvals were subject to conditions and it is unfortunate that the three ethics committees refusing approval would not consider any discussion or attempt to clarify or answer any problems. This is in contrast to the guidelines of the RCP which suggest a more open attitude and making available to an investigator a review of any adverse decision.

The developments in defining guidelines for general practice clinical trials and the need to obtain ethical approval for these trials are major moves in emphasizing the importance and necessity for this type of trial. General practice clinical trials are now regarded as valuable and essential clinical research for the evaluation of any new drug therapy. The publication of a Code of Practice for conducting clinical trials in general practice should leave no one in doubt as to the correct procedures to be followed. It would be helpful to all and perhaps allay the fears of many members of the public if ethics committees were more open in discussing their reasons for refusing a research project.

Media and pressure groups

The pharmaceutical industry is in a particularly vulnerable position regarding the media and the various pressure groups associated with the health sciences. The therapeutic discoveries of the past 30 years have not only resulted in a vast expansion of clinical research to test these new drugs, but also in the general public's interest in clinical trials and the marketing of drugs.

This interest may or may not have been fuelled by the media and such groups as the Patients Association, the Consumers Association and other pressure groups. Whatever the reason, the workings of the pharmaceutical industry are under intense scrutiny and this must be recognized.

Much of the comment from the media and pressure groups is thoughtful, useful and of benefit to the industry and physicians conducting clinical research. The various societies of medical ethics provide useful forums to discuss the difficult philosophical concepts that can arise in research. Yet the definitions of ethics used now are not the same as they were 20 years ago, and nor will they be the same in the year 2001. They are what is acceptable at a particular moment in time. Medical ethics, as everything else, are not immutable and they change as society changes. We must be wary of both thinking that our ethics are better than anyone else's or, what could be worse, acceptable to everyone else.[24]

There has been debate in Germany and in France about the morality and legality of randomized and placebo-controlled studies.[52,53] Whatever the reasons for this debate and the particular beliefs of the people putting forward the objections, it must be accepted that there will be variations in the approach to certain aspects of ethics. These variations in approach may be related to time, cultural or national differences, or even political persuasions. What may be regarded as ethical in one country may be unethical in another and so on. The presence of active media – be it radio, television or the press – and the internationality of certain pressure groups allows more rapid dissemination of and comment on any anomalies in the interpretation of medical ethics. The danger is, of course, that only one side of an argument may be reported, and then from a biased viewpoint with the minimum of facts. The airing of any gross anomalies in the interpretation of medical ethics is undoubtably of benefit. However, care must be taken when commenting on the more frequent subtle differences that may be much more closely related to interpretation of the legal system, cultural and ethnic backgrounds, or to the social environment.

Even where there is a comparatively tried and accepted format for reviewing the medical ethics of research, problems can arise. In a well publicized case[40] a patient died while taking part in a randomized controlled trial in the UK. The patient was suffering from cancer and was entered into a trial in which a cytotoxic drug was administered directly into the portal vein. The protocol laid down that a blood count should be taken every alternate day after the operation in order to detect any bone marrow depression. Unfortunately, the patient did not have this carried out for a period of about 7 days. During this time bone marrow depression occurred, other complications set in and the patient eventually died.

The trial was organized and run by experienced and eminent clinicians and the protocol was accepted by 11 area ethics committees. In each case the local ethics committee agreed that in view of the nature of the trial (for cancer) patients should not be informed of their participation, and so informed consent was not obtained either from the patient or a relative.

The inquest on this patient's death lead to an enormous amount of comment and criticism in the media. A barrister-at-law has commented that it was wrong not to obtain informed consent before entry into the trial and that 'the search for a cure for cancer, however laudable, must not be used to justify the abrogation of basic human rights'.

It is not the purpose here to comment on the rights or wrongs of the decisions of the 11 ethics committees to waive the need for informed consent. However, it is necessary to emphasize the problems that can arise if such a far-reaching and important decision is taken and the possible resulting effects both on that trial and subsequent trials if something goes wrong. Human error probably led to this patient's death. Yet it was not so much that error, but the failure to obtain informed consent from the patient, that made the headlines.

The development of medical ethics is now reaching an important and perhaps critical stage. It is a stage in which the decisions of ethics committees may well be thrown open to general debate, comment and criticism in the national and international media and by various pressure groups. If these decisions are open to general discussion tremendous problems in relation to confidentiality of data could arise. This may not only affect the pharmaceutical company involved if the research concerns a new drug, but also the doctors and patients. A careful watch needs to be kept on this development.

There is intense pressure to place more lay members on ethics committees and, in the future, it may no longer be acceptable to have ethics committees consisting entirely of doctors and members of associated health specialities. The next 20 or 30 years will probably see as many changes in the practice of medical ethics and ethics committees as have occurred in the last 30 years. The clinician conducting or sponsoring a clinical trial must be aware of these changes and adapt their research objectives to satisfy the current atmosphere.

References

1. (1949). *Trials of War Criminals Before the Nuremberg Military Tribunals under Control Commission*, Law No. 10, Vol. 11. Washington DC: US Government Printing Office: 180–2.
2. World Medical Association (1975). Declaration of Tokyo: Guidelines for medical doctors. *World Medical Journal* 22: 87.
3. Lambo TA (1979). Safeguarding human rights in medical experiments. *World Health Organisation Chronicle* 33: 326.
4. Breuer H, Fischer FW (1981). Role of ethical guidance committees in clinical trials. *Controlled Clinical Trials* 1: 421.
5. WMA (1964). Human experimentation: code of ethics of the World Medical Association. *British Medical Journal* 2: 177.
6. Statement by Medical Research Council (1964). Responsibility in investigations on human subjects. *British Medical Journal* 2: 178.
7. Report of the committee appointed by the Royal College of Physicians of London (1967). Supervision of the ethics of clinical investigations in institutions. *British Medical Journal* 3: 429.
8. Report of a WHO Scientific Group (1968). *Principles for the Clinical Evaluation of Drugs*. World Health Organisation Technical Report Series No. 403, Geneva.
9. *Report of the Committee on the Supervision of the Ethics of Clinical Research Investigations in Institutions* (1973). Royal College of Physicians of London.
10. DHSS (1975). *Supervision of the Ethics of Clinical Research Investigations and Fetal Research*. Health Service Circular (Interim Series) HSC (15) 153.
11. Working Party on Ethics of Research in Children (1980). Guidelines to aid ethical committees considering research involving children. *British Medical Journal* 280: 229.
12. Local Ethical Committees (1981). *British Medical Journal* 282: 1010.
13. Gutteridge F, Bankowski Z, Curran W *et al.* (1982). The structure and functioning of ethical review committees. *Social Science and Medicine* 16: 1791.

14. Royal College of Physicians (1990). *Research Involving Patients. A Working Party Report*. London: RCP.
15. Royal College of Physicians (1990). *Guidelines on the Practice of Ethics Committees in Research Involving Human Subjects*, 2nd edn. London: RCP.
16. Thompson IE, French K, Melia KM *et al.* (1981). Research ethical committees in Scotland. *British Medical Journal* **292**: 718.
17. O'Brien M, Mahadevan S (1980). A system for the ethical control of clinical research. *Public Health* **9**: 219.
18. Allen PA, Waters WE (1982). Development of an ethical committee and its effect on research design. *Lancet* **1**: 1233.
19. Denham MJ, Foster A, Tyrrell DAJ (1979). Work of a district ethical committee. *British Medical Journal* **2**: 1042.
20. Ethical Committee, University College Hospital (1981). Experience at a clinical research ethical review committee. *British Medical Journal* **283**: 1312.
21. Faccini JM, Bennett PN, Reid JL (1984). European ethical review committee: the experience of an international ethics committee reviewing protocols for drug trials. *British Medical Journal* **289**: 1052.
22. Ramsay LE, Tidd MJ, Butler JK *et al.* (1977). Ethical review in the pharmaceutical industry. *British Journal of Clinical Pharmacology* **4**: 73.
23. Royal College of Physicians (1983). *Guidelines on the Practice of Ethics Committees in Medical Research*. London: RCP.
24. Marsh BT (1981). The pharmaceutical industry. In *Ethical Committees for Clinical Research*. London: Medico-Pharmaceutical Forum: 103–16.
25. Leader (1986). Who's for bioethics committees? *Lancet* i: 1016.
26. Pearce JMS (1986). Ethics Committees. *Lancet* i: 1156.
27. Fost N, Cranford RE (1985). Hospital Ethics Committees. *Journal of the American Medical Association* **253**: 2687.
28. Browne A (1987). Ethics committees for what? *Canadian Medical Association Journal* **136**: 1149.
29. Lo B (1987). Promises and pitfalls of ethics committees. *New England Journal of Medicine* **317**: 46.
30. Health and Human Services Department, Food and Drug Administration (1981). *Standards for Institutional Review Boards for Clinical Investigations*. Federal Register 46, 8975.
31. Fost N (1979). Consent as a barrier to research. *New England Journal of Medicine* **300**: 1272.
32. The Lord Scarman (1986). Consent, communication and responsibility. *Journal of the Royal Society of Medicine* **79**: 697.
33. Griffin JP (1981). Medicines regulations. In *Ethical Committees for Clinical Research*. London: Medico-Pharmaceutical Forum: 27–44.
34. Vere DW (1981). Controlled clinical trials: the current ethical debate. *Journal of the Royal Society of Medicine* **74**: 84.
35. Dahan R, Caulin C, Figea L, *et al.* (1986). Does informed consent influence therapeutic outcome? A clinical trial of the hypnotic activity of placebo in patients admitted to hospital. *British Medical Journal* **293**: 363.
36. Myers MG, Cairns JA, Singer J (1987). The consent form as a possible cause of side effects. *Clinical Pharmacology and Therapeutics* **42**: 250.
37. Skegg PDG (1977). English Law relating to experimentation on children. *Lancet* **2**: 754.
38. Dworkin G (1978). Legality of consent to nontherapeutic medical research on infants and young children. *Archives of Diseases in Childhood* **53**: 443.
39. Stanley B, Guido J, Stanley M *et al.* (1984). The elderly patient and informed consent. *Journal of the American Medical Association* **252**: 1302.

40. Brahams D (1982). Clinical trials and the consent of the patient. *Practitioner* **226**: 1829.
41. Baum M (1986). Do we need informed consent? *Lancet* **ii**: 911.
42. Campbell JD, McEwin K (1981). The hospital ethics committee. *The Medical Journal of Australia* **1**: 168.
43. Harry JD (1987). Research on healthy volunteers – a report of the Royal College of Physicians. *British Journal of Clinical Pharmacology* **23**: 379.
44. Vere DW (1987). Research on healthy volunteers – a report of the Royal College of Physicians. *British Journal of Pharmacology* **23**: 375.
45. Royal College of Physicians Working Party (1986). Research on healthy volunteers. *Journal of the Royal College of Physicians* **20**: 243.
46. Darragh A, Kenny M, Lambe R et al. (1985). Sudden death of a volunteer. *Lancet* **i**: 93.
47. Fazackerley EJ, Randall NPC, Pleuvry BJ (1987). Three cases of illness during a drug trial in healthy volunteers. *British Medical Journal* **294**: 562.
48. Royle JM, Snell ES (1986). Medical research in normal volunteers. *British Journal of Clinical Pharmacology* **21**: 548.
49. Marsh BT (1981). Clinical trials in general practice from the point of view of the pharmaceutical industry. *Journal of Drug Research* **6**: 55.
50. Joint agreement between BMA, RCGP and ABPI (1983). Code of practice for the clinical assessment of licensed medicinal products in general practice. *British Medical Journal* **286**: 1295.
51. Ashford JJ (1987). Recent experience of ethics committee review of a multicentre research project. *British Journal of Clinical Pharmacology* **23**: 373.
52. Burkhardt R, Kienle G (1979). Controlled clinical trials and medical ethics. *Lancet* **2**: 1356.
53. Arpaillange P, Dion S, Mathe G (1985). Proposal for ethical standards in therapeutic trials. *British Medical Journal* **291**: 887.
54. NHS Management Executive (1991). *Health Service Guidelines – Local Research Ethics Committees*. HSG (91) 5.
55. General Medical Council (1987). *Professional Conduct and Discipline; Fitness to Practice*. London: GMC.

Appendix A

Since this chapter was revised two important UK reports have been published by the RCP of London,[14,15] and one by the UK Department of Health (DoH).[54] The first of the RCP reports deals with research involving patients and complements an earlier report on research in healthy volunteers.[45] The second report gives guidelines for ethical committees and is a revision and update of a similar report published in 1983.[23] Many of the issues covered are common to both reports and they should be read in conjunction. As all three reports are indicative of current UK medical attitudes to research in patients and to ethical committees their main contents are highlighted below.

Research involving patients

This report[14] addresses the special problems of conducting research on patients, both medical and surgical, and provides advice for all concerned. In particular, this report is intended to increase awareness of the need for research, but at the same time give guidance on the best ways to protect the patient and ensure public confidence in these procedures.

The main points covered are listed below:

1. Justification for research.
2. Role of research ethics committees and the assessment of ethics. It is suggested that ethics committees should report regularly and at least annually to the body which set it up and that the report be available to the press and public.
3. Assessment of quality of research, including risk/benefit analysis.
4. Patient selection.
5. Patient recruitment, in particular the consent procedures with patient information sheets and written, witnessed consent. Special consideration to be given to groups with limited comprehension such as children, the mentally handicapped and psychiatric patients. Justification for initiating research without the consent of the patient is also considered. Inducements to patients and investigations are discussed. The committee producing this report considers payments to an investigator on a per capita basis are unethical. This contrasts with the General Medical Council (GMC) guidelines[55] and also the report by the RCP on guidelines for ethics committees. Both the GMC and the RCP guidelines on ethics committees comment on the possible ethical problems of per capita payments, but neither states unequivocally that such payments are unethical.
6. Comments on the ethical problems of randomized controlled trials and placebos.
7. Responsibility for the conduct of research.
8. Ownership of results.
9. Monitoring the conduct of research and possible sanctions.
10. Legal implications and arrangements for compensation.

Guidelines on the practice of ethics committees in medical research involving human subjects

This report[15] points out that in the UK the practice of research ethics committees continues to vary in many ways. In addition, there is often no single correct answer to an ethical problem or question.

The main points covered are listed below.

1. Objectives of research ethics committees. These are to maintain ethical standards, to protect patients, to preserve subjects' rights and to provide reassurance to the public.
2. Definition of classes of research.
3. Recommendation for mandatory ethical review.
4. Terms of reference and scope of ethical committees.
5. Membership of ethics committees.
6. Method of working.

7. Applications to ethics committees and the suggested format of these applications.
8. Problems associated with therapeutic trials such as design, consent and placebos.
9. Responsibilities in law and the suggestion that members of ethics committees be indemnified against legal costs by the organization setting up the committee.
10. Consent and the information required.
11. Special classes of research such as children, pregnant women, mentally handicapped and unconscious or acutely ill patients.
12. Research involving foetuses, foetal material, *in vitro* fertilization and embryos.
13. The Medicines Act 1968.
14. Compensation.
15. Payments to subjects and investigators.

Local research ethics committees.

The UK DoH has issued a booklet on NHS guidelines on Local Research Ethics Committees (LRECs).[54] For the first time in the UK it is now obligatory for all research projects being performed on NHS premises or by NHS staff to be submitted to a LREC for approval.

Every health district is required to have a LREC and the District Health Authorities are responsible for establishing and maintaining these LRECs. The booklet gives advice and guidance on:

The establishment and function of LRECs and the administrative framework within which they work.
The ethical principles to which LRECs should have regard.
Particular groups as research subjects, such as children, women, prisoners and mentally disordered people.

Responsibility for deciding whether a research proposal should proceed within the NHS lies with the NHS body under whose auspices the research would take place.

These LRECs were to be in place by 1 February 1992. Any NHS body asked to agree to a research proposal falling within its sphere of responsibility has to ensure that it has been submitted to the appropriate LREC for research ethics approval as follows:

District health authorities, about research within their hospitals or community health services, or in private sector providers under contract to these authorities.
Special health authorities, about research within their units.
Family health services authorities, about research involving general medical, general dental or other family health services.
NHS trusts, about research within the units they control.

These bodies should take the LREC's advice into account before deciding whether the research project should go ahead. Projects that do not have LREC approval must not be agreed to.

Appendix B
Declaration of Helsinki: Recommendations Guiding Physicians in Biomedical Research Involving Human Subjects.

Adopted by the 18th World Medical Assembly, Helsinki, Finland, June 1964 and amended by the 29th World Medical Assembly, Tokyo, Japan, October 1975, 35th World Medical Assembly, Venice, Italy, October 1983 and the 41st World Medical Assembly, Hong Kong, September 1989.

Introduction
It is the mission of the physician to safeguard the health of the people. His or her knowledge and conscience are dedicated to the fulfilment of this mission.

The Declaration of Geneva of the World Medical Association binds the physician with the words, 'The health of my patient will be my first consideration', and the International Code of Medical Ethics declares that, 'A physician shall act only in the patient's interest when providing medical care which might have the effect of weakening the physical and mental condition of the patient'.

The purpose of biomedical research involving human subjects must be to improve diagnostic, therapeutic and prophylactic procedures and the understanding of the aetiology and pathogenesis of disease.

In current medical practice most diagnostic, therapeutic or prophylactic procedures involve hazards. This applies especially to biomedical research.

Medical progress is based on research which ultimately must rest in part on experimentation involving human subjects.

In the field of biomedical research a fundamental distinction must be recognized between medical research in which the aim is essentially diagnostic or therapeutic for a patient, and medical research, the essential object of which is purely scientific and without implying direct diagnostic or therapeutic value to the person subjected to the research.

Special caution must be exercised in the conduct of research which may affect the environment, and the welfare of animals used for research must be respected.

Because it is essential that the results of laboratory experiments be applied to human beings to further scientific knowledge and to help suffering humanity, the World Medical Association has prepared the following recommendations as a guide to every physician in biomedical research involving human subjects. They should be kept under review in the future. It must be stressed that the standards as drafted are only a guide to physicians all over the world. Physicians are not relieved from criminal, civil and ethical responsibilities under the laws of their own countries.

I. Basic principles

1. Biomedical research involving human subjects must conform to generally accepted scientific principles and should be based on adequately performed laboratory and animal experimentation and on a thorough knowledge of the scientific literature.
2. The design and performance of each experimental procedure involving human subjects should be clearly formulated in an experimental protocol which should be transmitted for consideration, comment and guidance to a specially appointed committee independent of the investigator and the sponsor provided that this independent committee is in conformity with the laws and regulations of the country in which the research experiment is performed.
3. Biomedical research involving human subjects should be conducted only by scientifically qualified persons and under the supervision of a clinically competent medical person. The responsibility for the human subject must always rest with a medically qualified person and never rest on the subject of the research, even though the subject has given his or her consent.
4. Biomedical research involving human subjects cannot legitimately be carried out unless the importance of the objective is in proportion to the inherent risk to the subject.
5. Every biomedical research project involving human subjects should be preceded by careful assessment of predictable risks in comparison with foreseeable benefits to the subject or to others. Concern for the interests of the subject must always prevail over the interests of science and society.
6. The right of the research subject to safeguard his or her integrity must always be respected. Every precaution should be taken to respect the privacy of the subject and to minimize the impact of the study on the subject's physical and mental integrity and on the personality of the subject.
7. Physicians should abstain from engaging in research projects involving human subjects unless they are satisfied that the hazards involved are believed to be predictable. Physicians should cease any investigation if the hazards are found to outweigh the potential benefits.
8. In publication of the results of his or her research, the physician is obliged to preserve the accuracy of the results. Reports of experimentation not in accordance with the principles laid down in this Declaration should not be accepted for publication.
9. In any research on human beings, each potential subject must be adequately informed of the aims, methods, anticipated benefits and potential hazards of the study and the discomfort it may entail. He or she should be informed that he or she is at liberty to abstain from

participation in the study and that he or she is free to withdraw his or her consent to participation at any time. The physician should then obtain the subject's freely-given informed consent, preferably in writing.

10. When obtaining informed consent for the research project, the physician should be particularly cautious if the subject is in a dependent relationship to him or her or may consent under duress. In that case the informed consent should be obtained by a physician who is not engaged in the investigation and who is completely independent of this official relationship.

11. In case of legal incompetence, informed consent should be obtained from the legal guardian in accordance with the national legislation. Where physical or mental incapacity makes it impossible to obtain informed consent, or when the subject is a minor, permission from the responsible relative replaces that of the subject in accordance with the national legislation.

    Whenever the minor child is in fact able to give a consent, the minor's consent must be obtained in addition to the consent of the minor's legal guardian.

12. The research protocol should always contain a statement of the ethical considerations involved and should indicate that the principles enunciated in the present Declaration are complied with.

II. Medical research combined with professional care (clinical research)

1. In the treatment of the sick person, the physician must be free to use a new diagnostic and therapeutic measure, if in his or her judgement it offers hope of saving life, re-establishing health or alleviating suffering.

2. The potential benefits, hazards and discomfort of a new method should be weighed against the advantages of the best current diagnostic and therapeutic methods.

3. In any medical study, every patient – including those of a control group, if any – should be assured of the best proven diagnostic and therapeutic method.

4. The refusal of the patient to participate in a study must never interfere with the physician–patient relationship.

5. If the physician considers it essential not to obtain informed consent, the specific reasons for this proposal should be stated in the experimental protocol for transmission to the independent committee (I.2.).

6. The physician can combine medical research with professional care, the objective being the acquisition of new medical knowledge, only to the extent that medical research is justified by its potential diagnostic or therapeutic value for the patient.

III. Non-therapeutic biomedical research involving human subjects (non-clinical biomedical research)

1. In the purely scientific application of medical research carried out on a human being, it is the duty of the physician to remain the protector of the life and health of that person on whom biomedical research is being carried out.
2. The subjects should be volunteers – either healthy persons or patients for whom the experimental design is not related to the patient's illness.
3. The investigator or the investigating team should discontinue the research if in his/her or their judgement it may, if continued, be harmful to the individual.
4. In research on man, the interest of science and society should never take precedence over considerations related to the well-being of the subject.

12

The pharmaceutical physician
Karen Summers

'Doctors [in clinical practice] can't produce modern drugs and scientists in industry can't treat sick people' Sir Derek Dunlop*

The prospectus of The Faculty of Pharmaceutical Medicine of the Royal Colleges of Physicians (RCP) in the UK defines pharmaceutical medicine 'as a discipline concerned with discovery, development, evaluation and monitoring of medicines and their marketing'. Other chapters in this book address in detail the principles of pharmaceutical medicine; this chapter will discuss the practice of pharmaceutical medicine as a speciality.

Background

Historical perspective
The speciality of pharmaceutical medicine has a relatively short history. The first pharmaceutical physicians (or medical advisers as they were then known) were recruited by the pharmaceutical industry, as full-time employees, after the Second World War. Their principal functions were to act as a source of medical opinion to assist and focus drug development, particularly as it related to clinical trials, and to advise on marketing issues.

As a response to the thalidomide tragedy, in the UK the Dunlop Committee was set up in 1963 to advise on new medicinal products. The introduction of the Medicines Act in 1968 and formation, by statute, of the Committee on the Review of Medicines (CRM) and Committee on Safety of Medicines (CSM) increased the need for physicians both within the pharmaceutical industry and government. The rate of growth in the number of pharmaceutical physicians has been impressive. In 1989 Chandler[1] reviewed this growth in the UK pharmaceutical industry between 1 January 1974 and 1 January 1989 and estimated that the total numbers increased from 265 to 498, a growth of 88 per cent. Compared with other UK medical specialities the growth between the years 1972 and 1987 in pharmaceutical medicine (75 per cent) comfortably outstripped other specialities such as dermatology (+40 per cent), cardiology (+41 per cent), neurology (+44 per cent), general medicine (+47 per cent), anaesthetics (+52 per cent) and rheumatology (+54 per cent).

As with most medical specialities its growth, development, establishment and acceptance within the ranks of mainstream medicine has been

---

* Chairman of the Dunlop Committee. Quotation from 1st edn of this book.

closely intertwined with the establishment of professional bodies, and this is well illustrated by the course of events in the UK. In October 1957 a group of 30 medical advisers within the industry met to form an association called The Association of Medical Advisers in the Pharmaceutical Industry (AMAPI). In broad terms it was initiated as a forum for medical advisers within the industry to meet professionally and exchange views. It later came to protect and promote the professional interests of its members as well as promoting pharmaceutical medicine, endorsing training and safeguarding standards.

A major milestone in the development of pharmaceutical medicine was the establishment of the Diploma in Pharmaceutical Medicine in January 1975. The history of this Diploma can be traced back to 1968 and the publication of two reports, The Royal Commission of Medical Training in 1968 and the Joint Committee on Higher Medical Training, and ultimately resulted in the three RCPs initiating the Diploma in Pharmaceutical Medicine in 1975 with the first examination being held in November 1976. In particular the syllabus of this examination helped to shape and define the speciality of pharmaceutical medicine and the standards of knowledge that might reasonably be expected of an established practitioner.

With the evolution of the development and regulation of medicines it became increasingly apparent that pharmaceutical medicine was becoming an autonomous speciality. In the UK this led to the establishment, in October 1989, of the Faculty of Pharmaceutical Medicine as part of the three RCPs of the UK. It is dedicated to the setting, maintenance and improvement in standards of pharmaceutical medicine and its establishment has firmly registered pharmaceutical medicine as a defined and recognized speciality of medicine.

Pharmaceutical medicine has therefore been conceived, shaped and established as a medical speciality in about 40 years. There is little doubt that it will continue to grow as a speciality and make sizeable contributions to the practice of medicine.

Introductory comments on being a pharmaceutical physician

The differences in practising pharmaceutical medicine, as opposed to other specialities, have been a source of consideration by pharmaceutical physicians for some time.[2,3] This section will review these differences and some of the difficulties of the speciality.

Pharmaceutical medicine is mainly an office-based speciality and is the study of diseases and conditions and their response to medicines rather than a study of individual patient responses, which is clinical pharmacology. Accordingly the aspiring pharmaceutical physician must realize that they will, by and large, have to relinquish contacts with patients and for the majority of their time will no longer be treating individual patients in the clinic or at the bedside, exercising their diagnostic skills, performing practical procedures or comforting relatives. (Having said that, many companies allow and indeed encourage pharmaceutical physicians to have half a day a week assistantships at local hospitals. This allows them to keep up-to-date with developments in clinical medicine as well as preventing the loss of clinical skills and knowledge.)

While not often overtly stated, many physicians derive satisfaction at the status they hold either with fellow physicians or in the community at large. While pharmaceutical medicine has come a long way in terms of being appreciated and valued by the medical profession and society, it is still perceived by some to be a less acceptable branch of medicine than others. Higson[4] describes unfavourable experiences while manning a Faculty of Pharmaceutical Medicine Stand at two Medical Careers Fairs and feels that the industry needs to communicate key messages to medical students; in particular, that pharmaceutical physicians are part of the ethical conscience of the pharmaceutical industry and that being 'commercial' does not imply that physicians are automatically greedy, unethical and unreasonably affluent. The physician entering the pharmaceutical industry must therefore be conscious of this and be continuously prepared to raise awareness of the benefits that the practice of pharmaceutical medicine brings to medicine and society.

Physicians must also realize that they will be working within a large organization and within an entirely different managerial structure. Traditionally doctors are trained to work autonomously and to make independent decisions, quite often with speed. However, within either industry or regulatory bodies decisions are usually made on a much more consultative basis and inevitably take longer to reach; to many physicians entering the industry this approach can be a source of irritation and frustration. However, it is important that pharmaceutical physicians have the ability to consult widely and to be viewed by colleagues as 'good team players'. New pharmaceutical physicians must also realize that not all decisions may be made entirely on medical grounds alone; all companies are commercial organizations and need to be profitable to survive. The pharmaceutical physician, without ever compromising his medical integrity, standards or ethics, has to understand the realities of commercial life. That having been said, it is perfectly possible to produce a new medicine which is a medical and commercial success: undoubtedly there is little in the life of a pharmaceutical physician more satisfying than contributing to an effective new medicine which is also profitable, enabling the company to research and introduce further new medicines.

During their training doctors, when working together, usually have a senior colleague heading the group who is the fount of all knowledge; thus, increasing seniority within the group is accompanied by an increasing depth of knowledge. In industry, more often than not, it is the newcomers who possess the greatest degree of expertise within a given area. While recently recruited pharmaceutical physicians may be able to use their specialist expertise they have to realize that promotion within the industry is usually accompanied by their spending less and less time in areas where they are medically familiar and more and more time in areas where they are not. They must, therefore, during their training in industry, acquire the skill of being able rapidly to familiarize themselves with areas of medicine in which they have little or no previous experience. It also follows that the converse should apply as well: namely, that, as a physician progresses up the managerial tree, he or she should have the confidence to accept and respect the advice of their juniors.

Because of the nature of their jobs and possibly training, doctors are not noted for their tolerance of criticism, especially from non-medically qualified personnel. However, the physician in industry must be able to see criticism (and questioning of judgement) in a constructive sense, and not react in a defensive or aggressive manner which will tend only to distance him- or herself from colleagues.

Finally, in nearly all other branches of medicine, on completion of a recognized training programme, the physician is usually able to find a position that will offer a lifetime's employment. Generally the only reasons for loss of employment are ill health, negligent practice or gross misconduct. In industry these reasons also apply but there are other circumstances as well which may seem unfair or inappropriate. Industry is not static and the pharmaceutical industry is no exception. Downturns in the economy, company mergers or redefinition of corporate strategy are all part and parcel of working within the pharmaceutical industry and all can lead to the pharmaceutical physician's loss of employment. Physicians who enter the industry must realize that they cannot regard their position with the same degree of job certainty as can, say, their colleagues in general practice.

In summary then, doctors who intend to pursue a career in pharmaceutical medicine should necessarily be drawn to therapeutics and be primarily interested in treating diseases or conditions as they affect mankind in general rather than individuals. They must possess the expected qualities of any practising physician but in addition be mature and confident enough to accept criticism and questioning in a constructive manner. They should also possess an epidemiologist's gift of overview, seeing illnesses in their widest perspective. Also, like the epidemiologist they must have the faculty of noticing and recognizing the importance of the unusual.

Recommended background training before becoming a pharmaceutical physician

Before applying to be a pharmaceutical physician the doctor should have learnt two branches of medicine: Medicine the Art and Medicine the Science. They need to know Medicine the Science because the development of new medicines requires full scientific rigour in their evaluation. However, the doctor in industry also has to understand Medicine the Art, since this aspect of medical judgement is frequently called upon. For example, in many cases the interpretation of adverse events requires medical intuition and experience.

Clearly then the doctor must have completed a course in medicine and be fully registered. As part of this progress an intercollated degree in a biological science is valuable although not essential. However, training in a biological science at some stage in the physician's career (be it as an undergraduate or postgraduate) is an advantage on several counts. First, it teaches scientific rigour, something not usually taught on the wards where clinical expertise is often rated higher than pure science. Second, it enables the physician to understand the way scientists view medicine and physicians. We raise this area because it is not uncommon for scientists to regard physicians either with envy (because of their relatively higher rewards and status), or disrespect (because of their generally lesser scientific training) or disdain (when they see physicians practising Medicine the Art rather than Medicine the Science). Certainly a good scientific training will help to establish better working relations with preclinical and development staff within the company and enable the pharmaceutical physician to offer more to the preclinical development of a medicine. Third, the physician will derive greater job satisfaction based on a more complete understanding of the basic science underpinning the project.

After graduating and completing preregistration positions physicians should spend 2 years or so practising general medicine in its widest sense, ideally combining it with a higher degree or diploma or Board certification. This time spent is essential for the pharmaceutical physician as it affords the opportunity to accumulate practical medical experience, which is one of the key features that distinguishes physicians from their scientific colleagues and is the main reason for employing physicians in industry in the first place. This experience is used by the industry in a variety of ways. For example, an experienced physician has the ability to recognize when a statistically significant result is a clinically significant result and when not. Experience also means that realistic trials are carried out, recruiting the right number of patients in the allocated time frame. Experience gives the physician the ability to recognize those trialists who have appropriate expertise and those who do not. Experience allows easier and freer communication with scientists, senior management and academics. It is not infrequent for the science of a new medicine to need to be tempered by clinical reality, something which can lead to friction between physicians and research scientists; this is made easier if physicians are respected because of their expertise. In addition, physicians sometimes have to quell overambitious expectations from marketing or senior management colleagues, which is also made easier if their clinical judgement is valued.

As well as a good general medical training many companies look to hiring physicians with specialist training. As discussed above, it is not infrequent for these specialist skills to be utilized only for part of the pharmaceutical physician's career; they do, however, facilitate the entry of the aspiring pharmaceutical physician into the industry or civil service, usually at an enhanced salary to reflect this additional experience.

Higher training in pharmaceutical medicine

As in all branches of medicine training in pharmaceutical medicine has two aspects: on the job training and formal study. Furthermore, while the speciality of pharmaceutical medicine is a relatively recent development, it is already following in the footsteps of many other specialities in developing a number of subspecialities. For example, just as in gastroenterology there are those who specialize in the upper or lower gastrointestinal tract or the liver, in pharmaceutical medicine it is possible to find those who specialize in Phase I work, Phases II and III or Phases III and IV. It is also possible to find those who specialize entirely in adverse effects of drugs and, within that group of subspecialists, a further group of subspecialists who specialize in the epidemiology of adverse effects.

Where then should pharmaceutical physicians begin in their training? It is our opinion that the best overall perspective and introduction to the pharmaceutical industry can be offered by starting in the Phase III and IV areas, i.e. just as drugs are about to be or have been registered. Physicians who start work in this area of drug research will see first-hand many of the issues involved in pharmaceutical medicine and will interact with a wide range of groups within the industry. Having been involved in the Phase III/IV areas for 2 years or so pharmaceutical physicians are then in a position to decide which area they would like to specialize in. This having been said, many people choose to join the industry and work in the very early phases of drug research as it is perfectly possible, if not quite so easy, to get a full perspective of the industry from this vantage point. It should be the aim of pharmaceutical physicians who have recently joined the industry to gain enough practical experience in the first 2 or 3 years to complete the syllabus either of the Diploma of Pharmaceutical Medicine or Associateship of the Faculty of Pharmaceutical Physicians.

In terms of courses to facilitate passing these examinations, the longest standing and most comprehensive course in the UK is organized by the University of Wales. The aims of the course are twofold. First, to provide a training programme for doctors to acquire the specialist knowledge and skills required by pharmaceutical physicians and second, to prepare them for the RCP Diploma in Pharmaceutical Medicine Examination. The course is organized on a modular basis and consists of 10 teaching sessions spread over 2 years with each teaching session consisting of one module. The training is overseen by the BrAPP (British Association of Pharmaceutical Physicians; see below) Services Sub-Committee who have appointed module coordinators. The 10 modules are designed to be compatible with the revised syllabus of the RCP and are designed to incorporate interactive teaching sessions, workshops and learning through problem solving.[5]

Examinations and diplomas in pharmaceutical medicine

Diploma of Pharmaceutical Medicine
This examination (which was the first of its kind in the world) was first held in November 1976 and examinations have been held annually since then. In order to be eligible for the examination, candidates must be fully registered in the British Medical Register or in the country in which their qualifications were granted. In addition, they will normally have undergone either 2 years of postgraduate general medical training or 2 years of training in pharmaceutical medicine or have 2 years of experience with a drug regulatory authority or 2 years in a suitable academic department

(the Board of Management may modify these conditions of admission). A fee is payable to sit the examination and successful candidates are required to pay a Diploma fee after which the qualification and diploma will be granted.

The syllabus is structured into 12 modules (although these are not of equal weight either in training or in the examinations): Discovery of new medicine; Pharmaceutical development; Toxicity testing; Regulatory legal and ethical issues; Development of medicines; Clinical trials; Medical statistics; Safety of medicines; Regulatory affairs; Information promotion and education; Economics of health care; and The medical department. While no separate module is allocated to clinical pharmacology and therapeutics, it is expected that the candidate will have an up-to-date knowledge in these areas.

The examination itself consists of two parts: a written and an oral session. The written test has three sections: the first section is an essay question, the second, a multiple choice questionnaire and the third section consists of 10 short answer questions. In the oral test (which is held the following day) candidates are examined for 20 minutes by two examiners.

Examinations of Associateship and Membership of the Faculty of Pharmaceutical Physicians

Physicians who have recently joined the industry (that is after 26 October 1989) can only achieve associateship and membership of the Faculty of Pharmaceutical Physicians by examination. At the moment candidates are eligible to apply for the examination of Associateship who are either fully registered with the General Medical Council (GMC) of the UK or hold a medical qualification which is recognized by the GMC and are registered in the country in which the qualification was granted. Candidates must also be able to provide evidence of general medical training over a period of at least 2 years postregistration. In addition to this general training, candidates would normally have undergone 2 years of training in pharmaceutical medicine either as a pharmaceutical physician in a pharmaceutical company (or contract research organization) or in a drug regulatory authority or an academic department.

Currently achievement of the Diploma of Pharmaceutical Medicine entitles the successful candidate to Associateship of the Faculty of Pharmaceutical Medicine. However, as of November 1993 the Faculty will introduce an associateship examination. This has an identical syllabus to the Diploma of Pharmaceutical Medicine although examinations will be held twice a year. Questions on all sections of the syllabus will be presented at each examination session although the examination may be taken in two parts, each part at a different session. The examination will be held over 2 days with written sections on day one and oral sections on day two.

Entry to Membership of the Faculty is examined by presentation of a dissertation and is usually open only to those who have met the requirements for associateship. In addition, candidates need to have completed 6 years since qualification of which 4 years should have been spent within pharmaceutical medicine, either within a company (or contract research organization) or a regulatory agency.

The dissertation needs to be on a subject relevant to pharmaceutical medicine and should normally be between 20 000 and 25 000 words in length. Acceptance of the dissertation and subsequent passing of an oral examination will entitle the candidate to apply for membership.

It should be noted that while all three of these examinations are coordinated by British medical institutions this by no means prevents applicants from other countries applying. Indeed, such is the standing of these examinations that there are many holders of the Diploma of Pharmaceutical Medicine and Members of the Faculty outside the UK.

The above perspective is a singularly British one and other courses in pharmaceutical medicine are also well established. For example, the Spanish Association of Pharmaceutical Physicians (Asociacion de Medicos de la Industria Farmaceutica Espanola) established training courses for pharmaceutical medicine in both Barcelona and Madrid. The training courses are for 2 years and the syllabus is spread over 200 teaching hours. It is similar to that in the UK and successful candidates are entitled to a Pharmaceutical Medicine Diploma.[6]

Professional bodies of relevance to pharmaceutical physicians

International Federation of Associations of Pharmaceutical Physicians
The first discussions leading to the formation of the International Federation of Associations of Pharmaceutical Physicians (IFAPP) took place in 1972, with the establishment of this federation by 1975. It has a President, Vice-President, Secretary and Treasurer as its officers and each affiliated association contributes one main delegate to its committee. Major symposia have been held since 1972 on a triennial basis, with the last one being held in 1990 in Madrid. The purpose of these events is to discuss issues of international importance within the field of pharmaceutical medicine; for example, the title of the conference in 1990 was 'Communications in Pharmaceutical Medicine'.

The financing of the IFAPP comes from affiliation fees and any surpluses from meetings. The monies raised are spent on organizing committee meetings, taking a stand at the triennial International Conference on Clinical Pharmacology and Therapeutics and producing a regular newsletter. Apart from holding the triennial symposium the Federation attempts to hold an event at the International Conference on Clinical Pharmacology and Therapeutics which is held the year before and a 1-day meeting on a suitable topic the year after.

The Faculty of Pharmaceutical Medicine of the RCPs of the UK
As discussed earlier, this Faculty was inaugurated in October 1989, its mission the setting, maintenance and improvement of standards in pharmaceutical medicine.

The aims on which the Faculty were founded were:

1. To develop and maintain high standards in the practice of pharmaceutical medicine.
2. To work for the benefit of patients by ensuring the highest standards of competence and ethical integrity.
3. To enhance the standing of the speciality of pharmaceutical medicine in both the scientific and public domain.
4. To promote for the public benefit the advance and knowledge in pharmaceutical medicine.
5. To act as an authoritative body for the purpose of consultation in pharmaceutical medicine.

In order to help accomplish these aims the Faculty intends to carry out the following activities.

1. Establish a roll of associate members, members and fellows engaged in pharmaceutical medicine.
2. Establish a system that will set standards of competence in pharmaceutical medicine through a properly constituted Board of Examiners and then conform with requirements of its parent colleges.
3. Facilitate four specialist registrations for appropriately qualified practitioners in the discipline of pharmaceutical medicine.
4. Set up an effective communications system to serve the needs of all members.
5. Disseminate information on pharmaceutical medicine to professions and the public.
6. Ensure that physicians, including those in training, are aware of the speciality and have the necessary information to consider pharmaceutical medicine as a career.
7. Establish working parties on important issues of pharmaceutical medicine and to publish the Faculty's recommendations.
8. Organize symposia and lectures for the purpose of education and provide an advisory role for the education of pharmaceutical physicians within the industry.

Admission to associateship and membership of the Faculty by examination has already been discussed. In addition the Faculty may also nominate Fellows who are usually doctors with at least 10 years of experience in the pharmaceutical industry and who have made a distinguished contribution to the speciality. There also exists the provision to appoint Honorary Fellows who may not necessarily be medically qualified.

The British Association of Pharmaceutical Physicians
Details are given on BrAPP as this organization is illustrative of the many national organizations that exist around the world. Founded in October 1957 as the AMAPI its numbers grew as pharmaceutical medicine evolved, changing its name to BrAPP in 1986. In November 1992 it had 673 members. Its main responsibility is for the training, education and development of its members. It also aims to improve the standards, practice and expertise of

pharmaceutical physicians in the speciality of pharmaceutical medicine and its interfaces with marketing, preclinical research, finance and human resources. One of the main functions of BrAPP is to organize meetings and symposia together with training courses and workshops focusing on the above interfaces.

In order to maintain standards it liaises with the Faculty of Pharmaceutical Medicine to ensure that members' wishes are duly expressed. Since its inception BrAPP has been closely involved with the postgraduate course in pharmaceutical medicine at the University of Wales to ensure that the course fully addresses the basic training needs of the pharmaceutical physician.

Finally, the Association publishes, on a bimonthly basis, the news magazine *Pharmaceutical Physician* to help keep members abreast of developments in the field of pharmaceutical medicine, mainly, but not exclusively, from a British and European perspective.

The pharmaceutical physician in drug discovery

The pharmaceutical physician can, in theory, make valuable contributions to preclinical research and drug discovery. Just how much is possible in practice depends largely on the company culture and size and the proximity of pharmaceutical physicians to their preclinical research colleagues. There is certainly no doubt that the earlier pharmaceutical physicians are involved in drug discovery, then the greater will be their focus when constructing the clinical development plan.

One of the key issues for the pharmaceutical industry is that the sequence of events between drug discovery and the registration and marketing is extremely long. In any company which markets products which involve multiple steps between inception and delivery of the final product the potential for error is directly related to the number of steps and people involved. Nowadays most drug research and development is a large-scale process usually carried out on a multinational basis and can involve several hundred personnel. The relative isolation of drug discovery from the clinical and commercial arenas means that commercially poor decisions can be made at the level of drug discovery and not be fully appreciated until the drug has been fully registered and found to be commercially less than viable. However, by this stage several tens of millions of dollars may have been spent. As will become clear, the pharmaceutical physician is in a strong position to help those in drug discovery.

Because they are doctors pharmaceutical physicians are able to provide overviews of any given therapeutic area and identify medical needs. For example, they might identify that a medicine is not available to treat a specific condition or that the medicines which are available have some prominent disadvantage in terms of safety, efficacy or cost. Transmission of these deficiencies and needs to colleagues in basic research can sometimes lead to successful crossfertilization of ideas and the initiation of fruitful new research.

Much time is spent in drug discovery departments trying to improve on existing molecules to produce second generation products. Again, the pharmaceutical physician is ideally placed to identify the problems associated with the first generation products and to advise on the new characteristics required for a second or indeed third generation product. Equally important is the need to identify whether a second generation product is actually required; all too often, at great expense, a new drug is developed for which there is no real demand and which fails to generate any significant return or even cover its development costs. Indeed, it has been estimated that only two out of ten products actually marketed make significant returns. Frequently many companies are in a race to produce second generation products and continuous feedback by the pharmaceutical physician may help to identify the current position of the company's variant in the race and advise either aborting the programme, or niching of the product in potentially profitable but neglected areas. Such timely advice can help to prevent pursuing a product which is doomed to the commercial doldrums and focus resources on more commercially and medically desirable products.

Occasionally pharmaceutical physicians are also in a position to identify new leads by following up on reports of unexpected effects in marketed drugs. For example, the clinical observation of euphoria in hydrazines (developed for the treatment of tuberculosis) led to the clinical development of monoamine oxidase inhibitors.[7] Such leads may not be immediately obvious to scientists in the drug discovery department simply because they are so isolated from the clinical arena.

Close liaison of the pharmaceutical physician with the medicinal chemist discovering the new molecules can help to identify issues that will need to be addressed later on in the drug development programme, for example similarity of the molecule with those known to have specific effects. Prior knowledge of this can help direct strategic planning to incorporate appropriate preclinical and clinical studies into the programme.

The process of drug synthesis is obviously closely coupled to assessment of the new molecules by pharmacologists, biochemists, molecular biologists and so forth. The pharmaceutical physician may well be called upon to advise on this assessment, for it is critical that the lead molecule is tested in systems that have clinical relevance. Pharmaceutical physicians frequently work with academic colleagues who run their own preclinical departments and are keen to carry out preclinical evaluation for companies. This can help build bridges between the company and academic groups and facilitate the passage of a molecule through into clinical assessment.

In general terms it is good practice to bring together the academic physician who will be evaluating the new agent in humans, and the pharmacologist responsible for the project, with the pharmaceutical physician acting as the bridging person. Together they should review the emerging preclinical data to identify what the data are implying from a clinical standpoint and what further work should be done either preclinically or early on in Phase I or II studies. There is no doubt that this sort of close cooperation facilitates drug development, motivates preclinical researchers within the company and gains the confidence of physicians outside the company.

The role of the pharmaceutical physician in preclinical drug development

Preclinical development begins when a lead molecule has been identified as a possible new medicine. This will usually be on the basis of its potency and activity in suitable test systems. The purpose of the development department is to organize a scale-up of production of the new agent; produce a viable assay to test the drug; coordinate issues in safety pharmacology; carry out toxicological assessment; and produce a suitable formulation or formulations of the drug.

Scale-up is not usually an area where pharmaceutical physicians can have much input although they should be aware of any difficulties being encountered as they may impact on clinical development timetables. Occasionally unexpected impurities may be produced during the scale-up requiring bridging toxicology and this information will need to be carefully documented in the clinical investigator's brochure and registration documents.

Assay development, however, is often an area where the pharmaceutical physician's advice is sought; in particular, the pharmaceutical physician is frequently asked to advise what sensivity is desirable. This may be a difficult judgement call, at least before pharmacodynamic data are available in humans. It is very tempting, especially with very potent agents, to be too demanding in terms of assay sensitivity, at least in the early stages of clinical development. However, with few exceptions, it is highly desirable to have an assay by Phase I studies and the pharmaceutical physician should communicate this need to ensure that a suitable assay is available on time.

Safety pharmacology may or may not have been carried out before the new candidate was recommended for development or there may be further work required to resolve issues arising. It is not infrequent for the pharmaceutical physician to be called in to advise on the emerging results and their implications for the drug or the new medicine in humans. Depending on the results the pharmaceutical physician may have to advise that the agent is not viable for further development or that it is only suitable for certain groups of patients.

Toxicology is a complex speciality and few pharmaceutical physicians would profess great expertise in this area. However, a thorough grounding in this science and the ability to liaise closely with toxicologists is essential. While it is usually the toxicologists who will dictate whether the data permit further development in humans or not, it is the toxicologist in conjunction with the pharmaceutical physician who decides on the range of doses to be tested in the first studies in humans. The selection of these doses is difficult but can be fundamental to the way in which the agent behaves in later clinical studies; on the one hand, too cavalier an approach could endanger life and is clearly reprehensible but on the other, too cautious an approach may mean that the doses used in early studies are too low to observe a pharmacodynamic effect, with a consequent abandoning of the project and possible loss of a useful medicine. Toxicology also embraces reproductive studies with which the pharmaceutical physician should be entirely familiar. The pharmaceutical physician must also have widely discussed its implications for drug development and the advice which should be given to women who become pregnant while taking the new agent. While it is the norm to exclude women capable of conception from clinical trials and to contraindicate the use of most drugs during pregnancy, the reality is that women can and do become pregnant during trials and after the new agent has been marketed. The pharmaceutical physician must, therefore, be able to advise the physician in charge of the patient to enable her to make an informed choice on the possible risks of proceeding with the pregnancy.

The whole issue of formulations is one of great interest to the industry since the history of pharmaceutical medicine is littered with examples where successful formulations of old products have added greatly to the versatility of the drug whereas poor formulations have been medical disasters. It is therefore good practice for the pharmaceutical physician to liaise with the development department at all stages of the new candidate's development to review the way the formulation is performing. For example, preliminary pharmacokinetic studies may show that the drug has a short half-life and that the development department should be aiming to produce a long acting formulation. Alternatively, an intravenous formulation may be an irritant and need further work to produce a more acceptable version.

The pharmaceutical physician in the clinical evaluation of medicines

The worldwide organization of medical research

Currently there is a move towards a globalization of drug development and registration. From the company's perspective such moves ought dramatically to reduce costs, speed up the time from drug discovery to registration (and hence extend the useful patent life of the medicine) and reduce unnecessary animal testing. This approach is being matched by the regulatory bodies culminating in the recent international conference on Harmonization of Technical Requirements for Registration of Pharmaceuticals for Human Use (ICH1). Held in Brussels in 1991 it marks a major step forward in harmonizing the regulatory requirements of the EC, Food and Drug Administration (FDA) and Japanese Ministry of Health. However, it is likely that this process will take some time to achieve and conferences are already planned for ICH2 in Washington in 1993 and ICH3 in Tokyo in 1995.

The way in which global drug development is coordinated varies from company to company. In one variation the centre for coordination is always based at the company's head office, not infrequently in the country where the company was founded. Another variation is to coordinate all research from the centre where the medicine was originally discovered and where the preliminary stages of drug development were carried out.

Wherever the coordinating centre may lie there are usually regional head offices based in the USA, Europe and Japan. This helps to facilitate the globalization of drug research and has as its primary aim the achievement of registration of new products in the USA, EC and Japan. Most development plans try to reflect this as far as possible, although globalization plans may put the USA and EC as one group and Japan as a separate entity. Careful and skilled coordination of research between these major economic blocs helps to overcome unnecessary duplication and to optimize the available expertise throughout the world.

In most international companies the organization of medical research within the USA and Japan presents little difficulty in terms of internal company structure and politics. It is within Europe, because it is a collection of separate states with their individual regulatory requirements and approaches to the practice of clinical medicine, that issues arise. In practical terms most multinational companies have a European head office and business units with medical departments in individual states. What varies between companies is the way in which research is actually executed, of which there are two possible approaches. In the first the European head office is fully staffed with medical and ancillary personnel and will directly send out staff to whosoever they think best to carry out clinical studies, wherever they may be in Europe. The perceived advantages of this approach are that it permits tight control of the research programme by, in effect, keeping all research staff under one roof, which greatly facilitates communication within the company. In addition, this approach permits having a team of staff dedicated to one scientific project, thus expediting drug development. There are, however, drawbacks to this type of approach. The first is that the practice of medicine varies widely throughout Europe and it is not particularly easy for a physician from one country to understand another's way of practising medicine. Second, it is important that the marketing departments of local business units keep abreast of new research in the company's products; this is far easier if it is conducted by the medical department of the local business unit rather than by a distant body. In addition, local marketing departments need to establish communications with investigators, since they are frequently national opinion leaders whose views are important and need incorporation into marketing plans. Third, investigators do not discriminate between various parts of a company and certainly rarely understand internal corporate structure. Unfortunately internal communication not infrequently breaks down and the medical department of a local business unit may be unaware that one of their opinion leaders is an investigator for the European head office, with consequent embarrassment all round. A fourth disadvantage is that the regional medical offices do not get to be involved with the research programme until quite late on in the drug's development. Indeed, they may have no involvement with the drug until it comes to submitting a research package to the regulatory bodies. Staff in the medical department, therefore, have only a minimal amount of time to familiarize themselves with the product before it is launched. This clearly puts the local pharmaceutical physician in a disadvantaged position when offering advice to other physicians and the marketing departments at product launch.

In the second approach the role of the European head office is to coordinate, rather than execute, the clinical trial programme through using the medical departments of the local business units. This method has a number of advantages. The first of these is that it builds very strong bridges between the medical departments of local business units and the regional coordinating centre. Second, because physicians in the local business units are working with the new compounds from a very early stage, they will be more familiar with the product and therefore of greater help to their marketing partners in developing a national promotional package. Third, early involvement with new compounds tends to be more exciting than working with them at a later stage and is more motivational for the local physicians and support staff involved in the project. Furthermore, news that the company is working with an exciting new compound rarely stays quiet for too long and seeps out to all areas of the company. The knowledge that the company has an exciting portfolio of compounds in its pipeline can be motivational to company staff, especially in one going through a commercially difficult or quiet period.

The main disadvantage to this style of management (best described as 'matrix management') is that it is difficult for a person to have two managers; the local manager may set priorities that follow a different agenda to that of the European head office.

The ultimate aim, whichever of the above two options is chosen by a company, is to take the shortest time possible to complete the clinical plan, since the longer studies take to run the shorter the drug's effective patent life; a compromise solution may have to be sought in a time of an evolving EC.

It is likely though that, because of the harmonization of regulatory requirements within Europe, there will be less need for regulatory expertise in the business units in the long term and companies will therefore be able to save on these costs by reducing staff and focus regulatory resources within one European coordinating centre. This could, of course, also apply in the long term to clinical research, although this will probably take such a long time that one of the above choices will still be viable for at least the next 10 years.

The medical department

The essential personnel and their reporting structures are given in Fig. 12.1. In general terms the following services are provided by the regional research department: medical expertise, clinical trial support, regulatory affairs, drug safety and, more recently, pharmacoeconomic support.

Medical expertise

This is ultimately provided by the pharmaceutical physicians working within the department. They alone must assume total responsibility

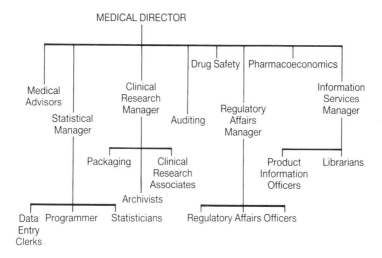

Fig. 12.1 Essential personnel and their reporting structures.

for all medical issues relating to the company's products and, in this aspect, all pharmaceutical physicians should carry adequate insurance against medicolegal complaints. Additional medical advice is given by the safety function, which will provide medical back-up on product-related safety issues. Finally, whilst not medically qualified, most of the staff carrying out clinical trials (clinical research associates) have an extensive knowledge of the drug they are investigating and usually can provide enough information when problems arise to enable investigators to make balanced judgements.

Clinical trials staff
In general terms the physician's time is expensive and it is simply not cost effective to use them to run all aspects of clinical trials. Many areas of drug development can be undertaken equally well (and arguably better) by scientists trained in relevant fields. Clinical trials staff can be considered under four broad headings: those who set up and run studies (clinical research associates); those who enter and analyse the data (statisticians); those who audit the procedures (quality); and those who store the data (archive).

Clinical Research Associates
Clinical Research Associates (CRAs) are usually scientists with a relevant background for clinical research such as pharmacy or pharmacology. The post of CRA is a highly respected scientific appointment and most advertisements attract many applicants of excellent calibre, frequently with higher degrees. Depending on corporate strategy and the individual's capabilities, it is perfectly reasonable for CRAs to be responsible for carrying out the majority of the work involved with clinical trials. This

may include writing protocols and case record forms, recruiting investigators, study site inspection, pharmacy liaison, monitoring the emerging data, closing down studies and writing the final report and papers for publication. In the early days of pharmaceutical medicine many of these duties were performed by physicians, although this was probably an unnecessary and wasteful use of the pharmaceutical physician's time. In clinical studies there are only a few areas where medical input is truly critical and where the pharmaceutical physician must have the ultimate say. First, they need to approve the final version of the protocol as this has medicolegal implications for which the pharmaceutical physician must bear responsibility. Second, the pharmaceutical physician must be closely involved with the recruiting of investigators as they are in the best position to assess the investigator. It is part of the EC Guidelines on Good Clinical Practice (GCP) that the investigator must be appropriately qualified and trained and experienced in research related to the clinical area of the proposed trial.[8] Third, the pharmaceutical physician must see and review serious adverse events to ensure that appropriate action is taken; this would include liaising with the safety director, if the position exists within the company (nearly always a physician). Fourth, in the unhappy event of fraud being suspected during clinical trials, the onus of taking further action should reside with the pharmaceutical physician and medical director. Fifth, the pharmaceutical physician should have the final editorial say in the production of the study report and any ensuing publications. This is to ensure that the correct clinical focus is brought to the study data. Other than these key areas, the running of clinical trials is best left to experienced CRAs, freeing time for the pharmaceutical physician to devote him- or herself to more medical duties.

The reporting tree for CRAs varies very much from company to company. In some companies physicians will have a team of CRAs reporting into them, in others, however, it is deemed best to have CRAs reporting directly to a CRA manager.

The statistical department

The statistical department is an essential element of the research group. In general terms there are three groups of personnel within the department: statisticians, data entry personnel and computer programmers, although in smaller companies some of these roles may be merged.

The Statistician

The statistician is involved with all aspects of the clinical study. Their input is essential in protocol design since they are in the best position to advise on sample sizes. Statisticians are invaluable in focusing physicians and CRAs alike onto the exact question that the protocol is attempting to answer. A fuzzy question invariably results in a fuzzy answer, whereas a focused question gives a focused answer which is both more desirable and easier to achieve. Statisticians also instil discipline into clinical trial design, bringing about concentration on areas that may affect the likelihood of adequately answering the questions in the protocol. For example, it may be that the biological variability of the measurement under evaluation is far greater than expected, with a subsequent increase in the number of subjects who need to be recruited for the study. It is also important that the statistician reviews the case record forms, not only from the point of accuracy but also to try and ensure that the data are recorded in the clearest possible manner.

Once the data are in-house and in a satisfactory format the statistician is then responsible for analysing the data and preparing statistical reports. As there is no such thing as a perfect clinical trial the statistician should highlight the inconsistencies and difficulties which were encountered during the study, which results were planned before the study commenced and which were *post hoc*. Frequently statisticians carry out interim analyses for a variety of medical and commercial reasons and these analyses, if they are to be carried out, should be planned at the beginning of the study, as interim analyses have their own set of statistical rules. The analyses also need to be carefully documented in the final report.

Data entry personnel and computer programmers

While facilities undoubtedly exist for the electronic transmission of data from investigators to the company the industry has been slow to adopt this routinely. Most clinical trial data is recorded on paper which is duly brought in-house by the CRA. The first task of the data entry clerk is to double check the case record forms to ensure that they are adequately completed and that all entries are legible. Thereafter the data entry clerk will enter the data onto specially designed screens. Frequently a process of double data entry is employed, i.e. two people independently entering the same data. This helps ensure that the number of transcription errors is as low as possible.

Personnel with a background in nursing are ideally qualified for this work since not only are they familiar with medical terminology but are also able to understand doctors' illegible handwriting! Finally, companies may have one person dedicated to computing who is required to produce screens for data entry.

Quality

This area has undergone considerable evolution in recent years and is destined to continue to do so for some time. Quality can be divided into: quality control (QC) and quality assurance (QA). The whole issue is fundamental to the concept of GCP and in the EC Guidelines a chapter is given over to quality assurance.

Quality control is defined in the EC Guidelines on GCP as 'the operational techniques and activities undertaken within the system of quality assurance to verify that the requirements for quality of the trial have been fulfilled'.

In most clinical research departments quality control falls upon those who are carrying out the various tasks and should be a self-policing process. In order to facilitate this each section of every medical department will have its own set of standard operating procedures (SOPs). The definition given in the EC Guidelines on GCP succinctly encapsulates the philosophy of SOPs, defining a SOP as 'sponsor standard, detailed, written instructions for the management of clinical trials. They provide a general framework enabling the efficient implementation of performance of all the functions and activities for a particular trial . . .'.

SOPs are invaluable in ensuring that all company members are 'singing from the same hymn sheet'. While this is important at any level it becomes particularly so in large-scale multinational and multicontinental studies. They are also a source of instruction and comfort for the newly recruited CRAs and help to prevent them feeling lost in the rigours of clinical research. In addition, they define standards that are to be expected of staff in the performance of their duty and therefore have disciplinary implications for company staff who are less than satisfactory in their approach to clinical research. They can also be an aid to dealing with truculent investigators who fail to see why they should comply with certain standards or adequately complete case record forms. Finally, it is essential to have in place a set of SOPs for dealing with cases of suspected fraud. Once the company has reason to believe that an investigator has behaved in a fraudulent manner the company has an ethical and medical obligation to follow this up to all bodies' satisfaction. In the UK this would include reporting a case of suspected fraud to the GMC (which is the body which licenses doctors to practise medicine). The GMC regards clinical trial fraud as an extremely serious act and has in place a disciplinary procedure for suspected fraud and misconduct for clinical research. The issue of fraud has recently been discussed by Shaw and the reader is directed to his article.[9]

Quality assurance is defined in the EC Guidelines for GCP as 'systems and processes established to ensure that the trial is performed and the data generated in compliance with good clinical practice, including procedures for ethical conduct, SOPs, reporting, personal qualifications, etc.'

The way quality assurance is carried out varies from company to company but certain principles are common. The first of these is that the department of quality assurance should be a separate entity, isolated from those departments carrying out clinical research. In Fig. 12.1 we have shown the quality assurance department (Auditing) reporting to the medical director but in many companies the manager of the quality assurance department reports to either regional or even supraregional authorities to ensure independence. Whether quality assurance should be performed by company personnel or outside contractors is a matter of debate. Advantages for the former include familiarity with company procedures and hence speed of audit. However, it is possible to argue that personal relations between members of the quality assurance department and other parts of the company on a purely social basis could compromise their stance on quality assurance under some circumstances and accordingly that quality assurance should be carried out by an outside body.

The way in which quality assurance is performed varies from company to company. At one end of the spectrum it is possible to audit every single procedure that is carried out, although this may be seen by some as excessive; the other end of the spectrum is where relatively few procedures are audited, and this would be judged by many as being inadequate. To help judge what are adequate amounts of audit some companies employ statisticians within their audit department to provide sample sizes for auditing procedures. Sample sizes should be so calculated as to pick up lack of quality at a reasonable level and in a reasonable number of instances. Whenever an audit has been performed, the quality assurance department will normally produce a certificate and it is an important part of the trial records.

Archive

The archive is the repository for all information data and documentation arising from a clinical trial. It is a requirement of EC GCP that all documentation, other than patient files and source data, should be kept by the sponsor for the lifetime of the product. This would include the protocol, audit certificates, adverse events and so forth. The final report has to be retained by the sponsor for 5 years beyond the lifetime of the product. Each clinical trial can generate vast amounts of data and it is essential that the clinical department has a well organized archive and designated archivist. The actual area designated for archives should ideally be fireproof as such information is irreplaceable.

Regulatory Affairs

The laws and regulations governing the development, licensing and promotion of medicines in Europe and beyond are covered by other chapters in this book; it is the responsibility of the regulatory department to ensure that such requirements are met. As can be appreciated, regulatory departments liaise with a wide range of personnel both within and outside the company.

Within the medical department Regulatory Affairs are responsible for preparing all the documentation required to permit clinical trials to proceed. They are also expected to coordinate the collection and collation of information for product licences and licence variations. The reporting of adverse events tends to be handled by Regulatory Affairs. This involves informing the regulatory bodies of their own country as well as passing on the information to other sections for reporting to other countries.

The regulatory affairs department of a local business unit is also usually responsible for the monitoring and checking of promotional material to ensure that it meets legal requirements and those laid down in the various codes of practice.

Finally, because they hold so much information about the company's products, personnel in regulatory affairs are frequently approached by members of the marketing and information services departments and from all parts of the company for information advice about products, especially at the time of product launch.

Information Services

The Information Services department plays a key role in product support. In former days Information Services were known as 'The Library' although this never fully described the department's true function.

First and foremost, Information Services remains the repository of all published information on the company's products, together with allied supporting publications be they books, papers or other written communications. Second, this department provides published information on whatever subject may be requested, together with appropriate computerized literature searches to focus this request.

Information Services is frequently the first port of call for outside enquiries. Such enquiries may come from a wide variety of sources, including physicians, pharmacists, the general public, other companies and even investment houses. Many of the enquiries are routine in nature and can be more than satisfactorily handled by appropriately trained staff; however, a pharmaceutical physician should always be available to assist in answering more complex issues. A percentage of enquiries are related to possible adverse events and it is important that the Information Services department be properly briefed as to how these should be handled; in particular, the pharmaceutical physician should be informed about enquiries concerning possible adverse events so that they can take the appropriate action. The department may also be contacted on issues of product quality. Again they need to be appropriately briefed on how to handle these issues and how to keep the pharmaceutical physician, registration and manufacturing departments appropriately informed.

Drug Safety

This department is one which is undergoing change. In a small company it would usually not exist as a separate unit but be undertaken by a physician in conjunction with the regulatory affairs department. In larger companies the department would consist of a dedicated pharmaceutical physician and support staff.

Pharmacoeconomics group

This is probably the most recent branch of pharmaceutical medicine and is in a state of rapid evolution. While not yet a regulatory requirement in most countries guidelines have been laid down by the Australian Regulatory Bodies for pharmacoeconomic evaluation and it is possible that other countries will follow suit, if not for actual registration then certainly for reimbursement, as already exists in Norway.

It is generally believed that pharmacoeconomic studies should be carried out by the clinical, rather than marketing, department and the pharmaceutical physician is well placed to head up this group. Because it is such a new speciality, debate continues as to the best modes of evaluation and whether such studies should be run individually or added onto ongoing Phase III and IV studies. Currently most companies are using the latter route, although adoption of the former may come about and would lead to a massive expansion of these departments.

The size of this department, if it exists as a separate entity, is usually small, consisting of one or two advisers familiar with the medicine and science of the company's products as well as health economics methodologies.

Role of the pharmaceutical physician in clinical research

All molecules put forward as development candidates are done so in the belief that the risks of developing the drug are less than the rewards and that a reasonable profit can be made by the company. This belief has to be accompanied by the power to obtain the funds to test the hypothesis; clearly the greater the collective belief then the easier it will be to obtain funding. Optimism, which is the prevailing sentiment in early drug research, will tend to exaggerate confidence in this belief. It has to be said, however, that many more times often than not this belief is usually wrong since only two out of ten molecules marketed (that is to say forgetting those that have fallen by the wayside during development) actually make a significant return on investment.

One of the prime purposes then of a clinical trial programme is to generate data to establish whether the initial belief continues to be justified, i.e. to replace enough of the belief with solid facts. Who should make decisions as to whether a drug is or is not effective is now currently very much a matter for debate. In the past this was left to physicians working within academia, industry and the regulatory bodies. However, patients' organizations are becoming increasingly vociferous and demanding that they too have a say in deciding when a medicine should be licensed; in general terms they are prepared to accept more risk and have a greater belief in the potential of a medicine than physicians have traditionally been prepared to do. This argument commenced in the USA where AIDS pressure groups have brought about a radical change in the way we assess and license medicines for HIV-related diseases. Currently there are signs that this approach may spread to other serious and life-threatening conditions.

If the reader has not already done so, they are advised to read the sections on clinical trials and adverse reactions in postmarketing surveillance before continuing, as these chapters extensively cover the practicalities of the clinical evaluation and surveillance of products. What follows is a discussion of the role of the pharmaceutical physician in these processes.

As already noted the whole point of a clinical trial programme is to collect data upon which decisions can be made. The clinical trial programme is run according to a clinical plan which has a variety of functions. The key point to emphasize about a clinical plan is that it is not cast in tablets of stone and should be continuously changing to reflect altering conditions, both within and outside the company. Table 12.1 lists some of these factors which may impact on the clinical plan.

A good clinical plan will chart the costs incurred in the product's development and the anticipated future costs. As the product moves successfully through its development the marketing departments will show an increasing interest and need to make necessary plans for the product's launch. An accurate estimation of the likely time of product registration is therefore important if resources are not to be wasted. The marketing department will also need to have studies evaluating the compound against competitor therapies and the fine-tuning of

Table 12.1 Factors which may impact on the clinical plan for a medicine's development

Internal	External
New toxicity data, e.g. carcinogenicity and reproductive studies	Pressure groups demanding early registration
Change of research priorities by Senior Management	Safety concerns about other members of the same family of compound
Data emerging from trials	Competitors coming onto the market
Marketing demand for different formulations	New methodologies developing, e.g. quality of life and health economics
Marketing demand for comparator studies	New registration needs
Company take-over or merger	Economic environment

these studies can only be done when the product is almost at the stage of being registered. Accurate dates are also required by senior management in their budgetary forecasts and presentations to investors and analysts.

Most companies now employ project teams to run a clinical trial programme. This team includes a pharmaceutical physician, an experienced clinical research associate, a statistician, a regulatory affairs officer and a project coordinator responsible for ensuring that the right things are happening at the right place and on time. Project teams should have the ability to coopt other members as appropriate; for example they may choose to have a pharmacologist in the team at the early stages to advise on interpretation of preclinical data and how they impact on the design of studies in humans. The role of the pharmaceutical physician is to ensure that the right safety and efficacy studies are carried out in the correct order to enable the product to be developed in the fastest possible time commensurate with sound clinical and ethical judgement. Another role in the project team is to produce the clinical investigators' brochure. This is a document which summarizes all the relevant data for the development of the medicine and is updated as the trial programme progresses. Finally, the pharmaceutical physician will review the way in which the emerging data affect subsequent studies. As the programme reaches its conclusion the pharmaceutical physician will be in close liaison with the marketing departments.

The pharmaceutical physician and the marketing of medicines

The successful outcome of a research and development programme will be the approval by licensing authorities to sell and promote the product. These activities are heavily regulated by most governments through acts of parliament and accompanying statutory instruments; within the EC there are a number of directives already in place or about to be enacted to control these activities.

Pharmaceutical physicians are heavily involved in these functions and have to be mindful of their status as physicians rather than marketeers or sales people.

Relations between medical and marketing departments

Relations between medical departments and marketing departments have traditionally not been easy. Viewed from the outside, a prominent broad-caster and journalist on consumer affairs stated that marketing depart-ments were the 'tail that wags the pharmaceutical physician dog'.[10] From inside the industry, a senior executive felt that, in the past, the medical and marketing departments did not appear to be working for the same company and 'medical staff are seen as blinkered fools who carry out trials that are expensive luxuries. Marketing people are seen as unethical, scientifically irrelevant, impatient and inconsistent'.[11]

That such a state of affairs can exist and has existed in the past is clearly a matter of concern and arises from the differing needs of the two groups. The marketing and sales departments see their role as promoting and selling products to the best of their abilities, which ultimately is measured by strength of sales. While fundamentally the medical department has the same company set of goals and ambitions, it must also serve a policing role to curb possible excesses by these departments. In reality, in compa-nies with well managed medical and marketing departments, there is little tension between the two groups since there is mutual respect of each other's professional capabilities. There will, however, always be disputed grey areas, especially when the competitive edge of one product over another is marginal.

Undoubtedly the best way to promote healthy relations between these two departments is to start involving the marketing department early on in drug development, as is now the case in most pharmaceutical companies. Involvement at an early stage should necessarily be minimal as a number of compounds will fail during subsequent late Phase II and early Phase III studies but, as the product progresses through its clinical development, marketing involvement is essential to enable the right studies to be in place to successfully launch the product. These studies in particular require a marketeer with vision, since it takes about 2 years to achieve results from conception of the study idea to receiving the final report. The marketeer must therefore have a sixth sense for those products likely to be competitor therapies in 2 years' time. A visionary marketeer will also anticipate product usage after launch and, in particular, whether this will be as a single agent or in combination with others. Finally, we are undoubtedly entering an era of global medical cost containment. For new medicines to succeed they will undoubtedly have to be innovative rather than 'me too' products and additionally represent good value for money. This does not necessarily mean that new medicines need to be cheap but, taken in the context of treating the patient and their condition as a whole, the medicine must justify its price; this has lead to the growth of the field of health economics. While such studies should be run by the medical department their commercial implications are obvious and the physician in charge of these studies has to know where the product is going to be positioned in the market; this in turn needs good relations with the marketing department.

Ultimately harmonious interactions between medical and marketing departments are synergistic and will benefit, as well as command the respect of, the immediate customer, the doctor, and the ultimate customer, the patient.

Promotional campaigns

Promotional campaigns occur at varying times during a product's life and are usually a time of intense frenetic activity. A successful promotional campaign, like a military campaign, depends upon extensive and careful planning; Wellington's success at Waterloo was due in no small part to the fact that he had planned this battle 1 year in advance. The experienced pharmaceutical physician will learn to anticipate these campaigns and allow sufficient time to devote to marketing and sales colleagues.

Probably of all promotional campaigns the most important is the first launch of the new chemical entity; an unsuccessful product launch will mean that a relaunch is required, though meanwhile valuable time has been lost when competitors are establishing or consolidating their position. Product launches can also be of new formulations to extend the product's useful life or market coverage. For example, the original product may have been brought out as tablets or capsules with later launches of other formulations such as soluble tablets, suppositories, injectable and topical formulations. Promotional campaigns may also need to be instigated when new indications are added to the product's licence or when new clinical trial data become available. In all promotional campaigns the medical adviser will be called in to provide advice on the product and its competitors and can be a major contributory factor to the success (or indeed failure) of the campaign.

Logistics and time scales

Using an initial product launch as an illustrative model we shall review the areas where the pharmaceutical physician has an important input.

The embryonic outline of the promotional campaign should be well defined by the time Phase III studies begin. At this stage the marketeers ought to have thought through the possible results and implications of Phase III studies. As results start to come through from these studies they should be thinking of the Phase IV studies required for further support (Phase III studies are to establish the product's safety and efficacy; Phase IV studies are to define the edge that the product has over its competitors). In the past many Phase IV studies were little more than poorly disguised seeding studies. The advent of GCP has largely helped put pay to these sort of studies, a fact which has been welcomed by responsible physicians, marketing personnel and academic colleagues alike. Such studies have been described as falling into two categories: the large and inadequate and the small and inadequate.[12] In the former category were large-scale studies, in effect seeding studies masquerading as postmarketing surveillance, whereas the former were studies carried out with small numbers of patients by so-called opinion leaders, and designed not to detect differences between products. Comparative studies are, of course, always required, but there is now a widespread realization that it is far better to have a small number of well designed studies published in premier peer review journals than a series of indifferently performed studies published in obscure or pay journals.

As part of their promotional campaign marketing personnel will wish to niche the product as having some advantage in terms of either efficacy, safety or cost; the problem with cost is the need to obtain as high a return on investment as possible consistent with price acceptance by the medical community. In order to justify their pricing strategy, which is an intrinsic part of the promotional campaign, marketing colleagues will request comparator studies with cost–benefit analyses included.

Having assisted the marketing department in developing their promotional platform for the new product before launch, the pharmaceutical physician will proceed to assist in the preparation of actual launch material, which can be divided into two broad categories; promotional material that directly relates to the product and material which is educational about the product's therapeutic area.

Direct promotional material (such as advertisements, videos, mailings and so forth) is subject to strict regulations. Well organized marketing departments will involve the pharmaceutical physician early on in the promotional campaign for, once up and running, it is expensive to have a volte-face if it is suddenly found to be in breach of the regulations; ideally, the pharmaceutical physician should inspect the early drafts of such material. Most companies have a copy approval system (sometimes with accompanying internal SOPs) to ensure that all promotional material is within the various codes of practice and laws. In the UK, the Association of the British Pharmaceutical Industry (ABPI) has a code of practice extending back to 1958 to ensure that not only will the promotion of a medicine stay within the appropriate UK regulations (the 1968 Medicines Act and accompanying statutory instruments) and EC Council Directive 92/28/EC[13] but also adheres to ethical standards and canons of good taste on the advertising of medicinal products for human use, which becomes fully operational on 1 January 1993. In the typical copy approval system information is generated in the marketing department and is then passed to the medical department for approval. This may involve Information Services to check that the typography and references are correct, the regulatory department to ensure that the relevant directives, acts and statutes have not been breached and the pharmaceutical physician to ensure that it is medically accurate and not misleading. Typically the copy may be circulated three or four times before being finally sent out. Any material distributed in the UK needs to be certified by a physician; certification of material that is in breach of the directives, acts and statutory instruments can have dire consequences.

As part of the new product launch activity there is often distribution of accompanying educational material for passing on to potential prescribing physicians; this material is usually welcomed by physicians as part of their ongoing education. However, as their time is valuable the pharmaceutical physician should ensure that such material is of a quality capable of commanding the time of the reading or viewing physician; marketing colleagues will therefore come to the pharmaceutical physician to seek advice on such educational material.

The launch of the new product is also usually accompanied by a launch symposium or series of symposia. While clearly these are dedicated to informing key members of the medical profession about a new product, they have to be carefully stage-managed; a launch symposium that is obviously intended to be promotional rather than informative is an embarrassment to the pharmaceutical physician and audience physician alike and is more likely to put off the very audience it is trying to impress. It is therefore the responsibility of the pharmaceutical physician to ensure that the company's good name and reputation are upheld at meetings. Following on from launch symposia there is frequently a series of publications. It follows that a well organized symposium, run to standards of academic excellence, should have no problems in being published in first-class journals. Frequently the pharmaceutical physician for the project has the pleasure of being an editor for the journal supplement, a very satisfactory conclusion to running a successful drug research programme.

After a product has been launched pharmaceutical physicians have an important role to play in the continuing dissemination of information about the product, as they are likely to be one of the most informed physicians about that specific product. In this postlaunch period it is part of the pharmaceutical physician's responsibility to spread this information to as wide a body of the medical community as possible and to ensure that the medicine is used in its safest and most efficacious manner. To this end the pharmaceutical physician may be asked to either produce or comment on product monographs and indeed give informative, but non-promotional, lectures on the product to selected audiences, bearing in mind all the time that such activities may be construed as being promotional and must always conform to the same standards that behoves any form of promotion.

The pharmaceutical physician and the sales department

If the marketing department are the generals overviewing the promotional campaign then the sales force are the field soldiers. In the military battlefield, the knowledge that there is good medical back-up is essential for morale and this could equally be said to be the case in a promotional campaign. The interaction of the medical department with the sales department starts, for an individual salesman, very soon after joining the company as shortly thereafter representatives are given intensive training. For seasoned representatives this will be about the new products they will have to promote. However, for the novice representative this will also include having to learn about basic medicine in order to pass the ABPI representatives' examination.

Because salesmen represent one of the key interfaces between the company and the prescribing physician, they are often the first to become aware of adverse events. It is an important part of the pharmaceutical physician's teaching role to transmit the necessity of feeding back information on adverse events to the company, as is now embodied in the EC directive on advertising and promotion of medicines.

A pharmaceutical physician who has established a good rapport with representatives will be rewarded by a representative who feels comfortable enough to ring up and ask for advice on questions from doctors; information which will in turn provide valuable insight to the company physician on how the new drug is perceived in the marketplace and how it is being used.

The future of pharmaceutical medicine

In 1785 William Withering (who discovered digitalis) said: 'The ingenuity of man has ever been fond of exerting itself to varied forms and combinations of medicines'. This holds true today and indeed the advent of complex computing techniques, coupled with developments in medicinal chemistry and biotechnology, means that the 'ingenuity of man' now seems endless.

However, medicine is now entering an era of cost containment and hard decisions are having to be made in the provision of health care facilities. Medicines are an obvious target for this cost containment despite the fact that, in the UK, they constitute only about 10 per cent of total NHS expenditure. Furthermore, many effective medicines have, or are about to have, come to the end of their patent life, with two implications. First, after the expiry of their patent the revenue that they generate is dramatically reduced, something which has, in some instances, threatened the very viability of the discovering company. Second, the introduction of new medicines, if they are to generate a significant return on investment, must be able to offer significant advantages in either safety, efficacy or cost above the effective and cheaper off-patent products.

It is clear then that the pharmaceutical industry must be innovative to survive, although the amount of innovative research in a company is not obviously proportional to its size. One way to increase the overall amount of innovation seems to have been set by the field of biotechnology, where there is a profusion of small but highly innovative companies. Many of these will not be successful although it is likely that enough of them will be for this trend to continue and grow. Larger companies, particularly those with pipelines short of innovative products, have in many cases taken up the option of forming strategic alliances with these smaller companies. This alliance may go further and result in the major company taking over the smaller company.

We are also likely to see changes in the field of clinical trial methodology driven by patient and consumer groups. This trend can be traced back to the AIDS activist groups who were not prepared to take placebos when they could be receiving an active medicine or to put up with the established development times for products. For drugs used in the treatment of AIDS, this has led to a trend towards earlier product licensing but with a greater emphasis on postmarketing surveillance. It seems likely that this concept will be carried into the treatment of other life-threatening diseases or serious illnesses.

The trend towards global harmonization in drug development is likely to continue from both the industry's and a regulatory point of view. Such harmonization ought to help reduce the number of animal experiments as well as speed up drug development times and reduce the number of clinical trials and hence overall costs.

So where does the pharmaceutical physician fit into these future trends and what will the pharmaceutical physician of the future be like? First, in purely numerical terms, it is unlikely that the speciality will enjoy the growth of former years. This is because of consolidation within the pharmaceutical industry as well as the fact that many of the jobs previously performed by physicians can be carried out just as well and more cheaply by experienced scientists. Second, because of the increasing number of small firms starting up there ought to be a widening of the range of pharmaceutical medicine that physicians can enjoy practising. For the physician who enjoys everything, then the small company will be ideal; for those who enjoy some specializing in, say, pharmacoepidemiology, then other opportunities will be provided by the large, postmerger companies. Cost containment measures by governments and their agencies will provide opportunities for pharmaceutical physicians skilled in health economics, which is therefore likely to become the fastest growing subspeciality in pharmaceutical medicine. The industry, to stay viable, must be innovative and creative and these then must be the qualities sought for in pharmaceutical physicians.

References

1. Chandler A (1989). Pharmaceutical medicine continues to expand. *Pharmaceutical Physician* **1**: 9–11.
2. Berde B (1985). Physicians as employees of the pharmaceutical industry. *European Journal of Clinical Pharmacology* **28**: 363–5.
3. Schmidt R (1991). The pharmaceutical physician – requirements for the position. *European Journal of Clinical Pharmacology* **41**: 387–91.
4. Higson D (1992). Experiences of a faculty rep. *Pharmaceutical Physician* **4**: 63–4.
5. Luscombe D (1992). New style postgraduate course in pharmaceutical medicine. *Pharmaceutical Physician* **9**: 72–3.
6. Ruiz Ferran J (1990). AMIFE (Spanish Association of Pharmaceutical Physicians/Asociacion de Medicos de la Industria Farmaceutica Espanola). *Pharmaceutical Physician* **2**: 70–72.
7. Weatherall M (1985). How are drugs discovered? In Burley DM, Binns TB (eds.) *Pharmaceutical Medicine*. London: Edward Arnold (Publishers) Ltd: 1–17.
8. EC Note for guidance (1990). Good clinical practice for trials in medicinal products in the European Community. CPMP working party on efficacy of medicinal products. *Pharmacology and Physiology* **67**: 361–72.
9. Shaw W (1991). Ignore . . . discord . . . blacklist . . . report – the evolution of the reaction to research fraud. *Pharmaceutical Physician* **3**: 26–31.
10. Medawar C (1992). Medicine and marketing – so close, yet so far apart.

Pharmaceutical Physician **4**: 30–35.

11. Jarrett A (1992). Call for war-game model of medics and marketeers to end as synergy brings new hope. *Pharmaceutical Physician* **4**: 28–9.
12. Nicholson P (1992). In: Inadequate studies expose patients to unacceptable risks; but better medical–marketing interaction is on the way, says senior industry physician. *Pharmaceutical Physician* **4**: 18–20.
13. Council directive 92/28/EC of 31 March 1992 on the advertising of medicinal products for human use. *Official Journal of the European Communities* **35(30.4.92)**: 13–18.

13

Introduction to the legal aspects of pharmaceutical medicine: a brief overview of some emerging issues
Diana Brahams

Currently the UK drugs bill is some £3 billion, yet successive surveys have shown many medicines to be ineffective: one US survey of 2000 drugs rated only 5 per cent as 'important', 15 per cent as 'moderately useful' and 80 per cent as having little or no therapeutic value.[1] Or as Dr Joe Collier[2] put it:

> 'As a nation we are hooked on medicines. Each year we blindly swallow millions of pounds worth of vitamins, sleeping tablets, sedatives, cough medicines, antibiotics, tonics and many more. Some of these undoubtedly relieve suffering and save lives; but most have little or no value.'

Some drugs undoubtedly also cause harm. Charles Medawar's book, *Power and Dependence*,[3] provides an eloquent critique on the monitoring and regulation of medicines and makes a strong case for greater lay involvement and public scrutiny.

It has been estimated that 80 per cent of all prescription drugs are issued by general practitioners in the UK. There is evidence of overprescription with concomitant non-compliance or only partial compliance by patients. However, of the several thousands of licensed prescription drugs on the market, most doctors admit prescribing from a fairly constant narrow list of between 250 and 300 products. Side by side with the high level of prescription drugs dispensed, sales of over-the-counter (OTC) preparations are booming along with sales of alternative or complementary medicines including vitamins, vitamin boosters, nutrients, health food supplements and dietary aids or reducing agents and so forth.

Let the buyer beware (*caveat emptor*)

English common law, which rests on a number of basic principles, has been developed by means of case-by-case decisions from which judicial precedents have emerged, fashioned in response (albeit delayed) to the demands of society and prevailing moral and ethical codes and the interpretation of the vast succession of statutes passed by Parliament. It is interesting to note that English contract law devolved from the position of *Caveat Emptor* – Let the Buyer Beware. Although a prudent buyer will always be wary, the Law now offers considerable protection to even the most unwary buyer and indeed, some would argue that it has reached the point of *Caveat Vendor* rather than *Emptor*. The era of laissez-faire and non-interventionism which at one time pervaded the moral and social climate is no longer acceptable today, at least in principle, in all aspects of life including the licensing, marketing and selling of medicines both OTC and by prescription. Whether the law achieves all that it could or might is highly arguable but it is certainly very much more protective of consumers' rights. Not surprisingly, among the watchwords for the 1990s are 'audit', 'accountability', 'lay scrutiny and representation of professional committees', 'watchdogs' and 'better complaints procedures'.

Litigation prompted by consumer dissatisfaction, most particularly with drugs and doctors, has dramatically increased over recent years.

Product liability

Compensating the injured patient: legal rights and remedies

Contract
Traditionally a patient may have a remedy in contract if its terms, express or implied, have been breached. A good example is the famous old case of *Carlill* v. *The Carbolic Smokeball Company* [1892] 2QB 484 affirmed [1893] 1 QB 256 in which the defendant manufacturers of a product called 'The Carbolic Smokeball' (price 10/-, refills 5/-) issued an advertisement in which they offered to pay £100 to anybody who succumbed to influenza after using the smokeball in the specified manner and for a specified period. They added that they had deposited the sum of £1000 with their bankers 'to show their sincerity'. The plaintiff, Mrs Carlill, relying on the advertisement, bought and used the smokeball as prescribed but caught influenza nonetheless. She sued for her £100.

Predictably, the Smokeball Company defended the claim vigorously, arguing ingeniously that the claim was a bet within the meaning of the Gaming Act, that the offer was a mere advertising 'puff' never intended to create a binding obligation, that there was no offer made to an individual person, and that if there were Mrs Carlill had failed to notify the company of her acceptance. The Court of Appeal, upholding the decision of the trial judge, found no difficulty in rejecting the argument that an offer cannot be made to the world at large. PER BOWEN LJ: 'It is an offer made to all the world which is to ripen into a contract with anybody who comes forward and performs the condition? Although the offer is made to the world, the contract is made with the limited portion of the public who come forward and performs the condition on the faith of the advertisement.'

None of the judges, however, saw fit to comment on the peddling of bogus or ineffective medicinal products, and it was only on a narrow contractual point that Mrs Carlill was able to obtain satisfaction.

The restrictions imposed by the rules of Privity of Contract

In the UK a patient or consumer of a medical product is in practice unlikely to have entered into a direct contract with the manufacturer of the medicinal product which they claim has injured them. This is first because medicines supplied under the auspices of the NHS do not create a contractual situation between the dispensing chemist and the patient even when money passes and most medicines are supplied in this way. However, even where the medicine is purchased directly, unless the seller is also a producer of 'own brand' medicines the manufacturer will not be a party to the contract for the purchase of the goods. There may be further exclusions on the part of the would-be plaintiff in that as with *Donoghue* v. *Stevenson* (discussed below) the purchaser may not be the ultimate consumer so that no direct contractual liability between him and the seller will have been created.

The duty of care – criteria for proof of negligence

It was not until the landmark House of Lords decision in *Donoghue* v. *Stevenson* [1932] AC 562 that a general duty of care was formulated as we would recognize it today and generally accepted and incorporated into the main fabric of the British legal system. The basic common law principles governing the creation of a duty of care (and which remain good until this day) were first authoritatively stated by Lord Atkin in his famous judgment [1932] AC 562 at page 580, as follows:

> 'In English law there must be, and is, some general conception of relations giving rise to a duty of care, of which the particular cases found in the books are instances. The liability for negligence . . . is no doubt based upon a general public sentiment of moral wrongdoing for which the offender must pay. But acts and omissions which any moral code would censure cannot in a practical world be treated so as to give a right to every person injured by them to demand relief. In this way rules of law arise which limit the range of complainants and the extent of their remedy. The rule that you are to love your neighbour becomes in law, you must not injure your neighbour; and the lawyer's question, Who is my neighbour? receives a restricted reply. *You must take reasonable care to avoid acts and omissions which you can reasonably foresee would be likely to injure your neighbour. Who, then, in law is my neighbour? The answer seems to be – persons who are so closely and directly affected by my act that I ought reasonably to have them in contemplation as being so affected when I am directing my mind to the acts and omissions which are called in question.*'

The facts in *Donoghue* v. *Stevenson* were that a manufacturer of ginger-beer had supplied his product in a sealed opaque glass bottle to a retailer who ran a cafe in a park in Paisley in Scotland. In August 1928 the plaintiff and a friend visited the cafe and Miss Donoghue's friend bought them both a bottle of ginger-beer to be served along with a slab of ice cream which was served up in a tumbler; the ginger-beer was poured over it. Miss Donoghue drank some of this concoction and her friend was topping up her glass with the ginger-beer that remained in the bottle when the remnants of a decomposed snail floated out. Miss Donoghue was very upset. She claimed that she had suffered shock and gastroenteritis. She was not, however, able to sue the cafe owner in contract owing to the rules of 'privity of contract' discussed above as her friend had bought the drinks and she had sustained the injury, so she took the then novel course of suing the manufacturer of the ginger-beer directly in tort claiming that he was in breach of the duty of care which he owed her.

The manufacturer tried to have Miss Donoghue's claim struck out by way of a preliminary issue on the grounds that no such duty of care existed in law. The case was fought to the House of Lords who, by a narrow majority of 3:2, said that such a duty existed. The case has formed the common law basis of our developing consumer law ever since and gave rise to Lord Atkin's famous statement of principle set out below.

Namely:

'. . . a manufacturer of products, which he sells in such a form as to show that he intends them to reach the ultimate consumer in which they left him with no reasonable possibility of intermediate examination and with the knowledge that the absence of reasonable care in the preparation or putting up of the products.'

The term 'product' is no longer limited to articles of food and drink and it includes cases in which the injurious element is not a foreign body but something which is intrinsically part of the product itself, and may cover cases in which there is no allegation that the product has been carelessly made but that it is dangerous to use without proper warnings or instructions which themselves may be actionable if carelessly expressed or produced.

Thus, it is clear that under British law manufacturers and marketers of pharmaceutical products owe (*inter alia*) their potential consumers a duty of care under the broad general principles laid down in *Donoghue* v. *Stevenson* which have since been expanded and broadened and applied in vastly different types of situation. (For further reading see *Street* (1988) and *Charlesworth and Percy on Negligence* (1990).)

Duty to monitor safety of a medicinal product; duty to supply additional information or to recall it from the market in whole or in part

Although a product may have been reasonably safe, or considered to be reasonably safe when it was sold or left the manufacturer or supplier's hands, it may be that further information comes to light which alerts or should alert them to previously unforeseen problems. There is a continuing duty on the part of the manufacturer and supplier of medicinal products to monitor their safety and to ensure that they are fit for their purpose and reasonably safe. On occasion a medicinal product, or a particular batch of the product, may have to be recalled and/or there may be a duty to issue further warnings or information about the product in the light of emerging knowledge and data. This may point to adverse drug reactions (ADRs) in certain vulnerable groups or when the medicine is taken along with certain other products or in certain circumstances, or the quality of a product may be adversely affected by its storage or age, etc.

It is important to point out that a plaintiff suing in negligence has to prove two elements in his case; first that he has suffered injury/damage and second that this injury/damage was caused by the defendant's negligent act. This may prove to be very difficult in practice on both scores, particularly in the realm of pharmaceutical medicines. For instance, the pertussis cases in the UK and Canada have all failed to surmount the first hurdle of causation. In the leading English case of *Loveday* v. *Renton* the pharmaceutical giant, Wellcome, a manufacturer of the pertussis vaccine under attack, was joined as a defendant at its own request ([1990] 1 MLR 117).[4-7] However a recent Irish decision awarded damages for causation due to injury caused by injection from a defective batch of pertussis vaccine in 1969 (see *Best* v. *Wellcome*, *Lancet*, May 1993). The case was settled for £2.5 million.

It is debatable whether the plaintiffs would have succeeded in proving negligence in the thalidomide cases, which would have required showing that the risks of the injury which occurred were reasonably foreseeable in the light of the then prevailing medical and scientific knowledge and practices for testing new products. The ensuing settlements were more probably a response to the pressure of a concerted media campaign and the feelings of moral outrage that some compensation should be given to the unfortunate victims and their families.

Group litigation

In the UK 'class' actions as such do not exist but where groups of people who have taken the same drug or been involved in the same disaster have been injured they may join together to form a 'group' action. The concept of the 'group' action is relatively new, and the rule and management of such actions is still developing. The first of these to be brought in England arose from the alleged adverse effects caused by ingestion of the prescription drug marketed in the UK as 'Opren' (benoxaprofen). Opren was a non-steroidal anti-inflammatory drug prescribed widely for sufferers of arthritis among whom numbered many elderly patients. The drug had not been tested specifically on elderly people, who were later found to be particularly susceptible to its unwanted side effects.

Publicity about the legal claim caused many potential plaintiffs to come forward and of these a number failed to qualify for legal aid because they had savings in excess of the small disqualifying sum. These privately funded claimants hoped that the main costs of the action would be funded by the legal aid fund on behalf of the legally aided claimants and that their costs would be minimal.

The manufacturers of Opren denied liability and the immense complexity of the case with its vast numbers of hours spent by the many professionals involved meant that the costs rapidly escalated. The Court of

Appeal ruled that privately funded clients could not ride piggyback on the investment made in the litigation by the legal aid fund and that each would be liable for a proportionate amount of the generic costs of running this litigation. The individual claims were mostly for relatively small sums and the fear of liability for costs including a potential proportion of the defendants' costs if the action failed caused panic among the privately funded litigants. But for the intervention of a property tycoon, Godfrey Bradman, dubbed the Fairy Godfather at the time, who underwrote their liability initially to the tune of £1 million but ultimately up to £5 million as the costs of continuing the case escalated, most of the privately funded litigants would have had to discontinue. In the event, a settlement was reached before the discovery of documents stage. The average award was between £2500 and £3500 with the usual discount reached on settlement. Even by this stage it is believed that the costs of pursuing and defending the claim heavily outweighed the total damages paid out.

Subsequently there were later Opren group actions formed, but the last two of these have run into serious difficulties with the limitation of time permitted for commencing a claim.

Since Opren there have been a number of other group claims. An action which aroused great public sympathy was that brought by haemophiliacs and other patients who were infected after being given HIV infected blood products during the 'window' period in the early 1980s when the risks of infection were known but not dealt with satisfactorily so as to protect recipients. Following *ex gratia* payments the claim was ultimately settled. The largest group claim yet to be launched in the UK has been the claims arising from the ingestion of a number of benzodiazepine drugs. These were narrowed down to Ativan (lorazepam), Valium (diazepam), Mogadon (nitrazepam), Librium (chlordiazepoxide), Serenid (oxazepam) and Halcion (triazolam). Each drug is the subject of a 'Master Statement of Claim', with the details specified in each individual claim contained in a subsidiary individual statement of claim attaching to the Master Claim. In all, some 5598 individual statements of claims were served by the 31 August 1992 deadline imposed by the judge presiding over the litigation, Mr Justice Ian Kennedy. The bulk of these claims related to claims made in relation to Ativan ingestion (3092) and Valium (1910). Most of the litigants received legal aid but claims in respect of Roche products were suspended in late 1992. An internal audit was carried out by the Plaintiffs initially on a sample of all the claims as agreed by the judge and the Defendants but latterly on Wyeth Products and Upjohn's Halcion with a deadline of 31 March 1993. As a consequence, legal aid support was withdrawn from claims against Roche products.

The number of claims in this kind of man litigation is so large that a strategy was evolved on the part of the Plaintiffs to divide their legal and medical teams roughly into two groups for the bulk of the work, namely 'generic' and 'case'. Although the steering group of solicitors remained contained and small, each individual plaintiff was entitled to approach their local or preferred solicitor, with the result that unprecedented numbers of firms of solicitors and an ever expanding team of case counsel and advising case medical experts had to deal under great time pressures with the large number of claimants notwithstanding the closing of the group at an early stage by the judge.

Another group action currently proceeding, although managed on a different basis, represents the claims of 'Myodil' patients and there are further potential group claims being currently investigated to see whether the medical evidence would support a claim for injuries allegedly suffered as a consequence of ingesting the drug concerned.

Second generation drug injury

The thalidomide cases were a good example of what have been called 'second generation' drug injury, and diethylstilboestrol (DES) is another such example. In both cases the drugs given to the pregnant women damaged the foetuses causing them to be born with injuries. In the thalidomide cases the injuries were obvious when the babies were born, but with DES they were not discoverable until puberty at the earliest and often much later.

Although no DES claims have ever succeeded in the UK and there are currently none underway, some claims brought by the 'DES daughters' have succeeded in the USA. Attempts by granddaughters to bring claims were recently struck out in New York. In December 1992 a court in Holland accepted that an action could be brought notwithstanding that the plaintiffs could not identify which manufacturer was responsible for the drug that injured them. A formula devised to get round this very real individual causation difficulty was accepted in the USA on the basis of market share.

When injuries caused by a drug prescribed, for example, in pregnancy are only discoverable as much as 15 or 20 years later, as with DES, this long passage of time makes litigation very difficult if not impossible. Individual doctors have died or left practice, companies have gone out of business, records have been destroyed or disappeared and so forth. This means that in most cases particular suppliers or manufacturers of DES may not usually be identified with certainty in a particular case, particularly since the drug was never subject to an individual manufacturer's patent and was widely produced by many companies. Predictably this led to the rejection of a multiplaintiff action in Holland (see below). In the USA and most recently in Holland some legal manoeuvring of the goal posts was allowed so that some groups of plaintiffs were allowed to proceed notwithstanding.

Second generation drug injury and the limitation periods

DES was developed by a researcher in the UK in the 1930s as an effective low-cost oestrogenic hormone. One view is that for altruistic reasons he chose not to patent it, but another explanation is that the research in developing the drug was paid for by government grant which at that time disallowed patenting of discoveries which had been publicly funded. Whatever the case, the drug was soon widely manufactured and marketed by many companies but with very little testing (if any as we would recognize it today) for efficacy and safety. However, the law of negligence takes into account the state of the art at the time the injury occurred and not with hindsight and in the UK even the new Consumer Protection Act 1987 (see. pp 328 and 330) allows the 'development risks defence'.

DES was extensively used in Holland (it was favoured by the Queen's gynaecologist) and in the USA for treating threatened abortion or preventing habitual abortion, but its efficacy is now regarded as highly doubtful for this purpose if not totally useless.[8] It was fortunately little prescribed in the UK. In Holland by contrast (population 12 million), it has been estimated that it was used in some 300/400 000 pregnancies. Tragically, some 12–15 years after the peaking of its prescription – the period between 1953 and 1967 – it was discovered that the female children of DES mothers tended to develop vaginal changes when reaching adolescence or maturity. These changes could become cancerous and also indicated a high rate of fertility loss through sterility and lost pregnancies. Estimates put the rate of defects at 50% or more. There are analogous changes in male children.

The effects on the DES daughters as they have come to be known are very serious, including possible impairment of their prospects of motherhood and propensity to develop cancerous tumours and malformation of bodily organs, lifelong monitoring to detect early vaginal or other forms of urogenital carcinoma which may require surgery.

Some courts in the USA may adapt the law in order to compensate victims

Many claims have been through the courts, most particularly in the USA, and actions have succeeded in some states (but not others) even though the plaintiffs cannot with certainty identify the manufacturers or suppliers of DES in the individual cases.[9] In *Abel* v. *Eli Lilly* the court relied on the theories of 'concerted action and alternative liability' because 'There are forceful arguments in favor of holding that plaintiff has a cause of action.'

'In our contemporary complex industrialized society, advances in science and technology create fungible goods which may harm consumers and which cannot be traced to any specific producer. The response of the courts can be either to adhere rigidly to prior doctrine, denying recovery to those injured by those products, or to fashion remedies to meet these changing needs . . .'

The court said: 'The most persuasive reason for finding plaintiff states a cause of action is that . . . as between an innocent plaintiff and negligent defendants the latter should bear the cost of the injury.' The court found that neither the plaintiff nor the defendants were at fault in failing to provide evidence of causation, but that the defendants' conduct in marketing a drug the effects of which were delayed for many years played a significant role in creating the unavailability of proof. Then with regard to policy, the court added, 'From a broader policy standpoint, defendants are better able to bear the cost of injury resulting from the manufacture of a defective product . . . . The manufacturer is in the best position to discover and guard against defects in its products and to warn of harmful effects; thus holding it liable for defects and failure to warn of harmful

effects will provide an incentive to product safety . . . . These considerations are particularly significant where medication is involved, for the
consumer is virtually helpless to protect himself from serious, sometimes
permanent, sometimes fatal injuries caused by deleterious drugs.'

DES claims rejected in Holland
In Holland, however, the court rejected a class action by DES daughters
in June 1988 because none of the plaintiffs could prove that the DES
tablets taken by her or his mother were produced and marketed by a
particular manufacturer, or even that one of the ten defendants named
must have been responsible. This was because at the time in question
most manufacturers, wholesalers and pharmacies could have imported
and sold the drug. (The defendants also fought the action on the grounds
that there was insufficient evidence that DES could or did cause the
defects complained of, but the court did not consider this part of the
case.) However since then a later ruling has accepted that an action
can be brought without the plaintiffs being required to identify each
manufacturer of each product taken (see p. 326).

In the UK the courts, however, will not adjust the substantive law on
the identification of defendants purely so as to admit claims by plaintiffs
whom they see as disadvantaged consumers. However, in the UK the
plaintiffs may sue the Department of Health (DoH) in negligence for
allowing such drugs on the market and any other body concerned as
well as the prescribing doctor.

In *Loveday* v. *Renton and Wellcome Foundation Ltd and others*[10] a pertussis
vaccine case tried in London in 1988, the judge found that the plaintiffs
had not proved causation of injury by the pertussis vaccine. Wellcome
had intervened at its own expense in its capacity as a big producer of
pertussis vaccine and because it had an interest in the outcome of the
decision. It was not sued, however, as a defendant, because the plaintiffs
were not in a position to identify the manufacturer of the vaccine used in
each case.

Limitation periods for personal injury claims
The normal period of limitation in the UK is 3 years from the date of the
incident complained of, but this may be extended in cases where it can
be shown that the consequences of the injury were latent and/or not
reasonably discoverable, or if there was fraud and concealment on the
defendant's part. In any event, the court has a discretion to extend the
period of limitation in all circumstances (see the Limitation Act 1980).

Where the injured person was at the time still a minor, the limitation
period will only run against from the date he achieves majority, which
is now age 18, i.e. a total of 21 years. If the injured party is mentally
incapable time does not run against him until he becomes lucid and
mentally competent; if his condition is irreversible, limitation is for his
lifetime plus 3 years; thus allowing for a claim to be brought by his
estate after death. These long and almost indeterminate limitation periods
for children and mentally incapable people have been criticized as a

breeding ground for stale claims and as putting an undue burden on the defendants, but recently a number have succeeded and attempts to shift the burden of proof in any way have been roundly rejected (see *Bull and Wakeham* v. *Devon Area Health Authority*; Brahams[11]).

Under the (British) Consumer Protection Act 1987, in force since 1 March 1988, there is a final cut-off period of 10 years, outside which the plaintiff must take his chance and sue in negligence. It is arguable that 10 years is too little, although it is a period designed to appeal to insurers; it would certainly exclude the kind of injuries suffered by DES daughters. Dispensing doctors as keepers of records, manufacturers and suppliers, as well as insurers, on the other hand are no doubt relieved that there is a 10 year maximum for the Act, which is of course, in any event, not retrospective. By contrast, the Swedish and Finnish pharmaceutical insurance schemes (also not retrospective from their introduction) have a 15 year cut-off period which would probably have cut through the DES claimants halfway if they had been able to qualify.

Foreseeability

To succeed in a claim in negligence the plaintiff will have to prove that the injuries/damages sustained were reasonably foreseeable at the time (see for example *Bolton* v. *Stone* [1951] AC 850). Accordingly, any claim will be judged by reference to prevailing standards of knowledge and practices, i.e. the state of the art, and it was for this reason that the thalidomide litigation was uncertain of success. The leading English case of *Roe* v. *Minister of Health* [1954] 2 QB 66 illustrates the protection that the state-of-the-art defence offers. There, a patient, Mr Roe, was admitted to hospital for a minor operation. An anaesthetist injected his spine with nupercaine that had been stored in glass ampoules that in turn were kept in a jar of phenol. Unfortunately, and unbeknown to the anaesthetist, the glass ampoule had developed cracks (which were not detectable by ordinary visual or tactile examination) through which the phenol had seeped and contaminated the nupercaine. As a result the patient was permanently paralysed below the waist. He sued in negligence but failed because the dangers were not at that time appreciated by doctors. As Lord Denning pointed out, the evidence at trial was that this was a risk that was first pointed out in 1951 and would not have been appreciated by an anaesthetist in 1947: 'Nowadays it would be negligent not to realise the danger, but it was not then.'

[It has been well argued in *Anaesthesia* that the ratio of the case developed from a misinterpretation of the evidence. The authors argue convincingly that it was a negligent and foreseeable failure to rinse away the cleansing agents and that it was the contamination by those agents which caused paralysis in the patient concerned and that the hairline cracks and the phenol in the ampoules played no part at all.]

The doctor's professional duty of care

A doctor owes his patient (and others whom he advises) a duty to use reasonable skill and care, but though British law imposes a legal duty, the standard of the skill and care provided is measured against prevailing medical standards. Accordingly, a doctor will not be found negligent if he followed a practice thought proper by a responsible body of medical opinion at the relevant time – this test was laid down by J. McNair in the seminal case of *Bolam* v. *Friern Hospital Management Committee* [1957] 1 WLR 582 later endorsed by the House of Lords. It has been expressed alternatively by Lord President Clyde in the leading Scottish case of *Hunter* v. *Hanley* [1955] SLT 213 at 217 from which the judge in *Bolam* drew 2 years later:

> 'In the realm of diagnosis and treatment there is ample scope for genuine difference of opinion and one man clearly is not negligent merely because his conclusion differs from that of other professional men . . . The true test for establishing negligence in diagnosis or treatment on the part of a doctor is whether he has been proved to be guilty of such failure as no doctor of ordinary skill would be guilty of if acting with ordinary care . . .'

'I would only add that a doctor who professes to exercise a special skill must exercise the ordinary skill of his specialty.' This was further endorsed by the English House of Lords in *Maynard* v. *West Midlands Regional Health Authority* [1984] 1 WLR 634.

The Consumer Protection Act 1987

For many years the consumer lobby had felt that British law was too protective of manufacturers and needed amendment to shift the onus of proof and render liability stricter. The impetus came from an EC Directive, which was incorporated (some would argue imperfectly) within the new Consumer Protection Act 1987. Part one of the Act, dealing with defective products, came into force on March 1988 (and is not retrospective).

The Act provides an additional basis for a claim for damages for personal injuries to an action in negligence or contract. It makes liability for a 'defective' product 'strict' subject to various defences, the most important of which is 'the development risks defence', often referred to as 'the state-of-the-art defence', and this substantially reduces its practical effect. It was left to member states to decide whether to include the defence, and its inclusion is an acknowledgement of the anxieties and demands of the forceful manufacturing lobby in the UK who argued that truly strict liability would seriously hamper the development of new products. This argument failed to convince many other members of the EC, however, who have not included it. Former West Germany in particular has imposed strict liability for injuries caused by pharmaceutical products since 1978 although the damages payable are on a more restricted basis than those available in a negligence claim.

Notwithstanding its limitations, the impact of the 1987 Act has been considerable, particularly with regard to pharmaceutical manufacturers, importers, suppliers, doctors and pharmacists. Improved record keeping is likely to be one bonus and, in particular, doctors and pharmacists will need to note the source of a particular drug, its batch number, etc. for at least 10 years (the limitation period imposed by the Act) if they are to be able to deflect a liability claim under the Act away from themselves.

This is because liability under the Act extends also to the person who manufactured the product (which for the purpose of the Act includes raw materials), any person who puts their name or trademark on the product as the manufacturer, and any person who imports the product. Because liability is not restricted to the ultimate supplier, a liability chain may be created which will increase the number of potential defendants to any claim. [Conventional product litigation whether under contract or in tort allows for the chain of liability to be extended by the addition of third (and even fourth and fifth parties etc.) to the original litigation at the behest of a defendant to whom the third party may have owed a duty in contract or tort.]

It seems likely that a product which is handed out free by a supplier or manufacturer to promote their business or the sale of the product or for the purpose of a clinical trial will fall within the provisions of the Act. Trials of products are carried out with the aim of extending the manufacturer's business, their range of marketable products – certainly the costs of funding a trial will form part of a company's expenses in its tax return to be set against its profits. But it is in this type of situation that the manufacturer if sued would be likely to try to invoke the protection of the development risks defence and it would depend on the circumstances whether a plaintiff would succeed. Obviously, even if the product was a relatively new one, if the trial data contained warning signals that were not collected up regularly and promptly or ignored, the manufacturer and the trialists could find themselves in serious difficulties in trying to defend claims in negligence or under the Act.

Trials performed on 'healthy volunteers' who are paid will also form the basis of a contractual agreement, although this will not necessarily be directly with the manufacturer but may be with an intermediary. Currently the Association of the British Pharmaceutical Industry (ABPI) recommendations suggest that all companies or individuals setting up trials on healthy volunteers should take out 'No Fault' insurance against unwanted and unexpected side effects and drug injuries.

Furthermore, on the legal 'neighbour' principle it would seem that a pharmaceutical physician who was involved in running a clinical trial (at whatever stage) would owe the patients or volunteers a duty of care (even if they were not directly under that physician's care) to ensure that it was competently and skilfully conducted within the confines of prevailing expertise (see *Donoghue* v. *Stevenson*, *Bolam* v. *Friern Hospital Management Committee* and *Hunter* v. *Hanley*, considered above). The pharmaceutical physician's company would be vicariously liable for any acts and omissions occurring in the course of that physicians employment in the normal way (see p. 330).

What is a 'defective' product?

The Act defines a product as 'defective' if its safety is not such as 'persons generally are entitled to expect'. This means that not only the nature and class of likely potential users/consumers of the product will be taken into account but also, and *most importantly in the pharmaceutical context, the manner and purposes for which the product is marketed and presented.* The packaging and any warnings and directions for use could be crucial in determining whether the safety of the product was as persons generally were entitled to expect. Presumably, the test of what people were entitled to expect will be objective rather than subjective, and is intended to refer to the consumer population rather than intermediate specialist groups, e.g. doctors. Members of the public will, of course, expect that drugs prescribed to them by their doctors will be reasonably safe to take and will rely on their doctors to provide a filtering process; presumably the filtering process will be taken into account in any litigation based on the Act.

Since patients can only sue their doctors in negligence (unless they were also fulfilling the dual role of suppliers and/or manufacturers of a product under the Act and could not pass on the liability), there will be some attraction in suing the manufacturer/supplier/importer directly under the Act, which does not require proof of negligence and, once causation is established, puts the onus on the defendant to satisfy the court that he should not be held liable.

It is also uncertain how far the role of the doctor/dentist/pharmacist as a 'learned intermediary' will affect the court's construction of what 'persons generally' are entitled to expect with regard to the safety of a particular product and whether in any particular case the doctor will find himself joined in the action as a third party by the manufacturer for failing in his duties as a 'learned intermediary'!

Safety is a relative term with regard to drugs

The Medicines Act 1968 and the common law accept that safety is a relative term in the context of medical treatment and drug therapy. The medical profession, the pharmaceutical industry and the licensing authority in the UK accept that registered medical practitioners and pharmacists should be supplied with fuller and more detailed information relating to the composition of and contraindications and potential side effects of prescription drugs than members of the general public, although there is an increasing demand from consumer groups for more information to be provided to the lay public.

As the 'learned intermediary' the doctor will decide whether and how much to prescribe of any drug and what warnings should be given in clinical practice. Another 'learned intermediary' interposed between the patient and the pharmaceutical industry is the licensing authority set up under the Medicines Act 1968. It will be the authority's primary duty to decide if a medicinal product is safe and effective and whether there is an appropriate and acceptable risk/benefit ratio; whether or not it should be licensed, or continue to be licensed and, if so, with what if any restrictions on its sale and warnings of contraindications in its packaging and promotion etc.

The consequences of withholding unfavourable data

If a manufacturer withholds information from the licensing authority and/or the medical profession generally as and when it becomes available (e.g. from clinical trials, monitoring or other sources), and this information if released might have prevented injuries and side effects in patients, the manufacturer and any physicians concerned with the withholding of the information may find themselves sued in negligence and/or under the Consumer Protection Act (because the product was not as safe as persons generally were entitled to expect). Depending on the circumstances, such conduct could lead to other more punitive legal consequences – for the doctor a charge of serious professional misconduct – and possibly an action in deceit against the company and even a criminal prosecution. If a patient were to die a charge of manslaughter could follow both against the physicians and the directors of the company. Corporate manslaughter looks to be a developing remedy to be used against errant companies who recklessly ignore the safety of the public.

Let us suppose that a manufacturer deliberately suppresses unwelcome evidence that a drug could be dangerous in certain circumstances and the risk materializes. In such circumstances US juries have awarded massive punitive damages and it is possible that exemplary damages could be awarded in the UK. In the UK civil claims for damages are generally intended to provide compensation not punishment, so as a general principle the fact that a treatment was outrageous in its incompetence (see *Lancet* and *AB Kralj* v. *CA* [1993]) does not allow extra damages to be awarded. The doctor may be erased from the register by General Medical Council (GMC), however, and if the patient dies due to the doctor's reckless disregard for the patient's safety, the doctor may be found guilty of manslaughter, as in the cases of *R* v. *Adamako*, *R* v. *Sargent*[12] and *R* v. *Salim and Sara*.[13]

The Consumer Protection Act makes it clear that the fact that a later edition of a product is marketed as 'improved' cannot be taken to infer that the earlier version was defective. The Act seems to take into account advertisements promoting the product as well as labelling and advisory leaflets that go with its distribution. Manufacturers under pressure from the Act and required by the EC from 1992 include patient information leaflets with single pack dispensing of prescribed drugs. If the manufacturer provides these but the supplier or prescriber removes them, then any consequent damage that may be caused owing to a misuse of the product which could have been avoided had the leaflet been left with the product is likely to fall on the supplier's or prescriber's head or at least have to be explained away to the satisfaction of the court.

As has already been stated, where a claim is brought under the Consumer Protection Act, once the plaintiff has proved that the defendant's product caused the injuries alleged then the onus will be put on the defendant to show that the product was not 'defective'. This is a considerable tactical and evidential advantage and will make the product's manufacturer the prime target rather than the clinician. The Act puts the onus on the manufacturer to consider in advance not only the *use* to which the product may be put over a short or a long term and whether it may be addictive, but also to what *misuse* the product could actually be put, e.g. overdosing or if taken in combination with alcohol or by children. It is for the defendant manufacturer to try to anticipate potential misuse by providing safer packaging or manufacturing processes and safety catches or stoppers; that said, the defendant is entitled to defend a legal claim by proving that the plaintiff was guilty of contributory or total negligence. As of December 1992 there are still no reported cases decided under the Act although a number are now progressing towards trial in the UK.

Defences

There are several defences listed in the Act, which include a plea that the injury was caused by compliance with legislation, that the defendant did not in fact supply the product or that the defect did not exist at the relevant time. However, the most important defence, and certainly the most controversial in concept, is the defence that 'the state of scientific and technical knowledge at the relevant time was not such that a producer of products of the same description as the product in question might be expected to have discovered the defect if it had existed in his products while they were under his control'.

For obvious reasons the development risks defence considerably limits the Act's protection of consumers and any future victims of a drug disaster could still find themselves without an effective legal remedy and without compensation. It would depend in each particular case whether the manufacturer could show that he had adequately tested out the drug at each stage on appropriate subjects (animal and human, young and old, male and female, etc.) for an appropriate period and that at each stage of testing and postevent monitoring that he had been vigilant and competent and honest in his appraisal of effectiveness and safety.

Damages under the Act include compensation for death and personal injury; personal injury includes any disease and any other impairment of a person's physical or mental condition (which would seem to include nervous shock) within the Act. Claims for less than £275 are excluded.

Prevention is better than cure

Obviously prevention is better than cure. It is a moot point as to whether the law is fulfilling its duty to protect consumers and patients from themselves, manufacturers, the medical profession and the pressures of life and contemporary fashions. Is our regulation system satisfactory in concept and in practice?

Dr Joe Collier's comments and other evidence suggests that the law in the West still does not adequately protect consumers from the promotion and prescribing of ineffective or unsafe medicinal drugs or 'foods'. In the Third World the law looks to be even less effective, with few if any controls in place and feeble or non-operable sanctions when injuries occur. So called self-regulation by the industry is not a substitute for firm, well supervised control of marketing and promotion.

At an 'ISPIC' meeting (International Society for the Prevention of Iatrogenic Complications) Charles Medawar of Social Audit pointed out that estimates suggest that as many people are injured by drugs as are injured on the roads, yet no equivalent strategy and legal framework existed to respond to this problem (see also Medawar[3]).

Obviously there has to be a workable balance between regulation and control on the one hand and innovation and experimentation on the other; few would wish to set rolling a choking bureaucracy of law in this area, but there is room for improvement in some respects.

That said, effective medicinal products which contain active ingredients cannot be guaranteed to be absolutely safe for everybody all the time in all circumstances. Safety in the context of drugs can only be a relative term. It follows therefore that medicines cannot be developed and tested and indeed prescribed for humans without some risk-taking, which must of course be kept to acceptable levels – as low as is reasonably possible. One cannot have the rose without its thorns, but at least the thorns should be as small and guarded against as possible.

There must be maintained a balance in the law between the risk and benefits or potential risks and benefits of the medicines and their applications; acceptance of the need for this balance to be held is inherent in the provisions of the Medicines Act 1968 and in its interpretation by judges and in the development of the common law to date.

The law starts with the premise that, unless otherwise stated, the results of medical treatment, including drug therapy, cannot be guaranteed. However, where an individual or a firm is unwise enough to guarantee outcome or provides misleading information, serious legal consequences and retribution may follow.

The licensing of medicinal products in Britain
The law has been slow to intervene over much in medical and scientific regulatory affairs. It was only in the wake of the much publicised thalidomide tragedy that the Medicines Act 1968 was passed. This created for the first time a comprehensive system for the licensing and regulation of prescriptive and OTC medicines in the UK.

The limitations of the Medicines Act 1968
The Medicines Act effectively regulates the licensing and testing of many pharmaceutical products and provides that medicinal products must be reasonably safe and effective before they can be licensed. It is not, however, all embracing and although all new medicinal products must be processed by reference to its licensing procedures, there are gaps and

weaknesses in its provisions which many feel should be plugged or at least strengthened to protect the consumer.

For instance, it only applies to a 'medicinal product' which is 'manufactured, sold, supplied, imported, or exported for use . . .' as *inter alia* for 'a medicinal purpose'. Many foods, although hyped as generally medicinal and helpful to people suffering from a variety of ailments, as well as vitamin supplements and so-called 'natural' products are excluded from its provisions. There is little control over homeopathic remedies and for many years so-called 'grandfather products', i.e. those in existence before the passing of the Medicines Act, escaped review whilst still remaining on the market.

The specialist committees set up under the Act *inter alia* advise the government on licensing – whether and in what form to grant product licences and whether an existing licence should be amended or withdrawn. The Act also restricts the nature of any advertising criteria, disclosures of risks, contraindications, the use of the product and its format. There are also provisions to punish false and misleading advertisements in the criminal courts. In *R v. Roussel Laboratories Ltd* and *R v. Good* (Dr Christopher Good was the medical director of Roussel) the defendants were held by an Old Bailey jury to have contravened s93 of the Act. They were fined respectively £5000 and £250 per each of the four counts with which they were charged and found guilty – negligible sums in the context of pharmaceutical turnover. (The legal costs no doubt totalled a great deal more than the fines and may have dented the defendants' pockets more effectively along with the adverse publicity.) Their appeals were dismissed.

In *Roussel* and *Good* the charges related to the advertising of tiaprofenic acid, marketed by Roussel as 'Surgam', a non-steroidal anti-inflammatory drug for the relief of pain and inflammation resulting from arthritis. Such drugs work by inhibiting the synthesis of prostaglandins, chemicals released at the sites of inflammation or injury, which among other things are responsible for the discomfort experienced by sufferers from arthritis. Most of these drugs have side effects, particularly gastric irritation which occurs because such drugs inhibit the prostaglandin which defends gastric mucosa (prostacyclin).

It was not disputed that Surgam was a useful drug, but the case against *Roussel* and *Good* arose out of a claim that Surgam operated in a special way by inhibiting the prostaglandin which caused pain without inhibiting prostacyclin. That was referred to as selective prostaglandin inhibition. The claim was based on experimental work, but it was challenged, and by 25 March 1983 Dr Good had serious doubts about it. Nonetheless, he allowed himself to be overrode and four advertisements appeared between April and June 1983 in respect of which the four counts were founded.

The criminal prosecutions produced a certain unease and wariness but, unfortunately, there is evidence that numerous breaches of the Act are ignored.[14]

The interpretation of the Medicines Act 1968 has been the subject of dispute between the licensing authority and the manufacturers with regard to the licensing of new and generic products and the procedures by which amendments may be made to existing product licences. Its provisions have also been affected and will continue to be so affected and amended by EC directives following the UK's entry into the Common Market.

In *SmithKline & French Laboratories Ltd* (on appeal from *R* v. *Licensing Authority*) [1990] AC 64,[15] the applicants, SKF, had undertaken the research and manufacture of cimetidine, used for controlling gastric secretion and healing peptic ulceration. The UK patents had been granted in 1972 and the applicants were granted a product licence to market the drug under s7(2) of the Act by the licensing authority established by the Act. In order to obtain their product licence SKF had supplied the licensing authority with details of their financially expensive research and testing which they regarded as highly confidential and which they did not wish to have exposed to their competitors.

Any company wishing to market the drug or a generic version of it in the UK is required also to obtain a product licence. The 1968 Act had been amended so that regard had to be given to the Council Directives from the EC Article 4.8 of Council Directive 65/65/EC, as amended by Council Directive 87/21/EC, which provided that an applicant for a product licence was not required to supply the licensing authority with results of certain tests if they could demonstrate that their product was essentially similar to a product already on the market.

A number of companies applied to the licensing authority for product licences of the drug, whereupon SKF applied for judicial review to prevent the licensing authority's proposed use of its confidential information in assessments of generic applications for licences of the drug. The judge granted SKF a declaration that the licensing authority could not use SKF's confidential data. The licensing authority, supported by two generic companies, successfully appealed against this ruling, with the House of Lords holding that the licensing authority was under a statutory duty to protect the public from the dangers inherent in the introduction and reproduction of drugs and to treat all applicants for product licences fairly and equally; that when considering applications for product licences for a particular drug it was necessary to compare the information supplied in any later application with that supplied with the original application so as to ensure that both products were similar, safe, effective and reliable; that the authority had therefore a right and a duty to make use of all the information obtained by it under the Act. Thus SKF had no right recognized in English law to prevent the use of their confidential material by the authority for any of the purposes for which it had been established, including the processing of applications for product licences for cimetidine.

Furthermore, since EC law operated *inter alia*, 'without prejudice to the law relating to the protection of industrial and commercial property', English law applied, and this did not protect SKF against the use of their confidential information by the authority for the purposes of the Act; there was no requirement to refer the appeal to the European Court of Justice under Article 177 of the Treaty.

Most importantly though, *per curiam*, the House of Lords said that *the licensing authority should not be deterred from exercising its rights and powers so as to ensure public safety and to ensure fairness to all applicants. The courts should be reluctant to criticize its practices or to grant injunctions or orders or declarations against it.* (In *SmithKline & French Laboratories Ltd* [1990] AC 64).[15]

While the SKF case was working its way through the appeals process another, and this time more successful, legal challenge was mounted against the licensing authority's procedures for reassessing the safety of Mianserin and amending its product licence.

Mianserin: Safety in overdose a relevant factor for Licensing Authority.

On 30 January 1990 the Court of Appeal held, in a reserved judgment, that comparative safety in overdose was a relevant factor that the licensing authority could (and impliedly should) take into account. The Court of Appeal dismissed the licensing authority's appeal against the decision of the Divisional Court.[16]

The genesis of the dispute lay in the requirements of s19, s20 and s28 of the Medicines Act 1968, that the licensing authority shall have regard to the safety of the product when deciding whether to grant, suspend, revoke or vary a licence. In the past there had been concern about the association between mianserin therapy and various haematological disorders and the product's data sheets had been varied by agreement.

More recently, however, new data gave cause for greater concern, especially with regard to patients aged over 65. Organon Laboratories challenged the provisional conclusions of the Committee on Safety of Medicines CSM (which, *inter alia*, wished to revise the drug's data sheet) on a number of grounds, and in particular, offered evidence of Mianserin's safety in overdose. Following legal advice, however, this was excluded on the basis that it was not a relevant factor when assessing the safety or harmfulness of a drug, which it was said should be judged by reference to its normal dosage. Referred to as 'safety in overdose' the evidence that the company wished to have considered indicated that Mianserin has a low toxicity when taken in excessive quantities, whether as a result of overprescription, accidental departures by the patient from the prescribed dosage, ill advised self-medication or attempts at suicide, and a particularly low toxicity by comparison with other drugs. The licensing authority, having at all levels excluded consideration of such evidence, indicated its intention to amend the drug's licence and data sheets as from 1 January 1989 and to issue a warning in its publication, *Current Problems*.

Organon Laboratories sought an injunction restraining the publication of warning and successfully challenged the licensing authority's decision which had, on the basis of legal advice given to the Department, excluded all or any evidence of 'safety in overdose'. The Divisional Court accordingly quashed the licensing authority's decision,[16] although for other reasons an amended warning went out in the Bulletin. The licensing authority's appeal was dismissed nearly a year later, but not before arguments on both sides had been considerably expanded and complicated with regard to interpretation of the relevant sections of the Medicines Act 1968 as amended and affected by the EC Directive 65/65, which 25 years on remained still unimplemented into the domestic legislation of the Medicines Act and in particular into s28(g) of the 1968 Act.

In the Court of Appeal[17] the case for the DoH was presented on the basis that the Divisional Court's decision made it mandatory in every case for the licensing authority to take into account the degree of risk attaching to the taking of that drug in excess and to perform in every case a comparison in relation to this risk between the drug under consideration and other drugs intended for the same purpose. This was not so.

Antidepressants and 'Safety' in Overdose
The Act allowed for the exercise of the discretion at two stages. First, it was for the tribunal to decide whether safety in overdose is the kind of material that could prove valuable in performing the 'judgmental' exercise called for by legislation. If the tribunal concludes that it could not be, then, subject to 'Wednesbury unreasonableness',[18] it is free to exclude it; the evidence never comes into the balance at all. On the other hand, if the tribunal decides that the material might be useful, then it is free to examine it, and to put it into the balance for whatever, if anything, it has proved on examination to be worth. Neither the Court of Appeal nor the Divisional Court held that the CSM or MC (Medicines Commission) were bound to admit the evidence or bound to attach a decisive or indeed any weight to it once admitted. Rather the Court held that by deciding in advance not to admit the material on safety in overdose the tribunals and hence the licensing authority had foreclosed the performance of the two stages described. This the tribunals and the authority could only do if, on its true interpretation, the relevant legislation posed a question to which safety in overdose could on no view of the matter be relevant.

The effect of EC Directives on the Medicines Act
The DoH had argued that the relevant sections of the Medicines Act 1968 had to be interpreted subject to the Council Directive 65/65 on approximation of medical products. That Directive, although expressed as mandatory, had, however, not been implemented and, although subsequent to it in time, the Medicines Act had been passed at a time when Britain was not a member of the EC (it joined in 1972). *While, for purposes of interpretation, amendments or legislation made subsequent to 1972 had to be interpreted in the light of the purposes expressed clearly and unconditionally in an EC Directive, the unamended sections of the Medicines Act 1968 were not subject to this overriding requirement of interpretation. Where the state had failed in its duty to carry the Directive into the local law, it could not seek to rely on its provisions.*

However, the Court of Appeal accepted Organon's argument that it and *any other 'citizen' engaged in a confrontation with the state or an emanation of the state in the context of an unenacted Directive was entitled to the best of both worlds. If the relevant UK legislation best suited its case, it need look no further; but if the Directive yielded a more favourable result, the company could rely on that instead of the Act although the State might not do so.*

In the present case Organon was content to rely on the Act and was entitled to do so and, thus far, Community Law did not materially affect s28 of the Medicines Act 1968.

Giving the leading judgment, Lord Justice Mustill said that the court had to treat the purpose indicated in the licence as the drug's uses against symptoms of depressive illness, i.e. relief or alleviation of those symptoms. When asking what test was to be applied when deciding whether Mianserin can 'safely' be 'administered' for the purpose of alleviating symptoms of depression, little was to be gained by considering the meaning of the word 'safety in isolation; indeed it was probably not possible to do so.'

Lord Justice Mustill continued:

> 'Thus, a drug which creates few hazards if marketed with appropriate warnings and recommendations may be much more dangerous if these are omitted. Again, there is no absolute standard of safety. Very few drugs are entirely free from the risk of inducing adverse side effects in some patients. The question must always be whether the degree of risk is sufficiently low to be acceptable, and this cannot be addressed without an appreciation of the benefits to be gained from taking a risk of that degree. Be that as it may, in the present context I think it clear that safety does not involve an immutable standard. Although section 28 is not a mirror of sections 19 and 20, it is quite plain that the section is concerned with a change in the balance of risk and benefit originally struck when consent was given for the marketing of the product, resulting from (inter alia) a recognition that the previous assessment of the risk can no longer be relied upon. I do not see how it can be decided whether the risk can now be regarded as unacceptably great, without considering what level of risk should be treated as acceptable, in the light of the benefits to be gained from the marketing of the drug.'

Following the start of the legal dispute with the licensing authority and the issue of the additional warnings with regard to the safety of Mianserin, sales dropped by 25 per cent by the date of the appeal judgment. It will be interesting to note if and how these marketing changes affect any reported instances of ADRs in patients taking this group of drugs.

Compliance with licensing requirements does not provide bullet-proof protection; the current trend is to join all possible parties as defendants (e.g. in the multiple actions made by patients injured by contaminated blood and blood products and pertussis vaccination claims). If there is no suggestion of malpractice by the doctor the plaintiffs' efforts are likely to be concentrated on the manufacturers, marketers, the DoH and the CSM who find themselves increasingly drawn into the litigation arena. One aspect of the claim may be that the manufacturers deliberately withheld data showing dangerous side effects or contraindications or that they failed to test adequately before and after marketing and that the government's watchdog role delegated to its specialist committees was inadequately, negligently or improperly performed.

In the UK expert and scientific medical evidence will be evaluated by a High Court judge sitting alone. Although no individual is infallible, such a judge may generally be relied on to assess the evidence that is presented with scrupulous care and without bias; the difficulty of establishing causation (the first hurdle) may prove a great burden, particularly when it must be followed by proof of negligence.

In the USA, by contrast, it will be lay juries of varying intellectual competence (described by one US economist as 'people who have nothing better to do with their time') who will be given the task of evaluating scientific and medical testimony. Allegedly all too often on the basis of emotional sympathy for a plaintiff and the demeanour and confidence of the expert witnesses in the courtroom.[19] This may make a nonsense of the scientific and medical data and negate the powers and protection given by the licensing authority, Food and Drug Administration (FDA). 'The FDA regulatory system is designed to maximize the attendant risks. Increasingly, however, manufacturers of medications that are approved by FDA experts as beneficial, and that are marketed and labelled in accordance with FDA specifications, are confronting state tort liability premised on theories of design, defect or warning inadequacy. This dual system of regulation jeopardizes the development and marketing of necessary medications, escalates the costs of health care, and undermines the objectives of the FDA.' This comment on the unsatisfactory turn of events in the USA issues not from the mouths of US doctors, but from American lawyers![20]

Are we in the UK likely to be faced with a similar situation? With judges rather than juries and the checks and balances imposed by the costs rules it is unlikely that the UK will run the full gauntlet of the US experience. But there are indications that British patients will be encouraged to exploit the spoils of the US system on occasion when the pickings are seen to be so much easier to gather and larger when you do.

Damages for personal injuries, although higher in the UK than in the rest of Europe, are well below the kinds of mega-sums available to plaintiffs in the USA. Furthermore, damages in the UK are usually compensatory only, whereas in the USA they may contain a massive punitive element. Where the manufacturer is a multinational corporation with US offices, plaintiffs injured in one jurisdiction – e.g. the UK – may understandably prefer to go forum-shopping to a more plaintiff-friendly system. Contingency fees (a share in the proceeds combined with a no-win no fee deal) are not yet permitted in the UK, but are common practice in the USA. What is not so generally known is that UK lawyers are perfectly entitled to appoint a US firm as their agents; the US lawyers will be retained on a contingency fee basis with the UK lawyers claiming a percentage of the US lawyers' contingency fees if the claim proves successful, thus allowing in contingency fees through the backdoor, and indeed encouraging the export of British claims to the USA, and an insidious import of the US system to the UK.

Obviously, if these manoeuvres are to the advantage of a particular plaintiff no lawyer can or should be criticized for maximizing his client's position. Indeed, the client may do better as part of a group or as an individual both in damages and funding – particularly if he does not qualify for legal aid and would find it difficult to fund a claim for which damages might be relatively low and the costs disproportionately high.

But the price of such litigation is high in both cost and choices of products and medical services. In the USA the costs of routine vaccination have rocketed to take account of potentially devastating potential legal claims. The fear of litigation may cause useful products to be withdrawn (there is only one interuterine device (IUD) left on the US market) and services to be withdrawn. Thus, although it may benefit a few individuals, the downside of the US tort system is very great and must be kept constantly in view.[21,22] The knock-on effects could be very high indeed for the National Health Service (NHS) and private medicine.

In the UK, however, we have no cause for complacency and radical changes and reforms are needed. The tort system is failing us both as a regulatory and compensatory mechanism and is slow and expensive. Claims for drug injuries would be better dealt with by a universal patient insurance scheme such as exists in Sweden, Finland and Norway.[21,23,24] Furthermore, our drugs need to be reviewed urgently in the light of existing consumer/patient dissatisfaction and professional concerns.

Informed consent and pharmaceutical trials

Introduction

How much information should patients be given? Clearly if the trial is on healthy volunteers who will not benefit personally from any treatment given, then the fullest possible information should be given. From this basic premise it follows as a good practice rule that the less essential the treatment the fuller should be the information offered, including details of risks and warnings of side effects and/or potential operational failure. This is in reality no more than another aspect of the risk/benefit equation. The most common situations that have been the subject of litigation and debate are those involving birth control measures and cosmetic treatments.[25–27]

Patients should not be pressurized or feel pressurized to join clinical trials if they do not wish to do so. At a Liverpool inquest in 1984 there was evidence that Mrs Doris Costello was unwillingly included in a trial for oral morphine tablets given following a routine gynaecological operation.[28] She died as a consequence of unexpected side effects of the tablets. The doctors initially called did not know she had received them and misdiagnosed her condition.

Where the patient suffers from a serious potentially terminal illness should they be routinely informed of this when a trial for new or to compare existing treatment regimens is set up? These may be a difficult question to answer, particularly when the prognosis is poor and treatment options are uncertain. However, anger may be generated by a failure to divulge essential information, to have obtained consent from the patient included in a trial when things go wrong or when the patient discovers that they have been in a secret trial. In 1982 at an adjourned inquest held in Birmingham it was revealed that an 84-year-old widow,

Mrs Margaret Wigley, had been an unwitting participant in a multicentre secret randomized controlled trial designed to compare the benefits of the treatment of bowel cancer after surgery with and without drug therapy. Eleven ethical committees had accepted that patients' consent should not be sought.[29]

Following the Wigley inquest there was considerable public criticism of the ethics committees' decisions and the ethics of secret trials in medical circles. The death of Mrs Costello in 1983 (the adjourned inquest was held in 1984) once again fuelled public and professional anxieties about clinical trial procedures with dangerous drug regimens. Furthermore, owing to faulty methodology, the results in the Costello study were shown to be valueless, highlighting the need for clear protocols, procedures and supervision in clinical practice at all stages.

Informed consent: A perceptible shift since 1982

Since 1982 and the publicity engendered by the Wigley and Costello cases, there has been a perceptible shift in ethical guidance and norms.[30] The latest Medical Research Council's Cancer Therapy Committee's recommendations issued in December 1986 entitled 'Investigations on Human Subjects, ethical considerations in the study of cancer therapy' reflect this and state that 'informed' consent of the patient ('the ideal') should now normally be sought where possible (see also the Report of the Royal College of Physicians[31] and the DoH[32]).

The standard clause for future Cancer Trial Centre clinical trial protocols requires all trials to be approved by the local ethical committee before patients are entered and that 'The patient's consent to participate in the study should be obtained after a full explanation has been given of the treatment options, including the conventional and generally accepted methods of treatment and the manner of treatment allocation.' And, furthermore, 'The right of a patient to refuse to participate without giving reasons must be respected. After the patient has entered the trial the clinician must remain free to offer alternative treatment if this is indicated and the patient to withdraw at any stage without giving reasons and without prejudice'.

On 9 and 16 October 1988 *The Observer*'s Open File columns published accounts of secret trials to assess different treatments for breast cancer in women; the design and ideological thinking behind the trials, however, related back largely to the pre-1982 period, with protocols designed as far back as 1979/80.

However, a patient, Mrs Evelyn Thomas (featured in *The Observer* articles) had in fact voiced complaints 2 years earlier in a letter to *The Lancet*[33] relating to the organizers' failure to seek consent. The principal trial in which she participated was a multicentre trial initiated by the Cancer Research Campaign launched in 1980. It was known as a 'collaborative trial for adjuvant systemic therapy in the management of early carcinoma of the breast'. The first results were published in 1988.[34, 35] The trial aimed at repeating a Scandinavian trial with cyclophosphamide and a UK tamoxifen study with a view to evaluating further the role of these two adjuvant regimens in patients with early breast cancer. The summary of results states that 'Two thousand two hundred and thirty women (aged under 75) were randomized into this trial between 1980 and December 1985 and preliminary analyses demonstrate a significant improvement in event-free survival for both regimens. Results from this study closely parallel the two trials it set out to repeat.'

As a matter of record, it is noteworthy that Mrs Thomas was randomized to receive tamoxifen, with hindsight, the preferred regimen.

Following primary treatment (surgery – and later to include the option of lumpectomy as compared with mastectomy), patients were randomized centrally into one of four treatment groups.

1. Control, no further therapy,
2. Tamoxifen 10 mg twice daily for 2 years,
3. Cyclophosphamide 30 mg/kg body weight (max. 2400 g) i.v. for 6 days postoperatively with approximately 5 mg/kg daily in one i.v. injection
4. Combination tamoxifen and cyclophosphamide at the prestated doses.

The protocol to the trial written in 1979 said on p. 13 that 'The Medical Reseach Council takes the view that informed consent need not be sought if either procedure compared in a clinical trial is fully acceptable to the physician in charge and satisfies the basic criterion that no-one is denied a treatment as good as the best available.'[35]

The working party felt that this approach was both ethical and compassionate. Ethical because all patients would be offered local therapy as good as the best available while the addition of cyclophosphamide or tamoxifen was unlikely to be harmful and could conceivably produce lasting benefit.

> 'Not to seek "informed consent" is compassionate also, as it would be very distressing for the patient to be made aware of the precise nature of her condition . . . half the patients would be left with the impression that they are receiving no treatment for the cancer left behind after mastectomy.'

The protocol continued,

> 'However, to protect the interests of the participating clinicians, it is recommended that the acceptance of the trial by the local ethical committee of each hospital is documented before patients are admitted.'

Yet, surely it must be a primary duty of an ethical committee to protect the interests of the patients?[36] It is when this is seen to be done that doctors stand protected from individual claims of ethical malpractice. Nonetheless, exactly how far the closed proceedings of medical ethical committees with their varied sizes, structures and methods of approving clinical trials are satisfactory is a matter for debate.[29,37] New guidance from the Department of Health and Social Security (DHSS) is expected shortly.

The final paragraph of the protocol says that physicians who are convinced that one treatment is better than another for a particular patient of theirs cannot ethically choose at random which treatment to give; they must do what they think best for the particular patient. For this reason physicians who feel that they already know the answer cannot enter patients into a trial. This is perfectly proper *in so far as it goes*. However, trials are usually conducted precisely because there is some evidence (theoretical or practical or both) to suggest that one or more treatments offer benefit, or that one should be discontinued as less beneficial but this may not be borne out by the trial at all, contrary to expectation.

In this case four different treatments were being conducted largely to reassess and re-prove the treatments and results gained from earlier trials. Although not 'convinced' (owing to the well accepted problems of unduly favourable bias inherent in first trials), many clinicians who took part must have had at least a view on what was the preferred treatment. Indeed, from 1 May 1984, after consideration of the results of the UK trial published many months earlier in 1983 (see also Report of the Royal College of Physicians[31]), clinicians 'were given the option to prescribe tamoxifen for all patients, with randomization only into the cyclophosphamide part of the trial.'

Moreover, since by then there was convincing evidence of the efficacy of drug therapy, was it really ethical thereafter to leave the option open of no drug therapy following surgery or for how long into the trial?

Another important ethical (and perhaps legal) point arises in relation to the trial physician who assures patients that when submitting themselves to his hands they will receive one of the best available treatments. While that may be true, the picture offered to the patient is incomplete, as the physician, but not the patient, knows that some of the treatments on offer are known to have more disagreeable side effects than the others (cyclophosphamide commonly induced alopecia (hair loss), afflicting 43 per cent of patients overall in the 3 months following the course, 20 per cent of whom required a wig, and nausea (20 per cent of patients)).

Nor will the physician tell them that those patients receiving drug therapy are, if this trial bears out the earlier ones, expected to gain a better chance of event-free survival. Indeed, proving this very point is of course the whole purpose behind the trial.

Furthermore, if the regimens vary widely in patient-acceptability (e.g. side and other effects) and there is a known or perceived advantage attributed to drug therapies, one of which may produce more unpleasant or toxic side effects than another, can the physician recommend them as all equally good in his informed view?

Experience has shown that where full information is offered on available options, equal numbers for the options cannot be found because many patients will self-select their perceived preferred choice of treatment and effectively vote with their feet.

Although the issues are by no means simple and straightforward, it seems difficult to reconcile secret randomized controlled trials such as this with patient expectations that medical advisers offer the treatment they believe is best tailored to patient needs – and with the doctor's duty to offer the treatment they believe to be best for an individual patient, given what they know or ought to know or think they know about the treatments available.

The price of randomized controlled trials operated secretly may be that perceived immediate best interests of some trial patients may be subjected to the best long-term interests of *future* patients? However laudable the ultimate end of evaluating most accurately the values of different treatment options, there remains a real danger that physicians (often the very best and most dedicated to the practice of better and more advanced medicine) will be tempted to tilt the balance in favour of the advance of knowledge rather than to offer the treatment he believes a particular patient would select given the choices? Yet without randomized controlled trials, now at risk from patient self-selection in key areas, advances in medical treatments (particularly cancer) may be seriously hindered.

Informed consent is often cited as the ideal, but many clinicians consider that in the real practical world there are many patients who would not want to be fully informed, particularly when their prognosis is poor; some patients cannot understand all the information that would need to be showered on them by this principle. However, most patients can, if properly counselled, grasp the key factors although they may very well not wish to become 'full partners' in their treatment with their doctors. On occasion, the blanket requirements of informed consent may be counterproductive and even go against the best interests of patients, present and future.[38] Indeed this was the prevailing gloomy mood at a meeting entitled 'Breast Trials Update' organized by the Cancer Research Campaign and held in Oxford on 7 October 1988.

Speaker after speaker stressed that in their view randomization was essential if medical treatments were to advance and ineffective or potentially harmful treatments were to be eliminated. Data gained from trials where patients themselves had selected treatment is very much less useful as the self-selection element introduces bias which cannot be accurately discounted. It is only the randomized clinical trial that offers doctors and statisticians sufficiently reliable and accurate results to evaluate relatively small percentage benefits (e.g. 5–6 per cent) between treatments. Yet these relatively small percentage treatment benefits could save the lives of hundreds of patients each year.

Unfortunately, informed consent requirements appear to create recruitment problems in certain types of cancer trials. Accordingly, the message from the chairman and other speakers, was sombre; 'uninformed' advocates of informed consent were posing a threat to the advancement of medicine by delaying, hindering and even preventing the implementation of important trials. However, the disturbing evidence is that even when trials show clearly the benefits of a particular therapy it takes many years for this information to percolate through to practitioners and often repeated and unnecessary trials are conducted when the evidence has already been gathered.[39]

Informed consent and the risks of imposing double standards

While a doctor in one hospital may be personally wedded to a particular regimen a colleague up the road may offer a different therapy, but the patient will not necessarily be told of the two or more options that exist when she consents to a valid treatment for her condition. The patient would be unlikely to win a negligence suit based on lack of information since although the doctor's duty to care for his personal patient is a legal one, the standard is set by the medical profession which endorses this limited disclosure when offering a valid treatment. To succeed the patient would need to persuade the Court that the information given was not sufficient to make a decision on whether or not to accept treatment.[40,41] Trialists claim with some justification, therefore, that the requirement to seek informed consent amounts to the creation of double standards which could threaten the demise of randomized controlled trials in cancer therapy.

It is notable that in *Sidaway* and *Bolam* the courts were not concerned with secret clinical trials of experimental procedures. In *R v. Mental Health Act Commission ex parte W*,[10,42] a patient appealed to the Divisional Court asking that his wish to receive an experimental treatment with a potentially toxic drug be honoured. STUART-SMITH LJ sitting in the Divisional Court said consent had to be 'informed' in that the patient knew the nature and likely effects of the treatment. Where the treatment was not routinely used and was not sold for the purpose contemplated, then it was important that the patient should know that the use of the drug was a novel one, investigations limited to animals and different age groups. The patient did not need to 'understand the precise physiological process involved before he can be said to be capable of understanding the nature and likely effects of the treatment or can consent to it.'

It is uncertain whether the law requires full disclosure of all available trial options when the randomized controlled trial has been set up to evaluate innovative but relatively established treatments perhaps with appropriately licensed drugs as this will depend on whether there remains a body of responsible medical opinion which would support limited disclosure.

Informed consent and vulnerable or incompetent patients

A child of 16 and above may consent to medical and dental treatment as if of full age (18); parents or those having taken on the mantle of parental responsibility may give consent on behalf of *children* too young or incapable of giving their consent if the treatment is for their benefit.

It is uncertain whether parents can consent on behalf of their children to experimental treatments that are not aimed primarily at benefiting them but more likely to benefit society at large and/or future generations. It is likely to depend on whether there is much risk or the treatment is invasive. Certainly if the treatment involves any serious risk without compensatory benefit it should not be given as this would seem to be both unlawful and unethical. Sterilization and other very serious, irreversible treatments which pose ethical problems should be referred to the court through the wardship procedures. In all cases parents should be given full details of the treatment options and not pressurized to consent.

Close relatives may not in law give consent to treatment on *incompetent adults*, although as a matter of evidence and convenience their opinions are likely to be sought as next best to knowing what the incompetent person would have wanted. For a long time, since the passing of the Mental Health Act 1959, it was thought that there was a lacuna in the law in this area and that there was nobody who could give a valid legal consent on the behalf of a mentally incapable adult outside an emergency situation. However, in the recent case of *F* v. *Berkshire Area Health Authority* [1989] 2 WLR 1025, the House of Lords held that the *Bolam* principle (see p. 330) of the reasonably competent doctor would apply as to what treatment might be given to the patient. Second, and on occasion, third opinions should be sought for serious non-routine treatments and a multidisciplinary approach adopted. The issue of medical decision making and comment has been extensively considered by the Law Commission and its Consultation Paper 129, published by HMSO in 1993 (see *Lancet*, 1993, April/May, Editorial).

Pharmaceutical drugs and crime

Pharmaceutical drugs may cause mood swings, disinhibit, lessen concentration and the ability to operate machinery, may stimulate physical activity or physical prowess and give rise to delusional states. Occasionally, the effects of prescription drugs may give rise to a criminal offence, either by being unlawful *per se* (steroids in sport to improve performance) or by affecting the individual's behaviour.[43,44]

In *R* v. *Hardie* [1985] 1 WLR 64, CA, the defendant who was splitting up with his mistress of long-standing took some of her valium tablets as he was distressed and she said they would do him no harm. Later he started a fire in the bedroom. His defence was that he had not realized what he was doing because of the effect of the valium but the trial judge refused to allow this defence to be put to the jury. His appeal against conviction succeeded as the Court of Appeal held that if the effect of a prescription drug is merely soporific or sedative, the taking of it, even in excessive quantities, cannot in the ordinary way raise a conclusive presumption against the admission of proof of intoxication for the purpose of disproving *mens rea* in ordinary crimes (as would be the case with alcohol). The defence should have gone before the jury.

(see also *R* v. *Quick* [1973] QB 910).

The taking of therapeutic drugs will provide no defence to the commission of a road traffic offence under the Road Traffic Acts because these are offences of strict liability. A person who drives after taking prescription medicines may therefore, in certain circumstances, be guilty of driving while under the influence of drugs; more likely, they will commit a road traffic offence because their driving ability has been impaired by the effects of the drugs. If they were reckless in taking the drugs and then driving then they would seem to have nothing to offer by way of mitigation, but as a rule, without recklessness, the effect of the prescription drugs can be pleaded by way of mitigation.[45,46]

If, in the light of current knowledge, it was foreseeable that there would be a risk of impairment to the intellectual function, control and physical coordination of an individual patient and, for example, that driving capacity or ability to use dangerous machinery was reduced then warnings should be given. A failure to provide a warning of the potential dangers could render the prescribing doctor, the pharmacist and the manufacturer liable in negligence to the patient. Furthermore, the drug in those circumstances could arguably be regarded as 'defective' under the Consumer Protection Act 1987; not as safe as might reasonably have been expected by 'persons generally'. Thus (see pp. 328 and 330), drugs that are likely to cause drowsiness, and/or confusion, and/or clumsiness should always carry warnings to the consumer. Similarly, contraindications such as consumption of alcohol or the effects of the drug if taken without an intake of food should be clearly labelled.

There is considerable evidence which has been surfacing in the UK that benzodiazepines when used over a period may induce dependency and are thus unsuitable for long-term prescribing. The data sheets have been altered to reflect this and litigation is now underway. However, benzodiazepines may, when used for sedation and/or anaesthesia during dental or medical treatment, have other unwanted effects and have been found to induce sexual fantasies in women patients and consequently cause them to believe they have been sexually assaulted.[47] On occasion, patients have accused the doctor or dentist of indecent behaviour.[48] If the doctor or dentist had no chaperone at the relevant time they may find themselves prosecuted in the criminal courts or before the relevant disciplinary body on a charge of serious professional misconduct. Accordingly, a warning of the dangers of sexual hallucination should be given by the manufacturers and/or suppliers to the health care professionals which, where appropriate, should probably be passed on to the individual concerned.

Propofol anaesthesia may produce similar fantasies,[49] and one anaesthetist told me[50] that in a series of 60 propofol anaesthetics for short gynaecological or orthopaedic procedures, he noticed mood elevation on recovery in 43 per cent. At interview on recovery to full consciousness, 50 per cent recalled dreaming. Five (8 per cent) of these patients admitted to dreams of a sexual nature. This practitioner suggested that susceptible patients be forewarned of the possibility of sexual fantasy and amorous behaviour in addition to assurances of a continuous third party presence before clinicians embark on the administration of midazolam or propofol.

References

1. Dean M (1992). London perspective: curbing the Drugs Bill. *Lancet* **340**: 1531–2.
2. Collier J (1989). *The Health Conspiracy*. London: Century Hutchinson: xiii.
3. Medawar C (1992). *Power and Dependence. Social Audit on the Safety of Medicines*. Social Audit Ltd.
4. Brahams D (1988). Pertussis vaccine on trial – the judge's conclusions. *Medico-Legal Journal* **56**: 167.
5. Brahams D (1990). Pertussis vaccine litigation. *Lancet* **i**: 905; (1988). **i**: 837.
6. *Rothwell and others* v. *Raes* [1988] 54 DLR 193.
7. Anon (1990). Vaccine damage cases. *AUMA Medical and Legal Journal* **i**: 13.
8. (1984). 343 Western Reporter, 2nd series.
9. Brahams D (1991). Diethylstilbestrol, third generation injury claims. *Lancet* **33**: 775.
10. *The Times* 31/5/88.
11. Brahams D (1989). Delayed birth injuries claim. *Lancet* **i**: 738.
12. Brahams D (1990). Two anaesthetists convicted of manslaughter. *Lancet* **336**: 431.
13. Brahams D (1992). Death of a remand prisoner. *Lancet* **340**: 1462.
14. Herxheimer A, Collier J (1990). Promotion by the British pharmaceutical industry, 1983–8: a critical analysis. *British Medical Journal* **300**: 307–31.
15. Licensing Authority (1989). The Licensing Authority – the use of drug manufacturers' confidential data. *Lancet* **i**: 395.
16. Brahams D (1989). Mianserin product licence. *Lancet* **i**: 452.
17. Brahams D (1989). Safety in overdose and drug licensing. *Lancet* **i**: 343.
18. Dictum of LORD GREEN MR in *Associated Picture Houses Ltd* v. *Wednesbury Corporation* [1948] 1 KB 223 at 230.
19. Miller DR (1987). Courtroom science and standards of proof in a leukaemia case. *Lancet* **ii**: 1283.
20. Anon (1990). A question of competence: the judicial role in the regulation of pharmaceuticals. *Harvard Law Review* **103**: 773.
21. Owles D (1989). Product liability. *New Law Journal* **Aug 11**: 1120.
22. Brahams D (1990). US litigation style in Britain. *Lancet* **i**: 847–8.
23. Mann RD, Harvard J (eds). (1989). *No Fault Compensation in Medicine*. London: Royal Society of Medicine.
24. Halley MM *et al.* (1989). *Medical Malpractice Solutions*. USA: Thomas.
25. Herxheimer A (1990). Duty to warn about likely adverse affects. *Lancet* **i**: 1151.
26. Brahams D (1989). What must women be told about the pill? *Lancet* **ii**: 285–6.
27. Mann RD (1990). *Oral Contraceptives and Breast Cancer. The Implications of the Present Findings for Informed Consent and Informed Choice*. Carnforth: Parthenon.
28. Brahams D (1984). Death of a patient participating in a trial of oral morphine for relief of postoperative pain. *Lancet* **i**: 1083–4.
29. Brahams D (1982). Death of a patient who was the unwitting subject of randomised controlled trial of cancer treatment. *Lancet* **i**: 1028–9.
30. Faulder C *et al.* (1983). Informed consent: ethical, legal and medical implications for doctors and patients who participate in randomised clinical trials. *British Medical Journal* **286**: 1117–21.

31. Report of the Royal College of Physicians (1983). *Guidelines on the Practice of Ethics Committees in Medical Research*. London: Royal College of Physicians.
32. Department of Health (1991). *Local Research Ethics Committees and HSG (91) 5*. London: Department of Health.
33. Thomas E (1986). Informed consent. *Lancet* ii: 1280.
34. Anon (1988). Research without consent continues in the UK. *Institute of Medical Ethics Bulletin* 40: 13–15.
35. Preliminary Analysis by the CRC Adjuvant Breast Trial Working Party (1988). Cyclophosphamide and tamoxifen as adjuvant therapy in the management of breast cancer. *British Journal of Cancer* 57: 604–7.
36. Report of the MRC (1963). *Responsibility in Investigations on Human Subjects, 1962–63*. London: MRC.
37. (1986). Research ethics committees. *Institute of Medical Ethics Bulletin* **suppl. 2.**
38. Baum M (1986). Do we need informed consent? *Lancet* ii: 911–12.
39. Antman E *et al.* (1992). A comparison of results of meta-analyses of randomised control trials and recommendations of clinical experts. *Journal of the American Medical Association* 8: 240.
40. *Bolam* v. *Friern Hospital Management Committee* [1957] 1 WLR 582.
41. *Sideway* v. *Board of Governors of Bethlem Royal Hospital etc.* [1985] AC 87.
42. Brahams D (1988). Voluntary chemical castration of a mental patient. *Lancet* i: 1291–2.
43. d'Orban P (1989). Steroid-induced psychosis. *Lancet* ii: 694.
44. Fenwick P (1989). Automatism and the Law. *Lancet* i: 753.
45. Brahams D (1987). Drugs and criminal acts. *Lancet* i: 874; (1991). i: 157.
46. Brahams D (1987). Criminal behaviour and medicinal treatment – iatrogenic crime. *Law Society's Gazette* **July 22**: 2175.
47. Dundee JW (1990). Fantasies during sedation with intravenous midazolam or diazepam. *Medico-Legal Journal* 58: 29.
48. Brahams D (1989). Benzodiazepine sedation and allegations of sexual assault. *Lancet* i: 1339–40.
49. Schaefer HG, Marsch SCU (1989). An unusual emergency after total intravenous anaesthesia. *Anaesthesia* 44: 928–9.
50. Brahams D (1990). Personal communication.

Further reading

Annas GJ, Law SA, Rosenblatt RE *et al.* (1990). *American Health Law*. Boston: Little Brown and Co.
Brazier M (1992). *Medicine, Patients and the Law*. Harmondsworth: Penguin.
(1990). *Charlesworth and Percy on Negligence*. London: Sweet & Maxwell.
(1989). *Chitty on Contract*. London: Sweet & Maxwell.
(1989). *Clerk and Lindsell on Tort*. London: Sweet & Maxwell.
Collins K, McLean SAM (in press). *Pharmaceuticals in the E.C.* London: Gower.
Dale JR, Appelbe GE (1989). *Pharmacy Law and Ethics*. London: Pharmaceutical Press.
Davies J, Jacob J (eds.) (1986). *Encyclopaedia of Health Services and Medical Law*. London: Sweet & Maxwell (loose-leaf).
Dukes MNG, Swartz B (1988). *Responsibility for Drug-induced Injury: A Reference Book for Lawyers, Health Professionals and Manufacturers*. Amsterdam: Elsevier.
Goldberg Sir A, Dodds-Smith I (eds.) (1991). *Pharmaceutical Medicine and the Law*. London: Royal College of Physicians.

Gostin LO (1986). *Mental Health Services: Law and Practice*. Crayford: Shaw & Sons (loose-leaf).

Jones MA (1991). *Medical Negligence*. London: Sweet & Maxwell.

Mason JK, McCall-Smith RA (1987). *Medico-Legal Encyclopaedia*. Sevenoaks: Butterworths.

Mason JK, McCall-Smith RA (1992). *Law and Medical Ethics*, 3rd edn. Sevenoaks: Butterworths.

McLean SAM (1989). *A Patient's Right to Know: Information Disclosure, the Doctor and the Law*. Aldershot: Dartmouth Publishing Company.

Nelson-Jones R, Burton F (1980). *Medical Negligence Case Law*. London: Fourmat Publishing.

Powers MJ, Harris NH (1990). *Medical Negligence*. Sevenoaks: Butterworths.

Smith JC, Hogan B (1988). *Criminal Law*. Sevenoaks: Butterworths.

(1988). *Street on Tort*. Sevenoaks: Butterworths.

Tolley LC (1992). *A Guide to Medical Negligence*.

(1989). *Winfield and Jolovicz on Tort*, 13 edn. London: Sweet & Maxwell.

Appendix I

Clinical trial compensation guidelines issued by the ABPI

Preamble

The Association of the British Pharmaceutical Industry favours a simple and expeditious procedure in relation to the provision of compensation for injury caused by participation in clinical trials. The Association therefore recommends that a member company sponsoring a clinical trial should provide without legal commitment a written assurance to the investigator – and through him to the relevant research ethics committee – that the following Guidelines will be adhered to in the event of injury caused to a patient attributable to participation in the trial in question.

1. Basic principles

1.1 Notwithstanding the absence of legal commitment, the company should pay compensation to patient-volunteers suffering bodily injury (including death) in accordance with these Guidelines.

1.2 Compensation should be paid when, on the balance of probabilities, the injury was attributable to the administration of a medicinal product under trial or any clinical intervention or procedure provided for by the protocol that would not have occurred but for the inclusion of the patient in the trial.

1.3 Compensation should be paid to a child injured in utero through the participation of the subject's mother in a clinical trial as if the child were a patient-volunteer with the full benefit of these Guidelines.

1.4 Compensation should only be paid for the more serious injury of an enduring and disabling character (including exacerbation of an existing condition) and not for temporary pain or discomfort or less serious or curable complaints.

1.5 Where there is an adverse reaction to a medicinal product under trial and injury is caused by a procedure adopted to deal with that adverse reaction, compensation should be paid for such injury as if it were caused directly by the medicinal product under trial.

1.6 Neither the fact that the adverse reaction causing the injury was foreseeable or predictable, nor the fact that the patient has freely consented (whether in writing or otherwise) to participate in the trial should exclude a patient from consideration for compensation under these Guidelines, although compensation may be abated or excluded in the light of the factors described in paragraph 4.2 below.

1.7   For the avoidance of doubt, compensation should be paid regardless of whether the patient is able to prove that the company has been negligent in relation to research or development of the medicinal product under trial or that the product is defective and therefore, as the producer, the company is subject to strict liability in respect of injuries caused by it.

2. Type of clinical research covered

2.1   These Guidelines apply to injury caused to patients involved in Phase II and Phase III trials, that is to say, patients under treatment and surveillance (usually in hospital) and suffering from the ailment which the medicinal product under trial is intended to treat but for which a product licence does not exist or does not authorise supply for administration under the conditions of the trial.

2.2   These Guidelines do not apply to injuries arising from studies in non-patient volunteers (Phase I), whether or not they are in hospital, for which separate Guidelines for compensation already exist.

2.3   These Guidelines do not apply to injury arising from clinical trials on marketed products (Phase IV) where a product licence exists authorising supply for administration under the conditions of the trial, except to the extent that the injury is caused to a patient as a direct result of procedures undertaken in accordance with the protocol (but not any product administered) to which the patient would not have been exposed had treatment been other than in the course of the trial.

2.4   These Guidelines do not apply to clinical trials which have not been initiated or directly sponsored by the company providing the product for research. Where trials of products are initiated independently by doctors under the appropriate Medicines Act 1968 exemptions, responsibility for the health and welfare of patients rests with the doctor alone (see also paragraph 5.2 below).

3. Limitations

3.1   No compensation should be paid for the failure of a medicinal product to have its intended effect or to provide any other benefit to the patient.

3.2   No compensation should be paid for injury caused by other licensed medicinal products administered to the patient for the purpose of comparison with the product under trial.

3.3   No compensation should be paid to patients receiving placebo in consideration of its failure to provide a therapeutic benefit.

3.4 No compensation should be paid (or it should be abated as the case may be) to the extent that the injury has arisen:

    3.4.1   through a significant departure from the agreed protocol;

    3.4.2   through the wrongful act or default of a third party, including a doctor's failure to deal adequately with an adverse reaction;

    3.4.3   through contributory negligence by the patient.

4. Assessment of compensation

4.1 The amount of compensation paid should be appropriate to the nature, severity and persistence of the injury and should in general terms be consistent with the quantum of damages commonly awarded for similar injuries by an English Court in cases where legal liability is admitted.

4.2 Compensation may be abated, or in certain circumstances excluded, in the light of the following factors (on which will depend the level of risk the patient can reasonably be expected to accept):

    4.2.1   the seriousness of the disease being treated, the degree of probability that adverse reactions will occur and any warnings given;

    4.2.2   the risks and benefits of established treatments relative to those known or suspected of the trial medicine.

This reflects the fact that flexibility is required given the particular patient's circumstances. As an extreme example, there may be a patient suffering from a serious or life-threatening disease who is warned of a certain defined risk of adverse reaction. Participation in the trial is then based on an expectation that the benefit/risk ratio associated with participation may be better than that associated with alternative treatment. It is, therefore, reasonable that the patient accepts the high risk and should not expect compensation for the occurrence of the adverse reaction of which he or she was told.

4.3 In any case where the company concedes that a payment should be made to a patient but there exists a difference of opinion between company and patient as to the appropriate level of compensation, it is recommended that the company agrees to seek at its own cost (and make available to the patient) the opinion of a mutually acceptable independent expert, and that his opinion should be given substantial weight by the company in reaching its decision on the appropriate payment to be made.

5. Miscellaneous

5.1 Claims pursuant to the Guidelines should be made by the patient to the company, preferably via the investigator, setting out details of the nature and background of the claim and, subject to the patient providing on request an authority for the company to review any medical records relevant to the claim, the company should consider the claim expeditiously.

5.2   The undertaking given by a company extends to injury arising (at whatever time) from all administrations, clinical interventions or procedures occurring during the course of the trial but not to treatment extended beyond the end of the trial at the instigation of the investigator. The use of unlicensed products beyond the trial period is wholly the responsibility of the treating doctor and in this regard attention is drawn to the advice provided to doctors in MAL 30 concerning the desirability of doctors notifying their protection society of their use of unlicensed products.

5.3   The fact that a company has agreed to abide by these Guidelines in respect of a trial does not affect the right of a patient to pursue a legal remedy in respect of injury alleged to have been suffered as a result of participation. Nevertheless, patients will normally be asked to accept that any payment made under the Guidelines will be in full settlement of their claims.

5.4   A company sponsoring a trial should encourage the investigator to make clear to participating patients that the trial is being conducted subject to the ABPI Guidelines relating to compensation for injury arising in the course of clinical trials and have available copies of the Guidelines should they be requested.

Index